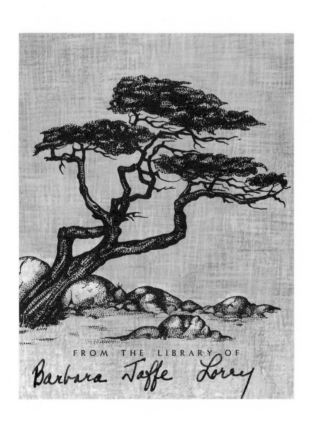

THE OBJECTIVE DIAGNOSIS OF MINIMAL BRAIN DYSFUNCTION

Other Books by Richard A. Gardner

The Child's Book About Brain Injury

The Boys and Girls Book About Divorce

Therapeutic Communication with Children:
    The Mutual Storytelling Technique

Dr. Gardner's Stories About the Real World

Understanding Children

MBD: The Family Book About Minimal Brain Dysfunction

Dr. Gardner's Fairy Tales for Today's Children

Psychotherapeutic Approaches to the Resistant Child

Psychotherapy with Children of Divorce

Dr. Gardner's Modern Fairy Tales

The Parents Book About Divorce

The Boys and Girls Book About One-Parent Families

THE OBJECTIVE DIAGNOSIS OF MINIMAL BRAIN DYSFUNCTION

RICHARD A. GARDNER, M.D.

Associate Clinical Professor of Child Psychiatry
Columbia University, College of Physicians and Surgeons

Creative Therapeutics   155 County Road   Cresskill, New Jersey 07626

Library of Congress Cataloging in Publication Data

Gardner, Richard A
  The objective diagnosis of minimal brain dysfunction.

  Bibliography: p.
  Includes index.
    1. Minimal brain dysfunction in children—Diagnosis
  I. Title.   (DNLM: 1.   Minimal brain
  dysfunction—Diagnosis.   WS340.3   G2280)

  RJ496.B7G37   618.9′28′58   79-11054
  ISBN 0-933812-00-0

Printed in the United States of America

10   9   8   7   6   5   4   3   2   1

To the late Morris Meister, Ph.D.
  founder and first principal of
  The Bronx High School of Science

for providing me with one of the richest educational
    experiences I have known,

for introducing me to the disciplines of science that have
    served as guidelines throughout this book,

and for opening doors whose very existence were previously
    unknown to me—thereby changing the course of my life.

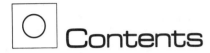 Contents

8   Visual Processing   185

☐○ Preface

The history of medicine is, to a large degree, the story of man's attempts to diagnose and treat illness. *Diagnosis* in Greek means to *know through* or to *know in depth*. When we are ignorant of a disease, we tend to be satisfied with applying a special label to a disorder and thereby may consider ourselves to have made a diagnosis. We may even use a term derived from another language (*cephalgia* for headache, *neuritis* for nerve inflammation) to give us the feeling that we are providing our patients with some special service. In true diagnosis we provide extra information beyond the observed (pneumococcal pneumonia, acute myelogeneous leukemia).

Reaching the point where we can make bona fide diagnoses has been a long and difficult process, dating back at least to the days of Hippocrates. One of the earliest phases in this process—and central to it—is sophisticated categorization. For example, we can envision a time when all people who exhibited sudden states of agitation were diagnosed as having *fits*. Then came a period when acute observers noted that not all people had the same kinds of fits. In one type, the individual would fall to the ground, foam at the mouth, bite his or her tongue, and become unconscious. Such people were called epileptics, and were considered to be possessed by supernatural forces. (Epilepsy is derived from a Greek word meaning *to take hold of*.) The Romans called it *Morbus Sacer* (Latin: sacred disease). Some fits were associated with periods of chills and fever and the onset followed exposure to swamps. They were considered to result from the bad air encountered in such areas and the disorder came to be known as *malaria* (Latin: *mala aria*, bad air). Another type was more frequently seen in women and was associated with loud, emotional displays of seemingly uncontrollable crying. The Greeks considered wandering of the uterus to be the cause of the disorder and it was therefore called *hysteria*. Clearly, such differentiations were crucial if one was to provide proper treatment.

For hundreds (and possibly thousands) of years, fever was considered a disease in its own right. We have come to appreciate that there is no specific disease that can justifiably be called *fever*. Rather, fever is a symptom of hundreds of different kinds of diseases, each one requiring its own form of treatment. There was a time when people were considered to have *heart disease*. We now have delineated dozens of different types of heart disease. Obviously, such differentiation has enhanced significantly our therapeutic efficacy. And the process is still going on. With increasing knowledge, each newly defined category becomes parent to a whole family of subcategories.

Our understanding of the disorder we presently call minimal brain dysfunction (MBD) is at that stage of development where heart disease was hundreds of years ago. Actually, we do better to view MBD as a group of disorders that have yet to be clearly differentiated from one another. When I use the term MBD the reader should appreciate that I am referring to a group of disorders of many etiologies, not one single entity. The impracticality of repeatedly using the term group of disorders should not leave the reader to conclude that I am describing a single entity. Some use the term *syndrome* when referring to MBD and, on occasion, we see the term *minimal brain dysfunction syndrome*. The *Blakiston's New Gould Medical Dictionary* (1952) defines syndrome as "a group of symptoms and signs which when considered together characterize a disease or lesion." Because there are many etiological factors that contribute to MBD, one cannot justifiably refer to it as a syndrome. If anything, it is a group of syndromes. Accordingly, the term I would prefer is *The Group of MBD Syndromes*.

When I use the term minimal brain dysfunction I am referring to a group of neurological disturbances in which the symptomatic manifestations are *mild* when compared to classical neurological disorders. Children with MBD have mild neuromuscular deficits, not the grosser abnormalities seen in those with cerebral palsy. They are generally less intellectually impaired than the retarded, but most often are not as bright as the normal. Accordingly, they learn better in school than educable retardates, but not as well as normal children. Their intellectual deficits are more isolated than those of retarded children, whose defects are more generalized. MBD children do not usually warrant the use of such terms as aphasia, anomia, alexia, and apraxia, but may exhibit varying degrees of dysphasia, dysnomia, dyslexia, and dyspraxia. These children are not deaf, yet auditory stimuli are not processed normally so they do not comprehend adequately what they hear. They are not blind, yet visual stimuli do not get properly utilized.

With such widespread symptomatic manifestations it is unreasonable to assume that we are dealing with anything less than a group of disorders. In addition, it is reasonable to view such deficits as affecting various parts of the brain. To consider one or a few focal areas of pathology is to take a simplistic view of MBD. Even though mild, one does well to consider the pathology widespread, affecting simultaneously various parts of the brain. Accordingly, the term *minimal* may be misleading. One does well to consider the term minimal as referring to the mildness of the pathology, but not referring to its extent. In the latter regard it may be far from minimal.

The term MBD is generally used in medicine today to refer only to a group of disorders in which there is a neurological component. Certain traditional symptoms of MBD, such as hyperactivity, impulsivity, and concentration impairment, can be psychogenic in etiology. However, most examiners (such as myself) believe that these same symptoms can *also* be manifestations of neurological impairment. (Of course, both organic and psychogenic factors can combine to produce such symptoms.) In this book I will discuss only neurologically based symptoms, even though some may also arise from psychogenic factors. I am aware that MBD children, like all children, may develop psychogenic problems. I am also aware that because of their handicap MBD children, like all handicapped children, are particularly prone to develop secondary psychogenic disorders. However, it is not my purpose to discuss these problems here. (The reader interested in my publications in this area may wish to refer to my articles on the subject listed in the References.)

Some readers may have wondered why I have chosen to use MBD in preference to other commonly used terms such as *hyperactivity* and *learning disorder*. I view hyperactivity and learning disorder to be two among many possible signs of MBD. It is unreasonable, in my opinion, to name a disorder with one of its common signs. It is the equivalent of calling appendicitis right lower quadrant abdominal pain. At this point, hyperactivity and learning disorders are rarely, if ever, seen in pure form. At most one can say that hyperactivity and/or learning disorders are common MBD manifestations, but that other signs and symptoms are usually present as well in the child with MBD. Many educators prefer the term learning disorder. They claim that the deficit is primarily educational and has nothing to do with neurological deficit. Although I cannot deny that MBD children most often have trouble learning in school, this does not mean that neurological problems are not operative.

Recently, the term attention deficit disorder has been introduced. My reasons for not utilizing this term are the same as those for rejecting hyperactivity and learning disorder. Only *some* children exhibit a basic attentional deficit. Even though they may comprise a majority of those who are considered to have MBD, the presence of many signs and symptoms unrelated to attentional deficits is great enough, in my opinion, to justify our not using the term in preference to the more encompassing MBD.

Occasionally, the terms neurological impairment (NI) and perceptual impairment (PI) are used synonymously with MBD. One can criticize the term MBD as being too all-encompassing. I believe that in time, as we define more clearly its various subcategories, the name MBD will fall into disuse. But the term neurological impairment is even more encompassing and could refer to neurological disorders outside of the brain. Although we are only beginning to learn about the various parts of the brain that may be implicated in MBD, we can at least say that the pathology is primarily if not exclusively in the brain and not elsewhere in the nervous system. I do not like the name perceptual impairment for two reasons. First, it uses one class of disorders to describe the whole group. Second, the term perception, as I will discuss in chapter eight, has become so loosely used and means so many different things, that it hardly serves any longer to communicate anything specific.

At this point, then, I believe that minimal brain dysfunction is the best term we have, its deficiencies notwithstanding. It tells us that the problems are not severe. It informs us that the disorder relates to pathology in the brain, and not elsewhere. And it advises us that this disturbance is organic in that the term *dysfunction* has traditionally been used in medicine to refer to this type of pathology as opposed to the psychogenic.

There are some who claim that there is no such thing as MBD, that the brain dysfunction exists in the heads of those who make the diagnosis and not in the children being so labeled. Some of the dubious are neurologists who take the position that a neurological sign is either absent or present, that there is no such thing as an intermediate or mild form. They deny the existence of soft neurological signs, and consider it "soft thinking" by those who use the term. Such doubters, however, will readily agree that the "all or none" principle does not hold in other branches of medicine. They will admit to the existence of subclinical infections, forme frusté variations of a disorder, and mild cases of a host of diseases. But somehow they do not accept the same continuum from health to severe illness with regard to this group of neurological disturbances. At the other extreme, there are those who are making the diagnosis in 75% or more of all children who are referred to them. It is almost as if the disorder were epidemic.

How did we come to this state of affairs? I believe that the answer can be found if one traces the history of psychiatric diagnosis in the past 100 years. In the late nineteenth century, our system of nomenclature was primarily that of Kraepelin and his followers. All psychiatric disorder was viewed as organic in etiology. In the early twentieth century, primarily as the result of the contribution of Freud and his followers, the importance of psychogenic factors in psychopathology was brought to light. Prior to World War II, the center of the psychoanalytic movement was in Europe where, interestingly, it has never enjoyed great influence in psychiatry. The movement enjoyed great receptivity in the United States (and to a lesser degree in England) during and after World War II with the flight of many European analysts. By the mid-1950s the movement had such great influence in the United States that most psychiatric disorders were considered to be psychogenic. By the mid-twentieth century, then, the pendulum had completely swung in the opposite direction from the totally organic orientation of Kraepelin to the strongly psychogenic orientation of the psychoanalysts.

It was in the late 1950s, especially after the publication of Strauss and Lehtinen (1947) and Strauss and Kephart's (1955) books that we begin to see the pendulum starting to shift back. Unfortunately, another factor operating in the shift away from the psychogenic orientation was the aversion of professionals in many areas to the self-assured, and even grandiose, attitude of many psychoanalysts. Such analysts seemed to have lost sight of the fact that Freudian theory was just that, a *theory*. It has been said (I wish I knew the author) that "psychoanalysis is a field in which one man's theory becomes another man's fact." Psychoanalysis shared (and still shares to some extent today), much in common with organized religious movements in which a leader surrounds himself with a coterie of the faithful who remain in favor as long as they espouse the beliefs of the leader and risk rejection from the fold if they disagree too strongly with the official doctrines. There were (and still are) many psychoanalysts who consider those who refute their theories to have unresolved neurotic problems. Such arrogance has, in my opinion, alienated many who might have taken a more receptive attitude toward psychoanalytic contributions. The condescending attitude of many psychoanalysts toward those who express healthy doubt has so alienated many that psychogenic theory in general has been discredited. I think that this has been unfortunate because we have much to learn from psychoanalysis. We should not reject it in its entirety because of the fanaticism, dogmatism, and arrogance of many of its adherents. Such blanket rejection has contributed to the exaggerated swing of the pendulum to close to where it was in the nineteenth century. (I speak here as an analyst myself, as someone who considers himself familiar with the strengths and weaknesses of the theory as well as the personalities of its adherents.)

So this is where we stand in 1979, at the time of this book's publication. The pendulum has to be brought back to a more moderate position. We cannot totally reject psychogenic etiology in learning problems as well as other types of childhood psychopathology. We cannot continue diagnosing MBD in most of the children we see. To do so is to substitute dogmatic adherence to an organic theory of etiology for a dogmatic psychoanalytical interpretation of behavioral abnormality. We must approach the diagnosis of children with an open mind, in order to be able to label an organic disorder with the same ease that we diagnose a psychogenic.

The primary problem that prevents us from doing this at the time is the paucity of objective diagnostic criteria for MBD diagnosis. A teacher will decide that a child is hyperactive because he is disruptive in the classroom. A child psychologist, a consulting psychiatrist, or a pediatrician may confirm the diagnosis even though the hyperactivity has not been directly observed by any of these examiners. MBD children are typically less hyperactive in the one-to-one situation where they receive individualized attention than in a group such as a classroom. Psychostimulant medication may then be prescribed on a daily basis over a period of years. Gross motor coordination deficits are diagnosed when the child does not catch the ball thrown by the examiner (the assumption here is that the examiner throws the ball perfectly each time). A neurologist asks a child to rapidly oppose his thumb to each of the other four fingers and considers a fine motor coordination problem to be present, not on the basis of any specific data, but on the basis of his "clinical experience." Children are labeled "dyslexic" because they are two years behind in reading. Social, cultural, educational, familial, interpersonal, and intrapsychic psychogenic factors may be totally ignored. Others are suspect for dyslexia because they appear to exhibit more letter reversals than their peers, but no normative data on reversals frequency is utilized to ascertain objectively whether the child's reversals frequency is indeed abnormal. It is subjectivity in diagnosis, more than anything else, that is responsible for the chaotic state of MBD diagnosis and treatment that exists at this time.

This book was written in the hope that it might play some role in rectifying this unfortunate state of affairs. It is a compendium of the MBD diagnostic criteria that I have collected over the last twenty years.

The one proviso that had to be satisfied for a test to be included in this battery was that normative data be available. Without such objectification, diagnostic instruments cannot be considered to be of much value. The tests here have been taken primarily from psychology (where the importance of objective measurement is often more appreciated than in psychiatry) and from pediatric neurology. However, much data here are my own. They were collected because, to the best of my knowledge, no data had previously been obtained. The battery presented here is not simple to administer nor can it be given in a short time. MBD is a complex disorder and it is unreasonable to believe that we can quickly diagnose it (in the true Greek sense of the word). I do not view the battery as something that should be routinely administered in *toto*. This is not only impractical (it might take 15 to 20 hours of testing) but unreasonable. The examiner should administer those tests that relate to the presenting symptoms as well as those assessing areas of suspected pathology. Many tests assess the same function. This prevents conclusions being based on one test only and provides the examiner with a number of instruments to either confirm or refute suspicions of pathology.

No test described in this book assesses only one function. Each test is presented in the section where its primary function is described. Other information obtained by the instrument is also discussed in the primary section and reference to the test is made in other parts of the book when applicable. All the tests need not be administered by one person. I, myself, have engaged the services of a psychologist who is knowledgeable about the traditional testing instruments, as well as some of the more specialized instruments used in MBD diagnosis. With one to two hours of MBD testing on my part and three to four hours on hers, we can usually provide a reasonably thorough description of the child's problems. The examiner should not just conclude that a child has MBD; he or she should describe in detail the nature of the deficits. Such information has proved useful to parents, teachers, and therapists. The more specific information the professional has about the exact nature of the child's deficits, the greater is his or her capacity to provide help.

The purpose of this book is to describe only the neurologic manifestations of MBD. MBD children, like all children with a handicap, almost invariably develop secondary psychogenic symptoms as well. It is not the purpose of this book to discuss these psychogenic problems (a book on this subject is planned for the future). The examiner should remember that there is not one test described in this book that cannot be affected by psychogenic factors. Tension and anxiety will usually increase hyperactivity. The obstructionistic child is so intent on thwarting the examiner that he cares little about poor test scores. The insecure and/or fragile child, who cannot tolerate failure, may refuse to continue a particular test once he senses that he is not getting most of the answers correct. Anxiety reduces concentration and when attention is impaired every test result must be suspect.

This book will only focus on the neurological information that can be derived from the tests described herein. There is no instrument discussed here that cannot provide psychodynamic information as well. The incorrect definition that a child gives to the words on the Vocabulary subtest of the WISC-R may be very revealing of psychopathological processes. The child may feel that the little boy in the center of the WISC-R Mazes subtest is trapped. When taking the Similarities subtest of the WISC-R he may say that the apple and banana are similar because they both can be used to feed a person poison. For the purposes of the MBD diagnostic battery described here, these are only listed as wrong answers. However, they are certainly noted and included in the section of this examiner's report devoted to psychodynamic issues.

The more observant the examiner is of the child's behavior and attitudes while taking a test, the more information he will be able to obtain and the more accurate will be his conclusions regarding the child's performance. For example, if one observes that a child's percentile rank progressively increases on each of the four subtests of the Purdue Pegboard, one should consider the possibility that the child's motivation increased as he went further along from subtest to subtest. This is not an uncommon phenomenon, as the child rises to the challenge and gets swept up in the task. In such circumstances, the examiner does well to repeat the earlier subtests while the child is in the mood of heightened enthusiasm. Recording both scores (even though a practice effect may be operating) provides the examiner and the reader of the report with a more accurate description of the child's capacity. The same phenomenon is sometimes responsible for a child's doing better on the Digits Backward than the Digits Forward section of the Digits Span subtest of the WISC-R. One can easily ascertain whether this has occurred by repeating the Digits Forward section with other numerical series of equal length to those that had previously been failed. Again, the experience should be recorded. One wants to know a child's true capacity, not merely his score. The former may not always be revealed by the latter. It is only with experience and careful observation of the child during the testing that one can arrive at the more accurate and useful conclusions to be derived from an assessment instrument.

Another important caveat. The examiner should not conduct his evaluation under time restrictions. Other than in emergency situations, physicians are not requested or required to perform their examinations within prescribed time limits. Most would not go to a physician who was under orders to limit all of his examinations to 15 minutes. Hardly anyone would submit to an operation when the surgeon was told that surgery had to be performed in a specific time. Yet many mental health professionals agree to limit their evaluations in just this way. Schools will advise a consulting psychiatrist that they will only pay for one or two consultation sessions, by the end of which a diagnosis and recommendations must be given. I do not accept referrals with such restrictions. Psychiatric residents traditionally conduct conferences in which a different attending is brought in each week for a one or one-and-a-half hour consultation. This may work well in other areas of medicine, but it has little place in child psychiatry, especially when the diagnosis of MBD is being considered. I no longer involve myself in such consultations. They are a disservice to the patient as well as the student who is trying to learn something about diagnosis.

I fully recognize that many who read this book work in settings where the case loads are such that a five-to-six hour evaluation is an impossible indulgence. This may be a source of frustration for the examiner working under such circumstances. He or she does well to impress upon those who impose such restrictions that the evaluation produced is being compromised. To the degree that one is free to conduct such an extensive evaluation, to that degree will one be providing the kind of in-depth assessment worthy of the term diagnosis.

Besides being of practical use in providing more accurate and objective MBD diagnosis, my hope is that this book will be of value in other ways. I believe that a greater understanding of minimal brain dysfunction can (and already has) enhanced our capacity to differentiate organic from psychogenic disturbance. And such knowledge cannot but shed light on such ancient controversies as nature vs. nurture and heredity vs. environment. Furthermore, it is my hope that this book will contribute to our knowledge of the various disorders subsumed under the MBD rubric. When this process of subcategorization has been satisfactorily accomplished, the term MBD will pass into disuse. And this will indeed be progress if each subcategory becomes parent to yet another generation of disorders as we delve deeper and deeper in our incessant quest to diagnose, or, as the Greeks said, *to know in depth.*

☐ Acknowledgments

I have a deep sense of gratitude to many people who have contributed in a variety of ways to this book.

The person who has had the greatest influence on me with regard to this book's basic philosophy is Dr. Martha Bridge Denckla, Associate Professor of Neurology, Harvard Medical School. I had the good fortune to meet Martha when she was teaching at Columbia. She impressed upon me the importance of normative data in MBD diagnosis and served as a model for the kind of investigator who, rather than just bemoaning the lack of such information, goes out and collects such data. In addition, her clinical reports were rarely confined to merely providing basic information about her patients. They were rich teaching instruments about her latest research. Many of her important contributions are to be found in various parts of this book, but her influence is present throughout.

Dr. Melinda Broman, Research Associate, Department of Psychiatry, Columbia University, College of Physicians and Surgeons, did most of the statistical work associated with the research studies that I conducted. My collaboration with her provided me with the fringe benefit of learning some important things about what had previously been to me a most arcane and confusing discipline.

Dr. Rita G. Rudel, Associate Clinical Professor of Psychology, Department of Neurology, Columbia University, College of Physicians and Surgeons, influenced me mainly through her publications. Like Dr. Denckla (with whom she often collaborated) she has served as a model of the kind of investigator who is most likely to provide us with the most meaningful and useful research. In addition, she provided me with occasional advice and guidance in perceptual psychology, a field in which she has made significant contributions.

Dr. Arnold Gold, Professor of Pediatrics and Neurology, Columbia University, College of Physicians and Surgeons, a dedicated and astute clinician, taught me much over the years via his informative reports. His parent questionnaire served as a useful model for my own.

Mrs. Katrina de Hirsch, formerly Director, Pediatric Language Disorder Clinic, Columbia-Presbyterian Medical Center, allowed me, during my residency days, to observe her while evaluating children with learning disabilities. She generously explained what she was doing and served as a model for careful and thoughtful observation of these children's difficulties.

Dr. Letty Pogul, Assistant Clinical Professor of Medical Psychology in Psychiatry, Columbia University, College of Physicians and Surgeons, many years ago introduced me to the value of various psychological tests in MBD diagnosis. She allowed me to watch her work and spent many hours explaining in detail what she was doing. Her sensitivity to children and her capacity to elicit the best from them has served as a model for me which has been difficult, if not impossible, to emulate.

Dr. Russell Asnes, Associate Clinical Professor of Pediatrics, Columbia University, College of Physicians and Surgeons, and Dr. Michael Weingarten, Clinical Assistant Professor of Obstetrics and Gynecology, New Jersey College of Medicine and Dentistry at Rutgers, provided me useful information relative to issues in my parent questionnaire that pertains to their specialties.

Mrs. Minna Genn, Supervising Psychologist, Division of Psychology, Columbia-Presbyterian Medical Center, has taught me much about MBD over the years through her thorough and informative reports.

Mrs. Dorothy Unger, Speech-Language Pathologist and Learning Disabilities Teacher Consultant, Tenafly, New Jersey, expanded my knowledge and appreciation of the role of auditory and speech deficits in MBD. Her reports have always taught me something.

Dr. Joseph Danto, Associate Professor and Director of Audiology, City College of the City University of New York, introduced me to the promising field of Dichotic Auditory Stimulation and provided me with vital information for my discussion of this subject.

My son, Andrew Gardner, Yale College, designed and built the original model of the motor steadiness tester. Alex Caemmerer, Tenafly High School, built an alternative model using digital logic and integrated circuits.

Dr. Melvin Schrier, optometrist, accepted my invitation to write the section on ocular dysfunction, thereby providing information in an area beyond my realm of competence.

Dr. Marilyn Birke, psychologist, Teaneck, New Jersey, actively collaborated with me in the administration of the MBD diagnostic battery described in this book. This not only lessened my work load but provided clinical substantiation for many of the diagnostic approaches presented herein.

Over 2000 children were involved at various times in the research studies described in this book. Although their anonymity must be preserved, my gratitude to them must be proclaimed. Testing these children would not have been possible without the active support and cooperation of many school personnel. In New Jersey: Mrs. Barbara Sugarman, Director of Special Education, Region IV and Mr. Leonard Margolis, Director of Special Education, Region III, Bergen County; Dr. Jane Sokoll, School Pediatrician and Dr. Herbert Gellis, Director of Special Services, Hackensack Public Schools, Hackensack; Mr. Dominic Grassano, Principal, Maple Hill School and Mrs. Mary Pramick, Principal, P.S. No. 6, Hackensack; Dr. Betty Ferraro, Learning Disability Consultant, Harrington Park Public Schools; Dr. Bernard Fidel, Chief, Child Study Team, New Milford Schools, New Milford; Dr. Joseph Cornell, Superintendent of Schools, Northvale; Mrs. Ruth Etzi, Psychologist, Midland Park Public Schools, Midland Park; Dr. Leo Sawitz, Chairman, Child Study Team, Mr. Louis O'Malley, Principal, Middle School, Mrs. Thelma Plender, Principal, Maugham School, Mr. Donald Miller, Principal, Smith School, Mr. Ernest Mueller, Principal, Stillman School, and Mr. Al Kane, Principal, Mackay School, Tenafly; Mr. David Dervitz, Superintendent of Schools, Dr. Hadassah Gurfein, Chief, Child Study Team, Mr. Joseph T. Ferrie, Principal, Dumont High School, Mr. Martin S. Rittenberg, Principal, Honiss School, Mr. Dale H. Genberg, Vice Principal, Honiss School, Mr. Dominick Pirisi, Principal, Selzer School, and Mr. James Gardner, Principal, Grant School, Dumont; Mr. Frank Pallante, Superintendent of Schools, Norwood; Dr. Harry Galinsky, Assistant Superintendent of Schools, Mr. Thomas Occhipinti, Director of Special Education, Mr. Joseph H. Roma, Principal, Parkway School, and Mr. Charles Mahler, Enrichment Teacher, Parkway School, Paramus; Mr. Raymond J. Albano, Superintendent of Schools and Mr. Robert D. Lynch, Principal, Charles De Wolf School, Old Tappan; Mr. Robert Lewis, Superintendent of Schools and Dr. William Dorney, Principal, Haworth Public School, Haworth; Dr. Reno Zinzarella, Superintendent of Schools, Mr. Harold Gottlieb, Psychologist, Westwood Public Schools, Mr. Thomas Olsen, Principal, Brookside School, Mr. Stanley Freeman, Principal, Ketler School, and Mr. Daniel Frost, Principal, Middle School, Westwood; Dr. Beatrice Lieben and Mr. Abner Strauss, The Community School, Englewood;

Dr. Adrienne Le Fevre, Psychologist, Bergen Center for Child Development, Englewood; Mrs. Toby Shor, Director, Paramus Cooperative Nursery School, Paramus; Mrs. Dulcie Freeman, New Jersey Association for Children with Learning Disabilities, Paramus; Miss Phyllis Jones, Director of the Pre-School Program, Hackensack Christian Schools, Hackensack; Mrs. Christine Sharp, Director, Marijude School, Bergenfield; Mrs. Louise Emory, Director, The Forum School, Waldwick; Mrs. Zelda Pollack, Director, Early Childhood Learning Center, Convent Station. In New York City: Mr. David Braunstein, Lotte Kaliski School; Dr. Miriam Michael, Stephen Gaynor School; Mr. Allan J. Blau, Executive Director, The Adams School.

The actual work involved in administering the various research instruments in my study was accomplished by Deborah Giannuzzi, Steven Glaser, Melissa Glass, Linda Gould, Martin Gottlob, Edythe Kornfeld, Marjorie Osborn, Diane Samuels, Shirley Shapiro, Rosa Sirota, Janice Snyder, Susan Teltser, Josephine Vaughan, and Theodora Waltman.

Mrs. Linda Gould, my secretary, ever-loyal and hard working, dedicated herself to the typing of the manuscript in its various renditions. Mrs. Frances Dubner, as she has done for so many of my previous publications, enthusiastically provided valuable and sensitive editorial advice. Mrs. Dee Josephson served in many capacities during the course of this book's publication. She edited the final manuscript for publication, designed the book, and admirably accomplished the formidable task of coordinating all phases of the book's production and manufacture.

1

The Parents'
Questionnaire

A detailed inquiry into the child's background can often provide the examiner with valuable diagnostic information. This is particularly true in the evaluation of children with minimal brain dysfunction. Often the only clue we may have regarding the etiology of such children's difficulties comes from the anamnesis because the examination itself often reveals little of specific value about history. In fact, at our present state of knowledge, we appear to be dealing with a *group* of disorders of various etiologies, which produce a variegated clinical pattern of symptoms. The clinical picture, however, is diverse, varying, and inconsistent from patient to patient. It is reasonable to hope that in the future, when the various etiological factors are more clearly identified and the MBD subgroups more accurately differentiated from one another, there will be more direct and well-defined relationships between etiology and clinical symptomatology. At this point, the best we can do is say that a child has MBD and then speculate on the probable cause or causes. Unfortunately, there are patients for whom the etiology still remains unknown, even after an exhaustive inquiry and evaluation. This should not be a reason, however, for doubting or discounting the diagnosis. If the clinical picture is definitely present (by utilizing the kind of "hard" and objective criteria presented in this book), then the diagnosis should be made. One should add in such cases that the etiology is unknown.

Because of the diversity of factors that have been etiologically implicated in MBD, a proper inquiry can be quite lengthy. Yet an exhaustive inquiry conducted with the parents is crucial if one is to avoid missing an etiological factor. In addition, such an inquiry can provide information of diagnostic value as well. Although one must use such data cautiously (parents are not always completely objective with regard to providing accurate information about their children) the information so gained can be useful in many ways in establishing the diagnosis.

Over the years, with increasing knowledge about the various etiological factors that have been implicated and with increasing appreciation of the importance of other anamnestic information that was important to gather, I found myself spending ever-increasing time in history-taking. Accordingly, I recently found it more practical to have the parents fill out an extensive questionnaire prior to the first session. I then had before me a wealth of important information which was available at a glance. I found that I could then spend more of my evaluation time doing things that could not be done outside the office.

In this chapter I will describe the questionnaire in detail. Throughout my discussion the text will refer to reproductions of the actual questionnaire. Besides providing the aforementioned information, the questionnaire may also have the fringe benefit of improving the relationship between the therapist and the parents. Many parents comment that the questionnaire is "thorough" and provides them with the feeling that the therapist is interested in going into great detail regarding the child's problems. Considering all the hostile, jealous, and rivalrous feelings that parents often develop toward the therapist—feelings that can undermine the child's treatment—anything that can impress the parents positively should be welcomed. An additional benefit of the questionnaire is enjoyed by the therapist if a report of the consultation or treatment is requested. It provides important background information in an organized fashion. A therapist's notes are rarely as systematic.

In my discussion of the questionnaire, I will not be providing specific references when referring to the various factors that have been considered to be of etiological significance in MBD. The literature on each is, however, voluminous. The evidence in support of some of the factors is strong and for others weak and speculative. It is beyond the purpose of this book to discuss the pros and cons of each agent's alleged etiological role in MBD. It is simply my purpose to alert the reader to those that have been suspected. The reader who wishes further information on many of the etiological factors mentioned here can refer to the following: Kawi and Pasamanick, 1958, 1959; Pasamanick and Knobloch, 1960; Pincus and Glaser, 1966; Knobloch and Pasamanick, 1966; Towbin, 1971; Cantwell, 1975c; Ross and Ross, 1976.

Generally, in the initial telephone conversation the parent is told that a questionnaire will be sent and that this is to be filled out prior to the first appointment. Because of the great value of the questionnaire at this time and because parents have not proven themselves completely reliable about completing it prior to the initial interview, the first statement on the first page (Figure 1.1) reminds the parents to bring the completed questionnaire when they come for the first time. Similarly, during the first telephone call, I suggest that both parents and the child come together for the initial consultation. As I have described in greater detail elsewhere (Gardner, 1975), I have not found the traditional approach, of seeing both parents alone during the initial interview and then seeing the child alone in the second, to be the most efficient and effective way of conducting the first interview. Seeing the parents alone without the child makes it more difficult for me to fully appreciate the child's problems. I feel that I am working in a vacuum, and that I am being deprived of my most important source of information—the child. I am not seeing the living human being who is the focus of my interest. In addition, I am being deprived of observing the various intra-familial interactions that are so important to witness in any psychiatric evaluation. With parents and child present, I can, of course, send one or two of the three parties out of the room if the situation warrants it, enabling me to have any combination of significant individuals that is indicated. Because of psychological resistance or disinterest, the calling parent may "forget" this aspect of my telephone instructions. The reminder is therefore given at the top of the first page of the questionnaire.

BASIC DATA

Most questionnaires request name, address, telephone number, etc. for the child and then for each of the parents. With the burgeoning divorce rate in recent years, fewer children are living in homes with both natural parents. Many other combinations are being seen and it is important that the examiner have a clear idea of the child's family structure and the exact nature of his or her relationship with the various adults who are involved in the child's care. Therefore, immediately after I get basic information about where the child is living (address, telephone number, school), the parent is asked to place checks in the appropriate places in the present placement table (Figure 1.1, middle) to indicate the child's relationship with the adults with whom he is living (column A), as well as those who are involved in his care but living elsewhere (column B). For example, a boy might be living with his natural mother and stepfather. Checks for these individuals would be placed in column A. His natural father might be living with his new wife, the child's step-

Figure 1.1

The Parents' Questionnaire

PLEASE BRING THIS COMPLETED FORM WITH YOU AT THE TIME OF YOUR

FIRST APPOINTMENT ON _____ AT _____

IT IS PREFERABLE THAT BOTH PARENTS ACCOMPANY THE CHILD TO THE

CONSULTATION.

Child's name_____ Birth date _____Age___Sex____
          last   first middle

Home address_____
          street   city   state   zip

Home telephone number_____
              area code   number

Child's school_____
          name   address   grade

Present placement of child (place check in appropriate bracket):

	Column A Adults with whom child is living	Column B Non-residential adults involved with child
Natural mother	( ) ___	( ) ___
Natural father	( ) ___	( ) ___
Stepmother	( ) ___	( ) ___
Stepfather	( ) ___	( ) ___
Adoptive mother	( ) ___	( ) ___
Adoptive father	( ) ___	( ) ___
Foster mother	( ) ___	( ) ___
Foster father	( ) ___	( ) ___
Other (specify)	_____ ___	_____ ___

Place the number 1 or 2 next to each check in Column A and provide
the following information about each person:

1. Name_____ Occupation_____
       last   first

   Business name_____ Business address_____

   _____ Business tel. No. ( )_____

2. Name_____ Occupation_____
       last   first

   Business name_____ Business address_____

   _____ Business tel. No. ( )

Place the number 3 next to the person checked in Column B who is
most involved with the child and provide the following information:

3. Name_____ Home address_____
                                street

   _____ Home tel. No. ( )_____
   city   state   zip

   Occupation_____ Business name_____

4

mother. Checks for these individuals would be placed in column B. The parent would then place numbers 1 and 2 next to the checks in column A for the natural mother and stepfather and the number 3 next to the check for the natural father in column B. More data on the nonresidential stepmother would generally not be obtained here (unless the situation specifically warranted its inclusion). Because the home address for the natural mother and stepfather has already been obtained, only their business addresses are requested. Then information about the natural father's home and business is requested. Although this type of inquiry may appear cumbersome at first, it is ultimately easier than the explanations that parents are required to provide when the questionnaire asks simply for data about the mother and father. In addition, columns A and B provide at-a-glance information about present placement.

Information about the referral source is then requested (Figure 1.2) as well as the reasons for the consultation. Just a few lines are available for this because I only wish the parent to make a brief statement here. To provide more space would probably result in a repetition of material to be obtained subsequently.

PREGNANCY

It is probable that many, if not most, of the causes of MBD exert their effects during pregnancy. Although genetic factors and those related to delivery and afterwards are certainly seen, it is probable that most of the cases of MBD are the result of interferences that occurred during the gestational period.

One should get further information about any of the complications of pregnancy that may have been checked off on the questionnaire. Most women stain during pregnancy. If, however, prolonged periods of bed rest were required, or hospitalization was necessary, then one could assume that this complication was in the pathological range. It is probable that many children's MBD is the result of maternal infections that get transmitted to the embryo and fetus. Sometimes such infections are subclinical and so we have no information about them. When they produce clinical symptoms, especially if severe, then the likelihood of their being of etiological significance is greater. The maternal infections that have most conclusively been demonstrated to produce fetal brain dysfunction are cytomegalic inclusion disease, toxoplasmosis, rubella, herpes simplex, and syphilis. Toxemia has been associated with MBD. One should, therefore, inquire about high blood pressure, seizures, and proteinuria. Most women vomit during pregnancy. Vomiting can cause dehydration that might result in fluid and nutriment deprivation to the

Figure 1.2
The Parents' Questionnaire

Business address_____Bus. tel. No. ( )_____

Source of referral: Name_____Address_____

_____Tel. No. ( )_____

Purpose of consultation (brief summary of the main problems):

_____

_____

_____

PREGNANCY
  Complications:
    Excessive vomiting_____hospitalization required_____

    Excessive staining or blood loss_____

    Threatened miscarriage_____

    Infection(s) (specify)_____

    Toxemia_____

    Operation(s) (specify)_____

    Other illness(es) (specify)_____

  Smoking during pregnancy_____average number of cigarettes per
    day_____

  Alcoholic consumption during pregnancy_____describe, if beyond
    an occasional drink_____

  Medications taken during pregnancy_____

  X-ray studies during pregnancy_____

  Duration_____weeks

DELIVERY
  Type of labor: Spontaneous_____ Induced_____

  Forceps: high____mid____low____

  Duration of labor_____hours

  Type of delivery: Vertex (normal____breech____Caesarean____

  Complications:
    cord around neck_____

    cord presented first _____

    hemorrhage_____

mother. The crucial question is how much vomiting is necessary to cause fetal deprivation? If hospitalization was required, especially for intravenous fluid replacement, then it is possible that the vomiting was excessive. This does not mean, however, that vomiting *was* the cause of the child's MBD. It would only be suspicious as an etiological factor.

Smoking during pregnancy has been associated with low birth weight, increased fetal and neonatal death rate, and impairments in the child's physical, neurological, and intellectual growth. And there appears to be a correlation between the amount of smoking and the incidence of these effects. Excessive alcoholic ingestion can cause what has recently been referred to as the *fetal alcohol syndrome.* These babies exhibit alterations in growth, facial dysmorphism and other disturbances of body morphogenesis, as well as low birth weight. MBD and mental retardation have been described in these children. Thalidomide has probably been one of the more widely publicized causes of congenital anomalies and intellectual impairment. Other drugs that have been known to cause brain dysfunction include aminopterin, diphenylhydantoin, methotrexate, and high doses of vitamin D. And there are probably many other drugs, as yet unimplicated, that will ultimately be shown to have such effects. A standard warning provided for a high percentage of drugs is that safe administration during pregnancy has not been established. Accordingly, any medication that was taken over a period of time during the pregnancy should be noted by the examiner. Exposure to X-radiation has also been implicated. The most common story is of a woman who presents with nausea, vomiting, and other gastrointestinal symptoms. Pregnancy may not be suspected, especially if the woman is single or over 40. The patient may undergo a number of radiological examinations (GI series, gall bladder studies, barium enema, etc.) in the attempt to ascertain the cause of the vomiting. By the time the correct diagnosis is made, the woman may have been exposed to significant amounts of X-radiation. (Most radiologists now inquire into the recent menstrual history to be sure that they are not exposing a pregnant woman to X-rays.)

One also wants to learn about the duration of pregnancy. Traditionally the mother's report on this has not been too reliable because many mothers do not know exactly when they became pregnant. One definition of prematurity (a term falling into disuse) used to be that a child whose gestation was less than 37 weeks was considered premature. Because of the unreliability of this figure, the child's birth weight was subsequently used and children under 2500 grams (5.5 pounds) were considered premature. Recently, this criterion has also been found wanting because there were some babies below this weight who showed none of the problems traditionally manifested by prematures. Accordingly, new criteria are being used to determine if the infant's birth weight is indeed a problem, and these will be presented below when I discuss the significance of the birth weight. The duration of pregnancy figure, however, can still serve as a clue (admittedly a poor one) as to whether there were problems regarding the pregnancy's duration. It is more significant if the *gestational age* has been determined by the physician, using recently developed physiological and neurological criteria. Only babies born after the early 1970s were so examined. In time, all knowledgeable mothers may refer to the child's gestational age at birth rather than the duration of the pregnancy.

DELIVERY

The delivery is another period when the child may be exposed to factors that can produce MBD. Inducing labor runs certain risks for the child, more so in the past than in the present. The physician may miscalculate the pregnancy's duration (especially if he or she relies too heavily on the mother's estimate) and deliver the baby before it can optimally thrive in the extrauterine environment. In the past oxytocin, the drug most commonly used to initiate and maintain uterine contractions, was administered by buccal tablet. One had no control over the duration of its action. Accordingly, uterine contractions might persist after it was determined that cephalopelvic disproportion was present and the fetus was being traumatized. In addition, drugs such as oxytocin can produce tetanic contractions of the uterus. These can cut off blood circulation from the placenta to the fetus and thereby cause anoxia in the child. In recent years such drugs can be given by intravenous drip, which can be carefully controlled. Once trouble is suspected, the oxytocin is immediately discontinued. Because there is no reserve of the drug present in the body (as is the case with buccal tablets) uterine contractions due to the drug can be quickly interrupted. The mother who was spontaneously delivered does not run the risk of these complications.

High forceps delivery is practically unknown today. Just about all obstetricians recognize the danger of its producing trauma to the infant. It is generally agreed among obstetricians that low forceps delivery is without danger, but mid-forceps delivery may cause some trauma. Most obstetricians will choose to do a Caesarean section rather than expose the child to the traumatic risks of mid-forceps delivery.

Mothers may not be completely reliable regarding the accuracy of their reports on the duration of labor. Considering all the things they have to think about during this time, they cannot be seriously faulted for such impairment in their recollection. Strictly speaking, labor is considered to begin when the cervix starts to dilate, and is considered to be continuing as long as there is progressive cervical dilatation. Most women enter the hospital already partially dilated so cervical observation and the more objective reporting of the onset is no longer possible. The clinical definition of the onset is the time when contractions begin to occur at a frequency greater than one every five minutes. Labor is considered to be going on as long as such contractions are *regular and continuous*. Normally, the duration of labor for the first pregnancy is 12–14 hours. Labors more than 16 hours should be considered prolonged, with an increased risk for fetal damage. The normal duration of second and subsequent labors is 8–10 hours, with more than 12 hours being considered prolonged. Of course, there is no exact cut-off point for defining prolonged labors. The longer beyond these figures the labor goes, the greater the likelihood there will be fetal distress and damage.

Head trauma incurred during labor is a common cause of brain damage. The most common manifestations of birth trauma that may be associated with brain injury are cephalhematoma, facial nerve paralysis, brachial palsy, phrenic nerve paralysis, fracture of the clavicle, and hematoma of the sternocleidomastoid muscle.

Breech deliveries are generally more traumatic than vertex. Caesarean sections, especially those that are resorted to because of complications that have interfered with delivery via the birth canal, have also been associated with MBD. It is probable that it was not the Caesarean section *per se* that caused the MBD, but the complications that caused the obstetrician to utilize this method of delivery. When a child is born with the umbilical cord around the neck, there may have been some compromise of blood circulation from the placenta to the fetal brain. When the cord presents first, there may be compression of the blood circulation to the child, with resultant impairment of circulation to the infant's brain. Excessive blood loss during labor may also reduce the amount of blood reaching the infant.

As mentioned, birth weight is no longer considered to be the criterion of prematurity. In fact, most neonatologists discourage the use of the term prematurity. Low-birth-weight babies, that is, those weighing less than 2500 grams, are divided into two categories: (1) those whose birth weights are appropriate for their gestational age (AGA) and (2) those whose weights are low, that is, they are small for gestational age (SGA). As mentioned above, we now have objective physiological and neurological criteria for determining gestational age and do not have to rely on a mother's recollection of when she thinks she became pregnant. The babies in these two groups are quite different. Consider, for example, two babies whose birth weight is 1500 grams. One baby is found to have a gestational age of 31 weeks and the other 37 weeks. Because 1500 grams is about normal for 31 week fetuses, the first baby would be considered AGA. The second would be considered SGA. The assumption is made that the second baby has only grown to the 31 week size in a 37 week pregnancy. Something has happened to retard the child's growth. The second child is more likely to exhibit difficulties that would include MBD. The first is more likely to develop normally in that nothing serious is considered to have happened to it, although its low birth weight is still an abnormality that may cause difficulty. The questionnaire asks the parent for the birth weight as well as whether it was an AGA or SGA baby. Many of the children now being seen were born before the utilization of these terms, but in time knowledge of them should become more widespread.

Babies of large size (over 9 pounds) are also at greater risk for the development of MBD, in that their deliveries are more likely to be traumatic. Babies of long gestation (over 42 weeks) are also likely to have complications such as MBD because the aging placenta becomes more inefficient in its functioning and meconium aspiration is also more likely in such infants.

POST DELIVERY PERIOD
(WHILE IN THE HOSPITAL)

The healthy child breathes spontaneously at birth. At most, the child requires some clearing of the nasal passages. The traditional slap to get the child breathing is considered by most obstetricians to be unnecessary. The usual nasopharyngeal aspiration provides enough stimulation to induce breathing. The longer the delay in breathing the greater the likelihood the child will suffer with cerebral anoxemia. The normal infant spontaneously cries at birth. A delayed cry is also an index of infant depression, especially of respiration and bodily response to stimulation. A fairly objective statement about the newborn's overall physical condition at the time of birth is the Apgar score (Apgar, 1953; Apgar et al., 1958). At one, two, and five minutes after birth, the child is given a score of 0, 1, or 2 on five items (Figure 1.3). The five physiological functions evaluated are heart rate, respiratory effort, muscle tone, reflex irritability, and general color. With a maximum score of 2 in each category, the maximum score is 10. A score of 1, 2, or 3 is considered severe depression; 4, 5, 6, or 7 is moderate depression; and 8, 9, or 10 is no depression. Most mothers are not aware of the existence of this figure, and many who are do not know what recording was made on their child. When the figure can be obtained, it is a valuable bit of information.

Figure 1.3

The Parents' Questionnaire

infant injured during delivery_____

other (specify)_____

Birth Weight_____

Appropriate for gestational age (AG)_____

Small for gestational age (SGA)_____

POST-DELIVERY PERIOD (while in the hospital)
Respiration: immediate_____delayed (if so, how long)_____

Cry: immediate_____delayed (if so, how long)_____

Mucus accumulation_____

Apgar score (if known)_____

Jaundice_____

Rh factor_____transfusion_____

Cyanosis (turned blue)_____

Incubator care_____number of days_____

Suck: strong_____weak_____

Infection (specify)_____

Vomiting_____diarrhea_____

Birth defects (specify)_____

Total number of days baby was in the hospital after the

delivery_____

INFANCY-TODDLER PERIOD
Were any of the following present--to a significant degree--
during the first few years of life? If so, describe.

Did not enjoy cuddling_____

Was not calmed by being held and/or stroked_____

Colic_____

Excessive restlessness_____

Diminished sleep because of restlessness and easy arousal_____

Frequent headbanging_____

Constantly into everything_____

Excessive number of accidents compared to other children_____

About 40% of newborns exhibit a transient physiologic jaundice (icterus neonatorum). There are two causes of this type of jaundice: (1) There is the increased destruction of red blood cells in order to reduce the high fetal red cell concentration (necessary for intrauterine existence) to the lower levels necessary after birth. (2) The immature liver is inefficient in its capacity to metabolize bilirubin and other products of red blood cell destruction. Generally, the jaundice appears on the second to fourth day and ends between the seventh and fourteenth. Jaundice due to Rh incompatibility (erythroblastosis fetalis) or ABO incompatability (icterus praecox) usually begins during the first 24 hours and is severer. Whereas transfusions are not necessary for physiological jaundice, they are for the treatment of Rh incompatability and severe forms of ABO incompatability. Recently developed immunological treatment with RhoGAM (an anti-Rh + antibody globulin) can prevent Rh incompatibility disorder in mothers who have not yet been sensitized. Less common causes of jaundice in the newborn are congenital obliteration or obstruction of the bile ducts, septicemia, hepatitis, and a variety of blood dyscrasias. The most common examples of brain damage caused by high bilirubin levels is the kernicterus resulting from icteric degeneration of the basal ganglia as well as other cerebral centers.

Cyanosis is a concomitant of anoxia, which may cause cerebral ischemia and nerve cell dysfunction and degeneration. Anoxia may be seen in prematurity in association with the respiratory distress syndrome (hyaline membrane disease), maternal toxemia, and any other condition in which the neonate is under stress. Intracranial hemorrhage (most often caused by birth trauma and hemorrhagic disease of the newborn), congenital atalectasis, hyaline membrane disease, and various congenital heart diseases can also cause cyanosis. The need for incubator care may be a clue to the presence of apnea, cyanosis, and a variety of diseases affecting respiration and circulation.

The normal baby has a strong suck. A weak suck at birth is generally suggestive of some pathological process. Often it is one manifestation of general neurological depression. Meningitis may be the result of infections in the newborn. Generally it is caused by organisms found in the mother's vagina infecting the fetus and producing septicemia in the newborn infant. Infected circumcisions, umbilical stumps, and otitis media, once common causes of mengititis, are less common today.

A variety of congenital anomolies may be associated with neurophysiological impairment. This is especially true of those disorders that directly involve the central nervous system and/or the tissues and bones in which it is encased. The most common disorders in this category are meningocele, meningomyelocele, meningoencephalocele, hydrocephalus, and spina bifida. Congenital cardiac anomalies may also be associated with cerebral nerve cell degeneration. This is especially true of the cyanotic forms that are associated with hypoxic spells such as the tetralogy of Fallot. In chapter 12 I will describe some of the minor external physical anomalies (stigmata) that have also been associated with minimal brain dysfunction.

If the child was in the hospital for more than five days, one should inquire about the reasons. Usually, a stay beyond that time was necessitated by some physical disorder that may be associated with MBD.

THE INFANCY-TODDLER PERIOD

The normal human infant enjoys being hugged and caressed. This desire is present from birth and the child who is deprived of such gratification may become listless, lose his or her appetite, withdraw interest from the environment, become marantic, and even die (Spitz, 1945, 1946a, 1946b). If a child, from the day of birth, does not respond to stroking and cuddling, then some interfering factor is usually present. Sometimes the mother herself is impaired in her desire and/or capacity to fondle her baby. Or she does so with such tension that the child does not find it a gratifying experience. Such mothers may consider breast feeding "disgusting" and may show other signs of inhibition in maternal capacity. Such a mother will generally react similarly to her other children. The child's hyporeactivity in such situations should be considered psychogenic.

If, however, the child is described as not having reacted to cuddling and stroking from birth and the siblings are described as having done so, then it is more likely that the child's impairment is due to some physical disease such as mental retardation, autism, and brain dysfunction. At times the MBD child may be differentiated from the retarded and autistic by its hyperreactivity to such stimulation. The autistic and retarded child may be described as lying in the mother's arms limp and unresponsive "like a sack of potatoes." The MBD child, however, may respond to stroking by becoming irritable, crying, and fighting off such stimulation. These reactions may be a manifestation of the same mechanisms that produce hyperactivity and impulsivity.

A history of colic is often described by parents of MBD children. They may look back upon the first year or two of the child's life as a nightmare in which they hardly slept. The cry of such children is often shrill and piercing, described by parents as "a sound like a siren," "an animal in acute distress," and "the high thin note of static on the radio" (Ross and Ross, 1976).

These children are often described as the "last to go to sleep at night and the first to get up in the morning." Their restlessness in bed may interfere with the sleep of others in the household. They may frequently knock themselves against the sides of their cribs or bang their heads. After they begin to walk, they are constantly into everything, and their curiosity is even greater than that of the normal toddler (whose curiosity is usually insatiable). Some parents say of MBD children that "their terrible twos started at nine months." They are heedless to danger and are accident prone. This does not appear to be on a psychogenic basis. They are not compelled by some deep neurotic or psychotic self-destructive need to harm themselves. Rather their accident proneness is the result of their neurophysiological impairments: their inability to learn well from experience, their intellectual deficits, their problems in adequately processing incoming stimuli, etc. They may be well known to the doctors at the nearby emergency room, and they may have a number of scars which serve to remind observers of their accidents, but not themselves.

DEVELOPMENTAL MILESTONES

Parents are not famous for the accuracy of their recollections regarding the times at which their children reached the various developmental milestones. Often, rather than saying that they do not recall, they give a figure that is no more than a guess. Obviously, such information is of little value to the examiner. Yet it is important for the examiner to get such data because developmental lags are commonly seen in children with MBD. Furthermore, the data provide vital information regarding the presence of the developmental type of soft neurological sign that will be discussed in detail in chapter 6. The questionnaire (Figure 1.4) allows the parent the face-saving "out" of being able to say that the information has been forgotten. In addition, three categories of response can be provided under the "I cannot recall exactly" heading: it occurred (1) early, (2) at the normal time, and (3) late. When developmental questions are so posed, the information the examiner does get is more likely to be useful.

The normal times at which the milestones occur is subject to significant variation, but the later beyond the normal range the capacity is reached the greater the likelihood that pathology is present. Smiling usually occurs by 2 months, sitting without support at 6–7 months, crawling at 7 months, standing without support at 10–11 months, and walking without support at 12–14 months. There is greater variability regarding the normal range for the onset of speech.

Figure 1.4

The Parents' Questionnaire

DEVELOPMENTAL MILESTONES
If you can recall, record the age at which your child reached
the following developmental milestones. If you cannot recall,
check item at right.

	age	I cannot recall exactly, but to the best of my recollection it occurred		
		early	at the normal time	late
Smiled				
Sat without support				
Crawled				
Stood without support				
Walked without assistance				
Spoke first words besides "ma-ma" and "da-da"				
Said phrases				
Said sentences				
Bowel trained, day				
Bowel trained, night				
Bladder trained, day				
Bladder trained, night				
Rode tricycle				
Rode bicycle (without training wheels)				
Buttoned clothing				
Tied shoelaces				
Named colors				
Named coins				
Said alphabet in order				
Began to read				

COORDINATION
Rate your child on the following skills:

	Good	Average	Poor
Walking			
Running			
Throwing			
Catching			
Shoelace tying			
Buttoning			
Writing			
Athletic abilities			

The words *ma-ma* and *da-da* are poor criteria for determining the age of speech onset because parents are likely to hear such articulations in the normal babbling sounds of the infant. (This is especially true for first babies.) Accordingly, the question for determining the age of onset of first words asks for words other than these. Nine to 14 months is generally the time for the appearance of single words. The appearance of first phrases and first sentences is very variable. First phrases appear at about 18 months and short sentences at about 24 months, but the normal range is so variable that the age of onset of these functions is of limited diagnostic value. However, it is important for the examiner to appreciate that there are children who do not speak at all until 3 and even 4 years of age who do not have any neurological impairment. I believe that the failure to speak between 2 and 4, when there is no demonstrable organic cause (such as MBD, severe hearing loss, retardation, autism or schizophrenia) is a manifestation of psychogenic problems. The period between 4 and 5 appears to be a crucial one for the onset of speech. My experience has been that if a child does not start to speak by 4 it may or may not be a sign of organic pathology. However, if a child does not utilize *intelligible* speech by 5 years of age it is almost invariably a sign of severe pathology. In such cases I generally consider mental retardation and autism or other forms of childhood schizophrenia. MBD children, although sometimes lagging with regard to the time of speech onset, are not generally so late that they do not start until 5 or after. In addition, the child who has not started to utilize intelligible speech by 5 may never do so. Such children must be differentiated from those with elective mutism. The latter know how to speak, but generally confine themselves to communicating verbally with certain people (usually their parents).

The general assumption is made that children cannot voluntarily control their bowel movements until they are old enough to walk. Accordingly, the parent who states that a child was bowel trained at 6 months and started to walk at 12 months is not providing valid information. One possibility here is that the child had a fairly regular schedule and the parent caught him or her at the right moment for placement on the potty or toilet. Bowel training for day and night usually occurs between 2 and 3 years of age. Bladder training occurs later and is more variable. Many children are bladder trained during the day (commonly established by 2½–3 years of age) before nocturnal control is achieved. So great is the normal variation for nighttime wetting that there is no good cutoff point in childhood which can be used to define the pathological. It is a disservice to a child to automatically assume that nighttime wetting after the age of 5 or 6, for example, is automatically a manifestation of psychiatric problems. It may be the result of neurophysiological immaturity or physiological hyperirritability. When bowel and bladder training are late in the MBD child, a number of factors may be operative: neurophysiological lag, hyperirritability, impaired attention to internal stimuli, and intellectual deficit.

Children of 2-2½ generally pedal a tricycle and by 6-7 ride a bicycle without training wheels. The ability to button clothing generally occurs at around 3½ and tying shoelaces at 5-6. At 4 most children can name the majority of major colors (I will discuss the complexity of this process in chapter 9) and by 5-5½ name a few coins. Most can repeat the letters of the alphabet at 4-5 years and start to read between 5 and 6. It is in the area of reading that the MBD child may exhibit his or her problems most dramatically. (More will be said about the MBD child's reading impairments in chapter 8).

COORDINATION

The evaluation of coordination may be quite subjective. This is not only true for the parent, but for the examiner as well. Accordingly, the coordination tests to be presented later in this book (chapter 5) use only objective criteria. The parents' views, however, often do have merit, especially if they are only asked to state whether the child is "good," "average," or "poor" compared to others with regard to the ability to perform certain functions that depend upon coordination capacity. The questionnaire (Figure 1.4) focuses on such functions that involve fine and/or gross motor coordination.

COMPREHENSION AND UNDERSTANDING

The questions in this section of the questionnaire (Figure 1.5) attempt to provide the examiner with information about the child's general level of intelligence. This may be a very highly charged area for the parents of the MBD child. They generally will see the child as brighter than he or she may be. They may use rationalizations such as, "His intelligence is really normal but he's *slower* to understand than other children." Others may even describe the child as "basically very bright" even though there is little if any evidence that this is the case. The parents may hold to the statement made by some professionals that "MBD children's intelligence is in the normal range." I do not believe that the average child who is correctly diagnosed as having MBD is of normal intelligence. Although there are many MBD children with above average and even superior IQs, there are many more in the low average and borderline range. The average MBD child in my experience has an IQ of about 90, that is, at the bottom of the normal range. The professional who says that the average MBD child has a normal IQ is ignoring all we know about the ways in which such children's deficits impair them on most, if not all, of the WISC-R subtests, the very test used to assess these children's intelligence.

The first question in this section of the questionnaire (Figure 1.5) is essentially directed to parents who are defensive about or denying their child's possible intellectual impairment. The second asks more directly about intelligence.

SCHOOL

It is in school, more than anywhere else, that the MBD child's deficits may reveal themselves. Many MBD children are not recognized as being different from others until they attend school. There the teacher has the opportunity to compare the child to others his or her age, and is generally knowledgeable enough about what is age appropriate to be able to spot atypical behavior quite readily. In addition, it is in school that the learning impairments, so commonly seen in MBD, may first become apparent. Lastly, it is in the school, more than anywhere else, that the child's capacity for self-inhibition is tested, and it is in school, therefore, that the MBD child's impulsivity is likely to cause him the most difficulty.

The questionnaire sections that refer to school (Figures 1.5 and 1.6) are divided into two categories: academic learning and behavior. In the academic section the questions attempt to provide the examiner with specific information regarding the child's level of performance. The questions have been designed to focus on information that will provide the examiner with as accurate a picture as possible of the child's academic functioning: specific grade levels in reading, spelling, and arithmetic; history of grade repeat; type of class (regular or special); and special therapy or remedial work.

The second section is devoted to school behavior. Again, the aim is to get information that is as specific as possible. The checklist in the middle of this section focuses on many of the most common complaints made by teachers about MBD children. These problems are manifestations of their hyperactivity (Doesn't sit still in his or her seat); impulsivity (Shouts out. Won't wait his or her turn); impaired concentration (Typically does better in a one-to-one relationship); and impaired ability to project oneself into another's situation (Doesn't respect the rights of others).

Figure 1.5
The Parents' Questionnaire

COMPREHENSION AND UNDERSTANDING

Do you consider your child to understand directions and situations as well as other children his or her age? If not, why not?_____

How would you rate your child's overall level of intelligence compared to other children? Below average_____Average_____ Above average_____

SCHOOL

Rate your child's school experiences related to <u>academic learning</u>:

	Good	Average	Poor
Nursery school			
Kindergarten			
Current grade			

To the best of your knowledge, at what grade level is your child functioning: reading_____spelling_____arithmetic_____

Has your child ever had to repeat a grade? If so, when_____

Present class placement: regular class_____special class (if so, specify)_____

Kinds of special therapy or remedial work your child is currently receiving_____

Describe briefly any academic school problems_____

_____

Rate your child's school experience related to <u>behavior</u>:

	Good	Average	Poor
Nursery school			
Kindergarten			
Current grade			

Does your child's teacher describe any of the following as significant classroom problems?

Doesn't sit still in his or her seat_____

Frequently gets up and walks around the classroom_____

Shouts out. Doesn't wait to be called upon_____

Won't wait his or her turn_____

Figure 1.6
The Parents' Questionnaire

Does not cooperate well in group activities_____

Typically does better in a one-to-one relationship_____

Doesn't respect the rights of others_____

Doesn't pay attention during storytelling_____

Describe briefly any other classroom behavioral problems_____

_____

_____

PEER RELATIONSHIPS

Does your child seek friendships with peers?_____

Is your child sought by peers for friendship?_____

Does your child play primarily with children his or her own age? ____younger_____older_____

Describe briefly any problems your child may have with peers

_____

_____

HOME BEHAVIOR

All children exhibit, to some degree, the kinds of behavior listed below. Check those that you believe your child exhibits to an excessive or exaggerated degree when compared to other children his or her age.

Hyperactivity (high activity level)_____

Poor attention span_____

Impulsivity (poor self control_____

Low frustration threshold_____

Temper outbursts_____

Sloppy table manners_____

Interrupts frequently_____

Doesn't listen when being spoken to_____

Sudden outbursts of physical abuse of other children_____

Acts like he or she is driven by a motor_____

Wears out shoes more frequently than siblings_____

Heedless to danger_____

Excessive number of accidents_____

Doesn't learn from experience_____

Poor memory_____

More active than siblings_____

Finally, both sections provide the parent with the opportunity to describe other school problems that may not have been referred to in the questions previously posed.

PEER RELATIONSHIPS

Information about peer relationships is less useful than school behavior, but more useful than home behavior in diagnosing MBD. The requirement for self-restraint is greatest in school, least at home, and somewhere in the middle of these with peers. Teachers will tolerate the least degree of antisocial behavior, parents the most, and peers something in the middle. The questions posed about peer relationships (Figure 1.6) attempt to focus specifically on the most common problems with friends that MBD children have. The most sensitive indices of whether the MBD child is relating well to peers is his or her degree of reaching out to them and whether they are seeking the child. The age of playmates (younger, older, same age) also tells something about the child's degree of success with friends.

HOME BEHAVIOR

Home behavior is a poor criterion on which to determine whether a child's behavior is pathological. Practically all siblings fight. Where does the normal degree of rather fierce sibling rivalry end and the pathological begin? All children exhibit poor table manners at times. Where does one draw the line between normal table sloppiness and the pathological? And, as mentioned, parents will tolerate greater degrees of atypical behavior than teachers and peers. Yet pathology can certainly manifest itself in the home. In order to ascertain whether the child's home behavior may be pathological, the parent is asked to check those items (Figure 1.6) in which the child's behavior is exaggerated or excessive when compared to other children the child's age. Included here again are those behavioral patterns that relate to some of the primary manifestations of MBD, viz., hyperactivity, poor attention span, impulsivity, and memory impairments.

INTERESTS AND ACCOMPLISHMENTS

Most of the previous items have focused on the child's deficits. Such emphasis may be upsetting to the parent who is filling out the questionnaire. For the parents' well-being, as well as providing the examiner with a more balanced picture of the child, a section (Figure 1.7) is devoted to the child's assets. An inquiry into hobbies, interests, and accomplishments may provide useful diagnostic information. Reading is obviously not likely to be the favorite pastime of the MBD child. Watching TV or listening to music may be (I don't claim these to be pathognomonic for the disorder). An MBD child may have deep involvement in sports and do well in them. Success in this area, then, provides information about the child's coordination. Others may do well in school but are abysmally poor in sports. In short, the areas of interest and pleasure may provide information about the child's healthy areas of neurophysiological functioning.

MEDICAL HISTORY

In this section of the questionnaire (Figure 1.7), an attempt is made to learn about any illnesses that occurred after the newborn child left the hospital, illnesses that might have been of etiological importance in the child's MBD. The traditional childhood diseases, such as measles and mumps, were occasionally associated with central nervous system complications such as encephalitis. Fortunately, with the advent of new vaccines, we are seeing much less of these disorders. A history of coma and/or seizures associated with such an illness is suggestive of central nervous system involvement even though medical attention may not have been sought. Operations may provide a clue to the etiology. For example, the child with frequent bouts of otitis media requiring myringotomies is suspect for hearing impairment which may interfere with speech and learning. There is hardly a child who does not sustain occasional head trauma. But when it is associated with unconsciousness or coma, then brain dysfunction (not necessarily permanent) must be suspected.

There was a time when a child who only had seizures with fever was considered to be neurologically normal. He was considered to have "febrile seizures," which were not taken as seriously as those that occurred in the afebrile state. One reflection of this relaxed attitude toward febrile convulsions was the view that such seizures did not warrant anticonvulsant medication. The traditional treatment of such seizures was to warn the mother to give the child elixir phenobarbital (or other anticonvulsant medication) as soon as the child showed signs of illness—especially a febrile illness. Unfortunately, children have a way of spiking fevers so rapidly that mothers were often unaware that the child was getting sick and so did not often give the anticonvulsant in time to prevent the convulsion. Many pediatric neurologists today

Figure 1.7

The Parents' Questionnaire

INTERESTS AND ACCOMPLISHMENTS

What are your child's main hobbies and interests?_____

_____

What are your child's areas of greatest accomplishment? _____

_____

What does your child enjoy doing most?_____

_____

What does your child dislike doing most?_____

_____

MEDICAL HISTORY

If your child's medical history includes any of the following, please note the age when the incident or illness occurred and any other pertinent information.

Childhood diseases (describe any complications)_____

_____

Operations_____

_____

Hospitalizations for illness(es) other than operations_____

_____

Head injuries_____

_____with unconsciousness_____without unconscious-

ness_____

Convulsions_____

_____with fever_____without fever_____

Coma_____

Meningitis or encephalitis_____

Immunization reactions_____

Persistent high fevers_____highest temperature ever

recorded_____

Eye problems_____

Ear problems_____

Poisoning_____

take such seizures more seriously. They hold also that in addition to the basic pathology that causes the seizures, a seizure *per se* can result in superimposed damage to the brain. A grand mal seizure includes an apneic phase and this can cause cerebral hypoxia. Accordingly, a child with febrile seizures may be placed on maintenance anticonvulsant medication if there is a family history of seizures, signs of organic cerebral dysfunction, or other factors indicative of a high risk of further brain dysfunction. I have seen a few children with MBD who had febrile seizures that went untreated because they were "only febrile." I believe that the extent of their brain dysfunction would have been far less had they been on medication to prevent their convulsions.

Meningitis and encephalitis, especially when associated with coma, is highly correlated with residual brain damage and is one of the more generally accepted causes of MBD. Encephalitides are also known to be a concomitant of untoward immunization reactions. There are some children who easily run persistently high fevers with practically any infection. Others may manifest such fevers without known cause. Children with fevers of unknown etiology may have some kind of neurophysiological dysfunction which is akin to and possibly a symptom of MBD. The same factors that have produced neurophysiological abnormalities in other parts of the brain may be causing impaired functioning of temperature regulatory mechanisms.

As will be discussed in chapter 8, reading difficulties can be the result of pathological processes anywhere along the pathway from the eye to the occipital cortex (as well as in neurological systems that are interconnected). Strabismus, squinting, tearing, holding the book at a distance, holding the book too close, inclining the head to the side while reading, and easy reading fatigability are all suspicious signs of ocular problems that can contribute to reading difficulties—problems that can usually respond to optometric and/or ophthalmological treatment. Such considerations are all too often neglected in the MBD workup and the parent's indicating a history of eye problems should alert the examiner to their presence.

Ear disorders, such as chronic infections, can involve the brain. The child who has trouble hearing or trouble understanding what he or she hears may not only have some disorder of the external ear but of the central auditory processing mechanisms as well. As will be discussed in greater detail in chapter 7, auditory examination is all too often neglected in the MBD workup. The parents recording a history of ear problems should warrant the examiner's further investigation.

Although lead has been implicated more than other substances as an etiological factor in MBD, the ingestion of other substances must be considered. The impulsivity, poor judgment, and intellectual impairment of MBD children makes them more likely to ingest drugs, poisons, and other dangerous substances. Accordingly, poisons should not only be viewed as primary etiological agents, but as potentially causing superimposed brain damage as well.

PRESENT MEDICAL STATUS

Most of the examiners for whom this book is written do not have scales in their offices for the purpose of measuring height and weight. Accordingly, it is useful to get these figures (Figure 1.8). They are not as likely to be significantly distorted by the parents as some of the other information provided, and the examiner, by merely looking at the child, can generally determine whether the figures provided are roughly accurate. In chapter 12 I will discuss the use to which the examiner can put such information.

It is also important for the examiner to know whether the child is presently suffering with any illnesses, as the symptoms of such disorders can affect one's findings. For example, acute allergic reactions can cause the kind of agitation that can sometimes be confused with hyperactivity. The allergic child, however, will manifest other signs of allergy (sniffling, rash, conjunctivitis, etc.) to help the examiner in the differential diagnosis. The medications a child is taking are also important to know about. We have a long way to go in learning about the various factors that can produce MBD. It is possible, and even probable, that long term use of certain medications might cause nerve cell dysfunction. In addition, the drugs a child is taking may affect performance on the diagnostic tests that are given. A child taking phenobarbital as an anticonvulsant (frequently the first choice anticonvulsant for children) is not likely to be as alert when taking the WISC-R, for example, as the child who is not taking barbiturates.

FAMILY HISTORY—MOTHER

One is interested in the mother's age at the time of the pregnancy with the patient because the older the mother the greater the likelihood she will give birth to a child with various kinds of anomalies and malformations. One is also interested in the past history of spontaneous abortion because it is reasonable to assume that if the mother tends to lose and reject embryos and fetuses, those that are retained may be subject to the same kinds of rejection processes. Accordingly, there may be a greater likelihood of impairment in such mothers' retained fetuses than

Figure 1.8
The Parents' Questionnaire

PRESENT MEDICAL STATUS

Present height_____Present weight_____

Present illness(es) for which child is being treated_____

_____

Medications child is taking on an ongoing basis_____

_____

FAMILY HISTORY - MOTHER

Age_____ Age at time of pregnancy with patient_____

Number of previous pregnancies_____Number of spontaneous abor-

  tions (miscarriages)_____Number of induced abortions_____

Sterility problems (specify)_____

School: Highest grade completed_____

  Learning problems (specify)_____grade repeat_____

  Behavior problems (specify)_____

Medical problems (specify)_____

Have any of your blood relatives (not including patient and
  siblings) ever had problems similar to those your child has?
  If so, describe_____

_____

_____

FAMILY HISTORY - FATHER

Age_____Age at the time of the patient's conception_____

Sterility problems (specify)_____

School: Highest grade completed_____

  Learning problems (specify)_____grade repeat_____

  Behavior problems (specify)_____

Medical problems (specify)_____

Have any of your blood relatives (not including patient and
siblings) ever had problems similar to those your child has?
If so, describe_____

_____

in fetuses of mothers with no previous history of spontaneous abortion. This is especially the case when chromosomal malfunctions habitually cause the abortions. In addition, one is also interested in the past history of induced abortions. A mother with a history of sterility problems may be rejecting fertilized eggs and providing an intrauterine environment that is not optimally conducive to the healthy growth and development of the fertilized ovum. It is reasonable to speculate that the embryo that does finally grow to maturity is being exposed to the same detrimental influences and has a greater likelihood of being malformed.

One does well to inquire into the presence of significant medical problems because many maternal illnesses (infectious, metabolic, toxic, etc.) can have a significant effect on the developing embryo and fetus. Lastly, one wants to learn if blood relatives of the mother had symptoms similar to the child's when they were younger. As mentioned, genetic factors are probably operative in some children with MBD and this aspect of the inquiry may elucidate this etiological factor.

It is also important to get information about the mother's school history. Genetic factors are often operative in MBD, especially the learning disabilities and hyperactivity. The questions on maternal history of school learning problems, grade repeat, and behavior problems are designed to provide information in these areas.

FAMILY HISTORY—FATHER

Sterility problems on the father's part may contribute to less than optimum sperm conditions for conception and a higher risk of embryonic abnormalities. One should give serious attention to the father's school history with regard to learning problems, grade repeat, and behavior problems, because present evidence suggests that the genetic factors appear more along the paternal than the maternal line. Although one should inquire into the father's medical problems, they are far less likely to be of etiological significance for the MBD child. Again, one should inquire into the presence of the child's symptoms in the father's blood relatives to evaluate the presence of genetic factors.

SIBLINGS

If the questionnaire (Figure 1.9) indicates that one or more siblings reveals symptoms of MBD, a detailed history of that child's disorder is also warranted. Such an inquiry can sometimes shed light on the etiology of the patient's disorder. If the clinical pictures are similar and the sibling is older, something may be learned about the patient's prognosis.

Figure 1.9
The Parents' Questionnaire

SIBLINGS

	Name	Age	Medical, social, or academic problems
1.			
2.			
3.			
4.			
5.			

LIST NAMES AND ADDRESSES OF ANY OTHER PROFESSIONALS CONSULTED

1. _____

2. _____

3. _____

4. _____

ADDITIONAL REMARKS

Please use the remainder of this page to write any additional comments you wish to make regarding your child's difficulties.

FINAL COMMENTS

Information from other professionals is most often useful. Many parents come with a folder of reports from previous professionals, and they can often provide valuable information. Lastly, the parent is invited to record any additional comments. Although the questionnaire attempts to be thorough, there are often special issues relevant to the patient that may not have been focused upon.

Although the anamnesis described here is lengthy and may be considered laborious by some parents, it is crucial to obtain if the examiner is to properly evaluate the child with MBD. It is important for the reader to appreciate that this questionnaire is designed to be of value only in the assessment of the MBD child. Although some of the information gained here may be of use in the evaluation of a child's psychogenic problems, it is of only limited use in this regard.

2

⬜ Hyperactivity

Hyperactivity has generally been considered to be one of the cardinal signs of minimal brain dysfunction in children and this author concurs. The association between hyperactivity and MBD is so deep that there are some who prefer the term *hyperactive child* to refer to children with MBD. The term hyperactivity, however, has been used loosely, and the most subjective criteria have often been utilized when employing the term. Many examiners have applied the label on the basis of teacher and/or parent impressions even though they may not have observed the sign themselves. (Hyperactive children are typically less active in the one-to-one situation, such as an office examination, when all attention is directed to them.) The professionals in such cases can be justifiably accused of putting their stamp of approval on a diagnosis made by nonprofessionals, of lending their authority to perpetuating a diagnostic label that may not be appropriate. There are few examples in medicine where physicians are as quick to take the word of others in making their diagnoses. The failure to use objective criteria for employing the term has added to the widespread confusion that already exists regarding MBD—its etiology(ies), diagnosis, treatment(s), prognosis, and even whether or not it actually exists.

THE SUBJECTIVE ASSESSMENT
OF HYPERACTIVITY

There are a number of criteria that have traditionally been used to determine whether a child is hyperactive. Most often these relate to historical material provided by the parents. Certain types of information provided by teachers have also been utilized, and direct observation by the examiner has often provided additional data. Although these sources are frequently utilized, they are poor criteria upon which to decide that a child is hyperactive. Few, if any, of them have been subject to rigorous well-controlled studies. The questionnaire described in chapter 1 was designed to elicit information regarding hyperactivity. Although such data are based on subjective impressions, they are useful to have because they suggest the existence of hyperactivity. When they are absent it is less likely that the child will be diagnosed as hyperactive.

Parents may describe the MBD child as having been more active in utero than the patient's siblings. Even the father may claim that the MBD child disturbed his sleep more than his siblings by kicking him as he lay close to the mother at night. At birth the MBD child is sometimes described as having been hyperirritable. Whereas normal children are calmed and quieted by soothing caresses, the MBD child may be made even more irritable. Colic is described as more common in these children and it is considered to be a manifestation of smooth muscle hyperactivity analogous to the child's skeletal muscle hyperactivity. MBD children are often described from infancy to be "the last to go to sleep at night and the first to get up in the morning." And even when they do sleep their restlessness keeps family members awake. Their "terrible twos" are said to start at nine months. They have more accidents than other children, ingest more inedible substances, and appear to be heedless to danger. They wear out their shoes more quickly than their siblings. At the meal table they jump up and down, wiggle in their seats, slop food all around them, sing and talk while eating, and prevent others at the table from relaxing enough to enjoy their meals.

In school the teachers generally report difficulty from the outset. The child does not sit still and listen to stories. He is out of his seat more than in it. He walks around the classroom, not only not doing his own work but interfering with others attending to theirs. He does not raise his hand and wait to be called upon; rather he blurts out his answers as soon as they come to mind. He does not cooperate well in group activities, but will do better in one-to-one relationships with the teacher. Especially during silent reading time is the child likely to be particularly rambunctious.

As mentioned, many MBD children do better in the one-to-one

situation. Accordingly, the examiner may not observe many of the manifestations of hyperactivity described by others. In the more severe cases, however, one may observe excessive talkativeness, fidgeting, frequent interrupting, climbing, swivelling in chairs, opening drawers, and inability to stick to any task as long as other children the child's age.

Such is the traditional picture of hyperactivity. How much of the above is fact and how much fantasy is difficult to say. All of the above is manifested to some degree by normal children as well as by those with psychogenic problems. Where the normal degree of such activity ends and the pathological begins is difficult to determine. The objective instruments described below were devised in the attempt to quantify such behavior.

**INSTRUMENTS DESIGNED
TO MEASURE
HYPERACTIVITY OBJECTIVELY**

Many instruments have been devised to quantitatively measure activity level in children. Irwin (1930, 1932) used a stabilimetric crib connected to a polygraph to measure the activity level of newborn infants from birth to two weeks of age. The studies were done in the early 1930s, prior to the introduction of the MBD concept, and so only normative data on 73 full-term infants is provided. Irwin found great variation among the infants, the most active being 290 times more active than the quietest. We cannot be certain that there weren't within his group some children whom we would today consider to have MBD. More recently, Lipsitt and DeLucia (1960) have described a stabilimetric crib combined with a photoelectric cell to measure activity level in the newborn. However, they do not provide normative data. Kessen, Hendry, and Leutzendorff (1961) used a technique of film analysis of newborns which quantifies activity. Displacement of various parts of the body were measured at specific intervals. Fifteen infants were studied in various ways, samples not large enough, however, to provide meaningful baseline data. These infant measuring instruments, like many of the others to be discussed, were designed as experimental devices for laboratory studies, and they do not lend themselves easily to widespread utilization in the office or clinic.

Sprague and Toppe (1966) used a stabilimetric chair to measure the activity level of 30 retarded children during a study in which the reinforcement capacity of low and high activity level youngsters were compared. One-quarter inch right-left or forward-backward movements of the child resulted in the depression of springs placed under the legs of the chair. These were connected to switches and counters that recorded the child's activity. Foshee (1958) employed a ballistographic chair to measure the activity level of 101 mentally retarded children in a study comparing the learning capacity of subjects with low and high activity levels. A schoolroom desk was secured upon a platform that was supported at the four corners by rubber stoppers. A mechanical lever arrangement connected to a transducer converted the longitudinal movements of the platform into an electric current for recording the chair movements. In both of these studies, no data is provided for either normal or MBD children, and the devices, although of interest and possibly of value to the clinical evaluation of children with MBD, do not lend themselves well to general utilization.

Ellis and Pryer (1959) studied the activity levels of 29 severely retarded children (mean IQ 17) in an 8 ft × 8 ft room crossed by six exciter lamp beams and pick-up photoelectric cells. Impulse counters recorded each interruption of the beam. The concept was described for possible future clinical utilization. Johnson (1972) attempted to use an ultrasonic device to measure activity level in retarded children and found significant drawbacks: it did not differentiate between fine and gross movements, distance from the device was an important determinant of whether it would record, and there was great variability among different units. He also used photoelectric cells to measure activity level and considered their main drawback to be the fact that activity that did not interrupt the beam (such as head and hand movements made while the subject was stationary) was not recorded. Montagu and Swarbrick (1974) were more optimistic than Johnson about the usefulness of the ultrasonic device for measuring activity level, but agreed that it measured total activity and did not discriminate among various types of activity (fine from gross motor, for example). For the measurement of locational activity they recommended the placing of pressure mats, of the kind used in burglar alarm devices, at various points under a carpet. Each time the subject stepped on one of the pressure devices a circuit was closed and a recording made. The method was relatively inexpensive (compared to the other devices thus far described) but no normative data was provided.

Lee and Hutt (1964) described a hidden camera technique for filming the activity of children in the playroom. Sainsbury (1954) found motion pictures to be useful in measuring the frequency of such movements as tics, nail biting, and nervous mannerisms and considered the method to have potential for measuring the frequency of other types of human body movement. Radio telemetry has shown promise for measuring activity levels, especially because it does not require any connection between the subject and the recording device. Rubenstein (1962) considered the movements between the trunk and the thigh to be representative of gross body movements in general. A transducer placed at this juncture activated a pocket radio transmitter whenever a trunk-thigh movement was executed of greater than 1° amplitude. Centrally located equipment recorded the transmitted radio signals on a chart and a magnetic tape. Herron and Ramsden (1967a, 1967b) designed a short range transducer-transmitter that can be placed in the heel of the subject's shoe and transmit signals related to leg activity. They considered such pedometers to be more reliable than mechanical devices. However, unlike the latter they require the subject to remain within the range of the central receiving apparatus. Again, no normative data was given, only descriptions of the device and recommendations for its potential use. Davis, Sprague, and Werry (1969) used a body transducer which, when moved, activated a transmitter to send signals to recording devices. They studied the effect of drugs on the activity level of nine severely retarded children (mean IQ 14). The transmitter was attached to a light hockey helmet and transmitted signals on both frontal and lateral head movements. The purposes of the study did not involve providing data for either normal children or those with MBD.

Pedometers have been particularly attractive as instruments for measuring a child's activity level because they do not require the child to remain in the laboratory, and so they lend themselves to more widespread use. Schulman and Reisman (1959) and Bell (1968) utilized actometers, viz., self-winding calendar watches that were modified to become activated by movement of the limb to which they were strapped. Pope (1970) used head and foot accelerometers to measure children's activity levels. Such devices generally record movement in one axis only, and one needs to strap instruments to various limbs in order to detect movement in all axes. Johnson (1971) raised serious questions about the value of actometers. He claimed that the reliability between and within watches varied greatly. Only the movement of the limb to which the device was attached was recorded, and even then the speed and acceleration of movements are also important if the instrument was to record properly. Most examiners agree also that it is not reasonable to expect a child to walk around with two to four such devices over a period of time without playing with, tampering, removing, or activating them for pleasure. Colburn et al. (1976) designed a small activity monitor that allowed the subject freedom of movement while continually monitoring and recording activity. The device, worn on the wrist, used a solid state digital memory to record movement and so the subject was not confined to a laboratory setting. Brown (1977) used the

Colburn device on hyperactive children and found that they played with the instrument and thereby artificially increased their scores. Placing it on the back of a special vest prevented this contamination of their studies.

In short, none of the aforementioned devices has ever enjoyed widespread utilization. Either they were too intricate, cumbersome, or expensive to be used outside of the laboratory setting or their particular drawbacks discouraged their utilization.

QUESTIONNAIRES DESIGNED TO MEASURE HYPERACTIVITY

A number of questionnaires have been designed to measure children's hyperactivity. These generally are of the rating scale type. They have the obvious advantage over the aforementioned mechanical devices in that they are inexpensive and capable of being used anywhere. The most well-known scales are The Werry-Weiss-Peters Activity Scale (Werry, 1968); The Bell, Waldrop, and Weller Rating System (Bell et al., 1972); The Conners' Teacher Rating Scale (Conners, 1969); The Conners' Parent Questionnaire (Conners, 1973); and Davids' Rating Scale for Hyperkinesis (Davids, 1971). I have serious reservations about these scales and have not personally found them useful.

One objection relates to rater reliability. When filling out such a scale the rater is often placed in the position of making almost impossible discriminations. He or she may be asked questions about whether a child's behavior falls into the category "just a little" as opposed to the category "pretty much" (Conners' Teacher Rating Scale and Conners' Parent Questionnaire). All six items of the Davids' scale (1971) ask the rater to differentiate "slightly more" from "more" and "much more" as well as "slightly less" from "less" and "much less." Especially on scales that have many items (The Conners' Parent Questionnaire has 94), the rater is going to fatigue and become less thoughtful regarding the answers. I would go further and state that if, immediately after completing one of these scales, a parent or teacher were asked to repeat his or her answers on a new blank, there would be significant differences, especially on the longer scales.

A number of years ago I conducted a study (Gardner, 1969) in which parents were asked to write their answers to 28 true-false questions. Immediately after the test was completed I verbally reviewed each question with the parent. I found that 10–15% of the responses had to be changed. Either the parent did not understand the question and yet marked an answer so as not to reveal his or her ignorance, or the question was understood but the parent placed an answer in the box inappropriate to the intended response. This was a simple true-false questionnaire, involving only a choice between two responses. The errors introduced into a scale that allows for four possible responses must be greater. Simpson (1944) found significant differences among raters when applying the category "frequently." Twenty-five percent of raters used the term to denote events occurring up to 40% of the time and another 25% used it to refer only to events occurring over 80% of the time. This so-called objective data is then fed into computers and serves as the basis for some of the most sophisticated statistical analyses. The conclusions derived from such studies must be suspect considering the questionable value of the data on which they are primarily based.

Subjective elements are introduced in other ways. The raters' own background and experience must contribute to whether he or she will consider many behavioral items unusual or excessive. People from European and Asian backgrounds consider just about all American children to be excessively active, and they consider the permissiveness of American parents to be the cause. Klein and Gittelman-Klein (1974) found that mothers tended to deny manifestations of hyperactivity when filling out such scales and to give their child lower scores than social workers. And most examiners agree that teachers are likely to see behavior as more severe when it causes trouble or conflict. By what criteria does one decide whether a child "talks excessively" (Werry-Weiss-Peters Activity Scale)? Where does the normal frequency end and the pathological begin for such behavior as "restlessness during church/movies," "restlessness during shopping," and "disrupt's other's play" (Werry-Weiss-Peters Activity Scale)?

My most important objection, however, relates to the basic validity of these scales—whether or not they actually measure hyperactivity. Some of the items are clearly related to hyperactive behavior, such as questions about wiggling, getting up and down from the seat, interrupting, and fidgeting. However, finding the point where the normal degree of such behavior ends and the pathological begins is often very difficult, if not impossible. In my opinion, it is the inclusion of items that have little or nothing to do with hyperactivity or minimal brain dysfunction that lessens significantly the value of such scales for diagnostic purposes, as well as for determining treatment progress. The Bell,

Waldrop, and Weller Rating System includes "emotional aggression" and "nomadic play" as two of the seven items in their hyperactivity scale. Although both of these *may* be seen in children with MBD, they are certainly seen with significant frequency in children with purely psychogenic problems. The Conners' Parent Questionnaire, which is purported to have diagnosed hyperactivity in 74% of 133 cases (Conners, 1970), has such items as headaches, stomachaches, vomiting, loose bowels, bullying, plays with sex organs, truancy, stealing, firesetting, pouts and sulks, perfectionism, shy, mean, and daydreams. These, and many of the other symptoms listed on the Conners' scale, are primarily, if not entirely, psychogenic in etiology. Because it may be true that MBD children, because of their basic handicap, are more likely to have such superimposed psychogenic problems than those without MBD, does not justify including such items in a scale designed to be used with children with this disorder. The tendency on the part of the rater has been to assume that these symptoms are an intrinsic part of MBD and not differentiate between those symptoms that are primary manifestations and those that are secondary psychogenic. Conners' scale mixes them all together.

Conners (1969) has factor analyzed the 39 items on his Teacher Rating Scale (which includes such items as selfish, daydreams, "tattles," steals, lies, appears to lack leadership, and shy) and has delineated five clusters: I, aggressive conduct; II, daydreaming-inattentive; III, anxious-fearful; IV hyperactivity; and V, sociable-cooperative. The factor IV group not only includes items that are traditionally associated with hyperactivity (sits diddling with small objects, hums and makes other odd noises, restless, and overactive) but others that I do not consider to be an intrinsic manifestation of neurological impairment (disturbs other children, teases other children and interferes with their activities, excessive demands for teacher's attention, submissive, and overly anxious to please.) Again, it is probably true that MBD children are more likely than normals to have these symptoms. However, the clear distinction between primary organic manifestations and secondary psychological problems is very important for etiological understanding as well as for therapeutic purposes. Scales that clump them together easily lead the user of the scale to forget about making this important differentiation.

Saxon et al. (1976) studied the construct validity of three of the aforementioned rating scales (Conners, 1969; Bell et al., 1970; Davids, 1971) by determining if there were any correlations between parents' ratings on the scales and two more objective laboratory measures of hyperactivity. Laboratory measurements of hyperactivity were determined by (1) actometers (self-winding calendar watches that had been converted to motion recorders), and (2) ultrasonic motion detectors (burglar alarm systems that quantitatively measured the amount of the child's movement in a 9 ft × 11 ft room). They found no significant correlation between the child's activity as measured by either of the two devices and activity level as determined by the parents' using any of the three scales. It is of interest that Saxon et al. used the total Conners Teachers' Rating Scale, not just the factor IV items, thus confirming my previously expressed belief that the more common use of the Conners' scale is to view all the items as being in some way correlated with hyperactivity. Ross and Ross (1976) share my views regarding the limitations of these four scales and provide an excellent discussion of their deficiencies.

In spite of their obvious drawbacks, these scales presently enjoy great popularity among researchers. They are frequently used in research on the efficacy of psychostimulant medication and often serve as the primary criterion for evaluating the potency of such drugs. Therefore, the value of a drug to reduce hyperactivity is being tested by scales that have not been well demonstrated to measure hyperactivity. Accordingly, the conclusions that are being reached by such studies are of dubious value. In short, I consider these scales to be of doubtful validity and questionable reliability. I much prefer the questionnaire that I provide parents at the time of my initial evaluation. It is designed to alert the examiner to the presence of the common etiological factors and basic neurological signs and symptoms of MBD. Such information provided by parents serves as a point of departure for a more detailed inquiry. The information so gained is far more valuable, in my opinion, than a pseudoscientific number that represents a composite of a wide range of often unrelated bits of information.

THE KLØVE-KNIGHTS STEADINESS TESTER

I believe that the steadiness tester holds promise to be one of the most sensitive, practical, and inexpensive tools for measuring hyperactivity. When a child is asked to hold a stylus in a hole, as steadily as possible, and contact duration with the hole's perimeter is electronically recorded, an objective measurement of steadiness is obtained. If the MBD child's hyperactivity is being "driven from within," i.e., a manifestation of central nervous system pathology, then it is reasonable to expect that there will be generalized hyperactivity, not merely of isolated parts of the body. (The MBD child is rarely described as exhibiting more activity in one part of the body over another.) Conners (1974) and Douglas (1972, 1974a, 1974b) provide good evidence that the MBD child's hyperactivity is not a primary sign, but secondary to a fundamental impairment in the ability to sustain concentration. Unable to maintain concentration on one goal, the child flits from one activity to the next—thus the hyperactivity (Pope, 1970). If this is the case, then a steadiness tester *that required prolonged attention* would pick up this deficit. Such a device would also detect the motor impersistence (Garfield, 1964; Garfield et al., 1966) also described in these children, because the child who would be required to hold the stylus steadily for a long period would falter as muscle contraction could not be sustained. Such a device would also detect the tremors and choreiform movements occasionally seen in children with MBD (Prechtl and Stemmer, 1962).

A steadiness tester is relatively simple to construct and more compact than many of the previously described instruments. It can be used in the office or clinic setting and need not be confined to the laboratory. Although it does not have the advantage of being taken home by the child, it cannot be tampered with or misused by the child either. Many of the scores obtained on the previously described devices depend upon the vicissitudes of the child's situation such as play interests, television viewing, distractions, etc. With a steadiness tester, one confines oneself specifically to a particular activity and so "purer" data are obtained. Lastly, the instrument is generally an attractive one to children—they often perceive it as a game and rise to the challenge of trying to hold the stylus as steady as possible. Accordingly, cooperation and predictability of response are enhanced.

Knights (1966) collected normative data for a steadiness tester devised by Kløve. The device used was the nine-hole steadiness tester manufactured by the Lafayette Instrument Company (catalogue no. 32011). The plate of holes consists of a top row of four progressively smaller holes and a bottom row of five progressively smaller holes (the first hole in the second row being smaller than the last in the first row). Children ages 5–8 use only the top four larger holes, whereas those 9–14 use all nine. The subject holds the stylus for 10 sec in each of the holes and the number of contacts with the edge of the holes as well as the total duration of contact with all holes is recorded. In Knights' original article, there were four to seven children of each sex in each of the age brackets. No information is provided regarding where along the stylus the child is permitted to hold it. This is of importance because the closer to the tip the child holds the stylus, the more steadily it can be maintained. Nor is anything mentioned about positioning of the hand, arm, or elbow. Obviously, if such positioning is not standardized it is difficult, if not impossible, to meaningfully compare children's scores. A child, for example, who is supporting his or her wrist on the table or elbow on the knee is going to perform better than one who is not benefiting from such support. Nothing is said about the duration of "resting time" between holes. Clearly, the longer the child has to rest between holes the better will be the performance. In later publications, Knights and Ogilvie (1967) and Knights (1973) state that there were significant differences between normal and brain-damaged children on the progressive-holes test, but specific data is not provided. Elsewhere, Knights and Moule (1968) provide further normative data for the test. However, in this study the scores of boys and girls at each age level are not separated; the assumption is made that there is no difference. The number of subjects at each age level ranges from 10–22 (average, 18.4). Smoothed normative data for the same group of subjects was subsequently provided by Knights (1970). Briggs and Tellegen (1971) have also published normative data using the nine-hole Lafayette instrument. However, their format was very different from that used by Knights et al.; 12 sec was required at each hole, and the data for boys and girls was separated.

THE GARDNER STEADINESS TESTER

Because of my reservations about the Knights' instrument and data, because of some of the operational problems intrinsic to the utilization of the instrument, and because of my belief that the steadiness tester has significant potential in both diagnosing and monitoring the treatment of MBD, my colleagues and I decided to work on an instrument that would attempt to correct the deficiencies of the Knights device while retaining its value. A. Gardner (Gardner et al. 1979) designed such an instrument (Figures 2.1 and 2.2). The device utilizes standard components (Figure 2.3 and Table 2.1). In an attempt to develop a more compact device, Caemmerer (Gardner et al. 1979) devised an instrument that utilizes integrated circuits (Figures 2.4, 2.5, Table 2.2, and Figure 2.6). Unfortunately, the Caemmerer instrument proved to be significantly more expensive to manufacture than the Gardner device and so it has not thus far been marketed.

Figure 2.1
Steadiness Tester Utilizing Standard Components (Examinee's View).

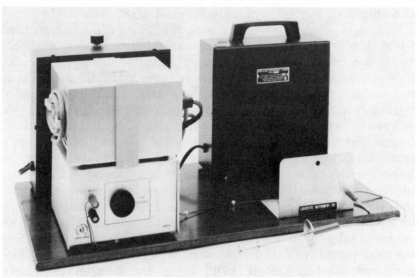

Figure 2.2
Steadiness Tester Utilizing Standard Components (Examiner's View).

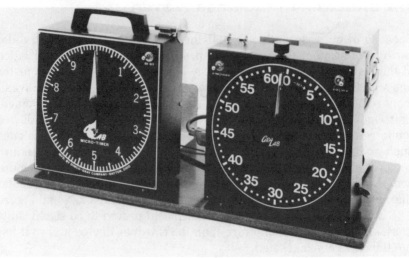

Figure 2.3
Schematic Diagram of the Steadiness Tester Utilizing Standard Components.

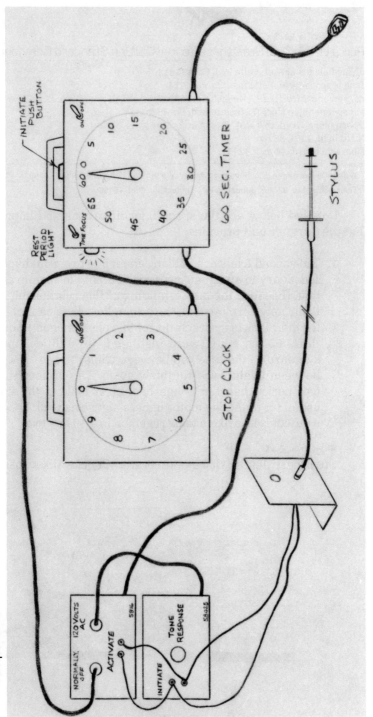

Table 2.1

Parts List for the Steadiness Tester Utilizing Standard Components

Stylus/hole tester (Lafayette Inst. Co. #32013)[a]
Tone response (Lafayette Inst. Co. #58025)
AC power control (Lafayette Inst. Co. #58016)
Micro-timer stop clock (Lafayette Inst. Co. #54011)
60-sec timer (Gra-Lab #400)[b]
Night light, 110V 60 Hz
Fiberesin board, 12 in. × 22 in.

[a] Lafayette Instrument Co., Sagamore Parkway & 9th Rd., Lafayette, Indiana 47902
[b] Dimco-Gray Co., 8200 S. Suburban Rd., Centerville, Ohio 45459

Detailed below are the specific modifications and improvements that the Gardner unit provides.

1. Ten-second trials are not long enough to bring out hyperactivity secondary to an impairment in the ability to sustain concentration. (Because the understanding of this relationship is a relatively new development, the original workers cannot be faulted for their lack of appreciation of this phenomenon.) Accordingly, three 60-sec trials were instituted. In addition, in order to standardize the time gap between trials, 15-sec "rest periods" between trials were routinely given. The prolongation of the test period has the fringe benefit of making the instrument useful for detecting motor impersistence as well, because such a defect is less likely to be revealed in a 10-sec trial.

Figure 2.4

Steadiness Tester Utilizing Integrated Circuits [Examinee's View].

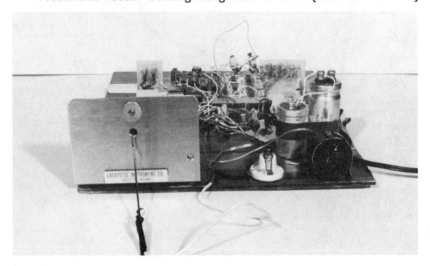

Figure 2.5
Steadiness Tester Utilizing Integrated Circuits [Top View].

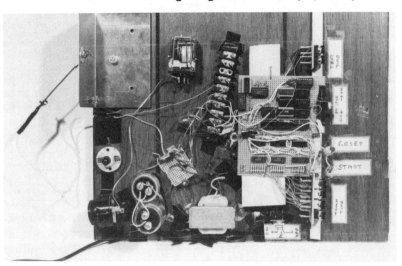

Table 2.2
Parts List for the Steadiness Tester Utilizing Integrated Circuits

C_1 100 pf	Q2 7805 5V regulator, 1A, heat sink required
C_2, C_3 C_2 + C_3 must equal at least 6,000 MFD	relay 5V, 10mA, coil
C_4 100 pf	R1 to R24 220 1/8 watt resister
D1 diode 20 PIV, 1A	R25 1K 1/8 watt resister
D2 bridge rectifier 20 PIV, 2A	R26 660K 1/4 watt resister
IC1 to IC3[a] 7447A	R27 1K 1/8 watt resister
IC4 to 1C6[b] 7490A	R28
IC7 7476	R29 1K trim-pot
IC8 7404	R30 to R44 220 1/8 watt resister
IC9[b] 7492A	S1,S2 normally open SPST push button
IC10 7414	S3,S4 STSP toggle switch (S3 rated at
IC11 74123A	120VAC, 1A)
IC12, IC13 7408	6 common anode 7 segment displays
IC14, IC15[a] 7447A	(DL 707)[a]
IC16 to IC19 7490A[b]	2 screw terminals for stylus and plate
Lamp, 1.5V bulb	1 wall socket power cord
L1 117VAC primary, 6.3VAC secondary,	Sonalert model #SC628 (P. R. Malory & Co.,
2A transformer	Inc.)
Q1 2N3414 (heat sink recommended)	

[a] Pin numbers for outputs IC1 to IC3 and IC14 and IC15 are as follows: a-13, b-12, c-11, d-10, e-9, f-15, g-14.

[b] Pin numbers for IC1 to IC3, IC14 and IC15 are identical to the ones marked on IC1. Pin numbers for IC4 to IC6, IC9, and IC16 to IC19 are identical to the ones marked on IC4.

Note: The outputs of IC1,2,3,14,15 are connected to the six DL 707 displays. The displays are not clearly marked on the schematic.

Figure 2.6
Schematic Diagram of the Steadiness Tester Utilizing Integrated Circuits.

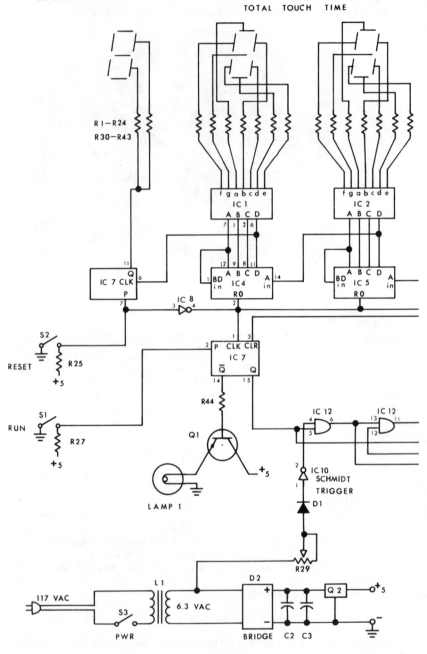

TOTAL TOUCH TIME

STEADINESS TESTER   MODEL TWO

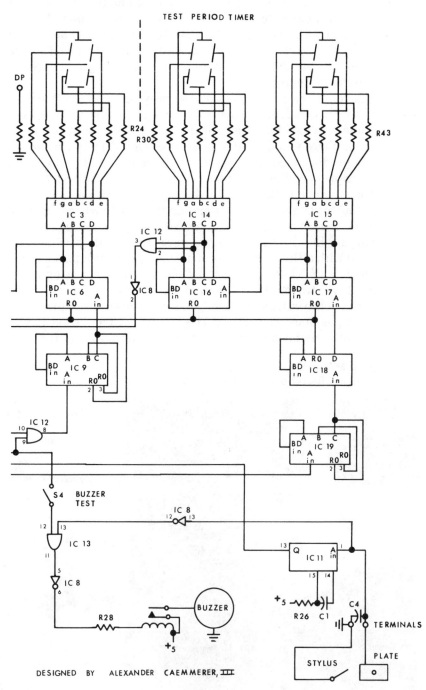

TEST PERIOD TIMER

DESIGNED BY ALEXANDER CAEMMERER, III

45

2. The use of four graduated holes for some children and nine for others appeared to be an unnecessary complication. Accordingly, a hole diameter of 9/32 (.281) in. and a stylus diameter of 5/64 (.078) in. were found empirically to provide a reasonable challenge for children from 5–15, as well as a good "spread" of data for analysis.

3. The tip of the stylus used by the previous workers is only a point. By withdrawing the stylus to a position slightly in front of the hole the child can "cheat." Accordingly, in the modified stylus there is a disc attached to the end of the stylus which will produce electrical contact with the hole plate if the child attempts to withdraw the stylus from the hole (Figure 2.7).

4. The distance between the stylus tip that is available for hole perimeter contact and the place on the handle where the child grips it has not been standardized by previous examiners. Varying the distance between these two points provides the child with different degrees of accuracy, because the closer to the hole the child's hand is, the smaller the arc a given movement will traverse, and the less the likelihood of contact. Accordingly, a stylus was designed with three discs placed at fixed positions (Figure 2.7). The function of the disc at the tip has already been described. A second disc, 1 in. in from the

Figure 2.7
Steadiness Tester with the Stylus Held in Hole.

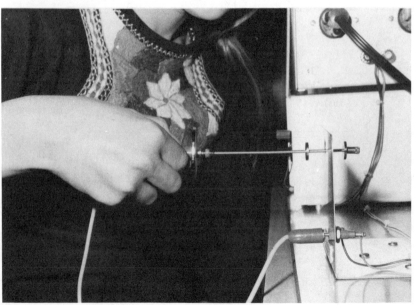

tip, prevents the child from pushing the stylus deep into the hole. (The two discs together serve to encourage positioning the stylus at a point about 1/2 in. from the tip.) A larger disc is placed exactly 4 in. from the tip and this acts as a shield, preventing the child from gripping the stylus closer to the hole. Lastly, the stylus handle is 1¾ in. long, thereby preventing the extra support and leverage that the child would gain from a longer handle that could be stabilized by resting it against the thenar eminence.

5. No standardization of wrist, forearm, and arm positioning is described by the previous authors. Clearly, leaning the hand on the table, the elbow on the table or the knee, or even pressing the arm against the chest can provide stability and thereby affect the child's score. In utilizing the Gardner instrument, the child is permitted to either stand or sit (younger children often choose to stand), but is told that all of the aforementioned forms of extra support are not permitted. A correctly positioned child is shown in Figure 2.8. (If a child provides himself or herself with such support during the testing period the trial is discontinued and then repeated in the proper manner.) Further standardization of positioning is provided by asking the child, prior to the test, which hand he or she prefers to use. The child is then so positioned in front of the apparatus (either when seated or standing) that the long axis of the child's arm and forearm are in the same plane as the stylus.

6. Two clocks are used—a regular clock and timer in the device using standard circuitry (Figure 2.2) and digital clocks (Figure 2.5) in the instrument using integrated circuits. One clock records total touch time and the other the duration of the trial. The clocks are so positioned that they cannot be seen by the child during the testing period. This prevents the child from being distracted by them (Figure 2.9). Counting the number of stylus contacts was omitted because it was decided that this figure is not too meaningful. A 1/10-sec touch, for example, would be counted the same as a 1-sec contact (10 times longer) —clearly a source of misleading data.

7. Instructions and administration of the test are also standardized. As the child approaches the unit he or she is told: "This is a test to see how still you can hold your hand. Which hand would you like to use?" The examiner then demonstrates how contact between stylus and hole produces a sound and then, after positioning the child so that no extra support is gained, provides the subject with a practice period of 15–60 sec. The three 60–sec trials are then conducted.

Figure 2.8
Correctly Positioned Child Using the Steadiness Tester.

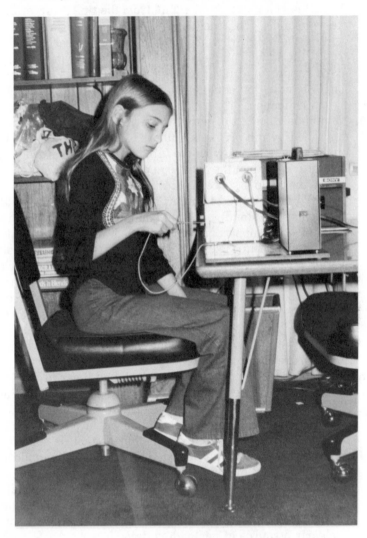

The number of children included in the aforementioned studies was not large enough to provide examiners with the security that firm normative data had been obtained, especially over a broad range of ages for each sex. In order to provide such data, 500 normal children (25 normal boys and 25 normal girls at each age level from 5–14) were

Figure 2.9
Steadiness Tester with a Child and Examiner Correctly Positioned for Testing.

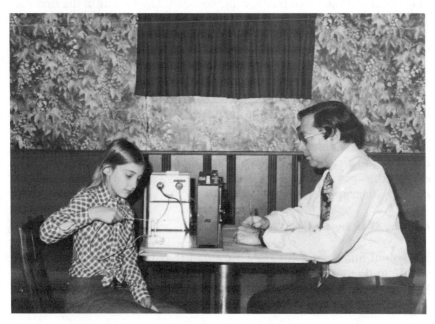

administered the steadiness test. In addition, data was collected from 356 children with MBD (250 boys and 106 girls, ages 5–15) for comparison purposes. The normal subjects were all students in northern New Jersey public schools. Attempts were made to include only children in the 90–110 IQ range. All children in regular classes with a history of significant academic difficulty, grade repeat, hyperactivity, poor concentration, or other manifestations of MBD were excluded from the study. Children in the MBD group were all in either special classes or schools designed for their education. MBD children "mainstreamed" in regular classes and those on medication were not included. The number of children at each age level in the normal group is large enough to warrant considering the data as standard for this group. The MBD group data were collected primarily for comparison purposes and the number of children at many age levels (especially for girls) is not large enough to justify utilizing the MBD data as "normative" for this group. Furthermore, the range for MBD children is much wider than for normals, further lessening the standardization of their data.

RESULTS

Each child's cumulative touch time, obtained by summing the touch time of each of the three trials, was recorded. The results of the findings on the 500 normal children are summarized in Table 2.3, which enables the examiner to compare a child's score with others his or her age utilizing means, standard deviations,[1] and percentile ranks. For the purposes of comparison, data was also obtained on 356 children with MBD. The findings for this group are shown in Table 2.4.

When I began the study, I was completely prepared to conclude either that MBD children did or did not differ from normals with regard to their performance on the steadiness tester. The comparisons of the two groups are summarized in Figure 2.10 where the mean touch times for boys and girls in each group (normals and MBDs) are presented for each of the ages studied. Figures 2.11 and 2.12 present the accumulated data in bar-graph form.

Age by Sex by Group Comparisons

Statistical analysis of the data revealed that the two groups differed significantly at all age levels, supporting the generally held belief that MBD children are more active than normals. Touch-time scores totaled across trials 1, 2, and 3 were entered into a three-way analysis of vari-

[1] For the reader who may not be familiar with this term, one way of viewing standard deviation is to consider it a measure of the concentration of measurements around the mean figure. For a distribution of measurements that form a bell-shaped curve, 1 standard deviation distance from the mean (represented by the fiftieth percentile level) includes approximately 34% of the measurements on either side of the mean. Accordingly, values from the 16% (50% − 34%) to the 84% (50% + 34%) levels are included. This is usually considered to be the average range. It includes the central 68% (34% + 34%) of the measurements. It is the central block of figures around the mean figure. Any measurement lying within ± 1 standard deviation (S.D.) from the mean is considered normal. Two standard deviations include approximately 48% of the measurements on either side of the mean. Therefore, the ± 2 S.D. range goes from the 2% level (50%−48%) to the 98% level (50% + 48%). Figures lying between 1 and 2 standard deviations from the mean are generally considered atypical enough to be abnormal. They roughly correspond (again, in the bell-shaped curve) to the 2% − 16% level and the 84% − 98% level. Similarly, 3 standard deviations include all measurements falling approximately 49.9% on either side of the mean, that is, from the 0.1% (50% − 49.9%) level to the 99.9% (50% + 49.9%) level. The greater the number of standard deviations from the mean, the more atypical the figure.

To calculate the number of standard deviations that a particular measurement differs from the mean, one determines the difference between the measurement and the mean and divides this figure by the standard deviation. For example, a 7½-year-old boy obtains a steadiness tester score of 32.5. Referring to Table 2.3 we note that the mean score for boys in the 7-0 to 7-11 age bracket is 13.93 ± 9.53. The difference between this boy's score and the mean is 18.57 (32.5 − 13.93). To determine the number of standard deviations that 32.5 differs from the mean, one divides 18.57 by the standard deviation 9.53. The figure we obtain is 1.95. Accordingly, we can conclude that this boy's score is deviant enough from the mean (almost 2 S.D.) to warrant our considering it extremely atypical or pathological.

Table 2.3

Steadiness Tester: Total Touch Time

Age	N	Mean	S.D.	Percentiles								
				10	20	30	40	50	60	70	80	90
Normal Boys												
5-0 to 5-11	26	39.03	20.95	74.40	56.75	47.87	45.75	34.25	31.30	24.60	19.85	11.57
6-0 to 6-11	30	25.45	16.59	47.32	38.85	30.67	24.30	22.25	17.85	16.72	11.55	7.42
7-0 to 7-11	27	13.93	9.53	26.90	22.95	17.20	14.80	12.50	11.10	6.55	4.90	3.15
8-0 to 8-11	28	8.23	6.06	20.32	10.95	9.50	8.65	6.75	5.60	4.25	3.25	2.20
9-0 to 9-11	27	10.43	7.18	17.05	15.10	14.05	12.60	9.75	7.55	5.55	4.50	2.70
10-0 to 10-11	28	8.80	7.33	20.17	12.45	10.15	7.50	7.00	6.30	5.02	2.85	1.72
11-0 to 11-11	25	3.97	3.78	10.25	4.45	4.05	3.30	2.50	2.50	2.25	1.80	1.50
12-0 to 12-11	26	5.40	5.79	13.55	9.05	7.10	3.25	3.00	2.70	1.80	1.45	0.85
13-0 to 13-11	27	3.77	3.25	9.30	6.50	5.00	4.25	2.75	1.85	1.25	0.75	0.25
14-0 to 14-11	12	4.99	5.83	16.90	9.50	7.20	3.15	1.75	1.75	1.42	0.65	0.15
	256											
Normal Girls												
5-0 to 5-11	27	30.37	22.63	71.25	40.70	31.80	28.45	26.75	21.60	16.50	13.85	6.90
6-0 to 6-11	29	22.05	14.40	48.25	40.00	29.25	19.25	16.25	14.00	13.00	9.50	7.50
7-0 to 7-11	25	13.77	9.74	29.95	24.60	19.25	15.65	11.50	7.95	5.50	4.70	3.55
8-0 to 8-11	27	5.77	5.77	13.70	9.45	6.20	5.35	4.00	2.75	2.25	1.90	1.00
9-0 to 9-11	25	5.75	5.54	16.55	10.75	5.00	4.55	3.50	3.00	2.70	1.65	1.15
10-0 to 10-11	25	5.01	3.72	9.50	7.40	6.25	5.15	4.25	3.05	2.60	2.00	1.55
11-0 to 11-11	25	2.10	1.88	5.80	3.75	2.50	2.05	1.25	1.10	0.75	0.50	0.50
12-0 to 12-11	25	1.87	1.47	4.60	2.75	2.05	1.75	1.75	1.20	1.00	0.75	0.25
13-0 to 13-11	25	1.17	1.05	2.85	2.00	1.80	1.15	0.75	0.60	0.45	0.25	0.15
14-0 to 14-11	11	3.25	2.86	9.65	4.25	4.10	3.20	2.50	1.70	1.40	1.25	1.05
	244											

Table 2.4
Steadiness Tester: Total Touch Time

Age	N	Mean	S.D.	10	20	30	40	Percentiles 50	60	70	80	90
MBD Boys												
5-0 to 5-11	10	87.00	37.26	150.35	108.40	106.65	98.80	91.25	89.85	63.52	45.30	28.87
6-0 to 6-11	16	74.66	53.91	159.40	131.05	105.85	95.10	78.87	33.80	30.77	19.35	10.50
7-0 to 7-11	28	45.79	30.58	87.02	65.80	59.62	45.55	41.87	33.15	30.02	21.85	10.80
8-0 to 8-11	29	43.04	41.98	115.00	100.00	45.50	37.75	26.50	16.00	12.75	11.00	8.50
9-0 to 9-11	32	33.98	33.71	63.12	56.15	42.87	35.50	23.37	17.00	12.22	8.50	4.40
10-0 to 10-11	28	18.30	17.45	55.57	28.00	23.65	17.15	11.00	8.35	6.55	4.60	1.95
11-0 to 11-11	26	29.97	33.02	89.27	46.90	31.47	26.25	15.62	12.15	7.60	5.50	4.15
12-0 to 12-11	26	18.09	26.77	51.20	24.90	15.20	13.10	9.00	7.50	5.55	3.00	1.25
13-0 to 13-11	28	14.69	18.24	50.50	27.15	12.95	10.40	7.12	5.60	3.17	2.40	0.97
14-0 to 15-7	27	15.07	22.60	46.35	19.35	13.80	11.25	8.50	4.80	2.85	2.45	1.25
	250											
MBD Girls												
5-0 to 5-11	2	114.00	22.63	—	—	—	—	—	—	—	—	—
6-0 to 6-11	8	99.00	56.48	—	167.35	—	120.64	—	71.45	—	50.15	—
7-0 to 7-11	15	60.45	45.37	152.60	94.35	76.95	53.55	40.50	40.20	32.50	21.50	16.05
8-0 to 8-11	11	60.38	40.70	145.20	90.50	70.55	61.15	58.25	46.05	29.95	23.95	17.45
9-0 to 9-11	15	38.73	40.64	121.80	68.80	46.00	38.85	32.50	14.00	9.25	5.25	1.95
10-0 to 10-11	9	48.69	48.81	—	81.25	—	62.00	—	19.25	—	11.75	—
11-0 to 11-11	16	39.16	51.66	142.80	84.30	41.57	28.25	8.25	7.60	6.32	5.70	3.02
12-0 to 12-11	10	30.63	38.19	120.80	41.85	39.10	32.85	18.50	11.35	6.57	3.80	0.80
13-0 to 13-11	13	15.52	17.29	49.15	25.15	23.40	13.15	8.00	6.65	4.20	3.20	2.70
14-0 to 15-9	7	21.32	31.73	—	67.40	—	6.60	—	2.60	—	0.55	—
	106											

Figure 2.10

Steadiness Tester: Mean Total Touch Time for All Subjects.
Normal Boys: N = 256; MBD Boys: N = 250. Normal Girls: N = 244;
MBD Girls: N = 106.

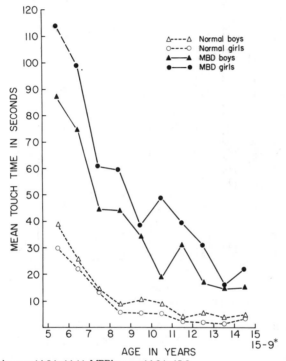

AGE IN YEARS

* Normals: ages 14-0 to 14-11. MBD's: ages 14-0 to 15-9.

ance, age (10 levels, 5 through 14–15 years) by group (2 levels, normals
vs. MBD children) by sex (2 levels, males vs. females). All three main
effects were highly significant: age ($p < .001$),[2] reflecting a linear decrease in touch-time scores with increasing age; sex ($p < .005$), reflecting
longer touch-time scores for girls; and group ($p < .001$) reflecting longer
touch-time scores for MBD children compared to normal children. Two
significant interactions—age by group ($p < .001$) and sex by group
($p < .001$)—indicated that age as well as sex differences varied according to group. However, age and sex did not interact significantly.

[2] For the reader who may not be familiar with the statistical symbol p, it symbolizes the
probability that a given event or relationship is due to chance. In this case the relationship
being considered is between age and total touch time. Here the term $p < .001$ indicates
that the likelihood that the relationship found to exist between age and touch time could
have been due to chance alone is less than 1 in a 1000. Or, stated another way, the chance
that the two are related is greater than 999 in a 1000.

Figure 2.11

Steadiness Tester: Ranges for Boys. Normal Boys: N = 256; MBD Boys: N = 250.

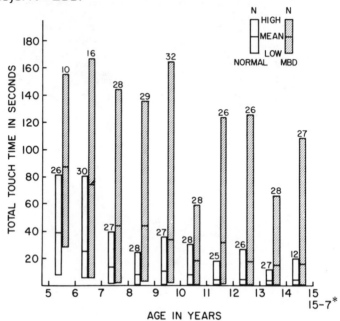

AGE IN YEARS

* Normals: ages 14-0 to 14-11. MBD's ages 14-0 to 15-7.

Individual age, sex, and group means were compared by the Duncan Multiple Range procedure (Duncan, 1955) in order to elucidate the meaning of the significant interactions.

Comparisons Among Age Levels According to Group

Within the normal group, 5-year-olds and 6-year-olds obtained longer touch-time scores than all other succeeding age levels (all p's < .05). Differences among age levels 7 through 14–15 years in mean touch-time scores were nonsignificant. Within the MBD group, 5-, 6-, and 8-year-olds differed significantly from all succeeding age levels (all p's < .05). Seven- and 8-year-olds did not differ, nor did 9- through 11-year-olds, nor did 12- through 14–15-year-olds; but differences among all of these age groups were significant (all p's < .05).

Comparisons Between Groups According to Age

Comparisons of means obtained by MBD and normal children at every age level indicated a superiority for the normal group throughout the range of ages tested (all p's < .05). If one accepts the author's premise

Figure 2.12

Steadiness Tester: Ranges for Girls. Normal Girls: N = 244; MBD Girls: N = 109.

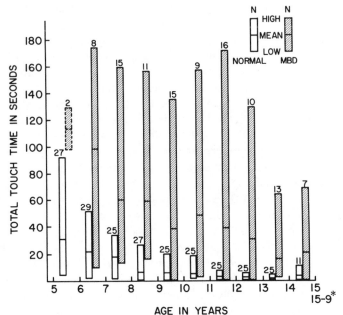

* Normals: ages 14-0 to 14-11; MBD's: ages 14-0 to 15-9.

that the steadiness tester is a sensitive gauge of hyperactivity, then the view that hyperactivity is more frequently seen in MBD children than normals is substantiated by this study. To conclude, as well, that hyperactivity is a manifestation of MBD is, in my opinion, also warranted. Otherwise one must postulate that hyperactivity is a separate disorder, unrelated to MBD, that happens to appear more frequently in MBD children than normal children. The two-disease postulation is, in my opinion, less preferable than the one-disease explanation.

Comparisons Between Sexes
According to Group

Comparison of scores obtained by MBD boys and girls revealed a significant superiority for boys ($p < .001$); however, although mean touch-time scores for normal girls were superior to those obtained by normal boys, this difference was not significant. The sex difference in the MBD group was consistent across age levels, as shown by the nonsignificant age by sex and by group interaction.

This finding raises an interesting question. Why should MBD girls do more poorly than MBD boys at every age level on the steadiness tester? It is well known that females not only live longer but appear to be more resistant to most diseases (except, of course, with the exception of disorders of the breast and the female reproductive system). Does such resistance extend to those factors that are of etiological significance in MBD? Most observers agree that there are far more boys being diagnosed MBD than girls (and this was certainly our experience). Perhaps the female's greater resistance is an explanation for this. With such heightened resistance a female would have to be exposed to a higher intensity of the etiological factor in order to acquire the disorder and, when acquired, it might manifest itself in severer form. On the other hand, one could accept the basic thesis that the female is more resistant and yet postulate that she might develop only milder forms of the disorder when afflicted. Her greater resistance, then, would lessen the likelihood of the disease process causing severe damage.

Another possible explanation for this finding is that it is an artifact of selection. In our society, we tend to be more protective of girls than boys. A girl might have to exhibit a far more severe form of MBD before being transferred to a special class or special school for the education of such children. This is another possible explanation for the higher representation of boys over girls in such classes. It might also explain our finding that the MBD girls do significantly worse on the steadiness tester at all age levels. Only the sickest girls were being represented. The mild to moderately severe MBD girls were not being transferred to such classrooms. Boys, however, in these categories were being so transferred.

CLINICAL UTILIZATION
OF THE STEADINESS TESTER
IN THE MBD BATTERY

The steadiness tester is not designed to be a simple test for the presence of minimal brain dysfunction. It is not even designed to be a simple test for hyperactivity. As mentioned, the instrument also measures impaired ability to sustain attention, motor impersistence, resting tremors, and choreiform movements. An MBD child's high score may be the result of a combination of any of these factors, as well as others to be described below. One can ascertain whether the other neurological factors are present by utilizing the specific tests designed to detect such impairments. If, for example, the child does not appear to have an attentional deficit on the basis of normal scores on the concentration tests that I will describe (chapter 3), *and* if the same holds true for the tests for motor impersistence (chapter 6), *and* if there is no clinical evidence for resting tremors and choreiform movements (chapter 6), then one *may* conclude that hyperactivity is *probably* present.

However, there are other factors, unrelated to MBD, that may contribute to a high score on the steadiness tester. The most common of these, in my experience, are tension and anxiety. On the basis of initial pilot studies (without enough data for meaningful statistical analysis) I believe that children with purely psychogenic tension and anxiety do not produce scores as high as those with MBD. Children with phobic symptoms, somatic complaints, obsessions, compulsions, and generalized insecurity are often quite anxious. Their scores tend to be high, but not as high as the higher scoring MBD children. It is likely that some of the higher scorers in my normal group were tense children, who are inevitably to be found in any normal group. Since no attempt was made to screen them out, their presence in my normal group is just about certain. In addition, the tension and anxiety that MBD children are likely to have must be considered to be contributing to their scores, especially those at the higher levels.

Differentiation between psychogenic and organic hyperactivity is sometimes difficult. The problem is further compounded by the fact that psychogenic hyperactivity can be superimposed on the organic. Most of the generally used differentiating criteria are subjective and of some, but not solid, reliability. Often organic hyperactivity is more constant; the psychogenic tends to occur when the child is tense, from either external or internal causes. The presence of clear-cut psychogenic symptoms such as phobias, tics, and compulsions suggests a psychogenic etiology, whereas the presence of traditional neurological signs such as coordination deficits, visual and/or auditory processing problems suggests a neurologic basis for the hyperactivity. The history can be useful in differentiating the two forms of hyperactivity. Hyperactivity from birth and the presence of some of the possible etiological factors described in chapter 1 would support an organic basis for the hyperactivity.

Some of the high scoring children are probably in the high-activity-level category of temperamental patterns that Thomas et al. (1963) have described. These authors have delineated nine behavioral patterns that they consider inborn and unrelated to environmental factors or brain dysfunction. A child whose high activity level has been present from birth *and* who shows no other evidence for MBD might be considered to fall in this category. Obviously, one must be cautious when making such a determination because it is very difficult to say with certainty that psychogenic tension and anxiety factors are not likely to be present, considering the ubiquity of such factors. It is easier to rule out the presence of other signs of MBD. I would generally not make the diagnosis of MBD with only hyperactivity being present. In such cases I would tend to attribute the hyperactivity to psychogenic factors or, if there was very good evidence that psychogenic factors were not operative, I would then conclude that the child falls into the category of high-activity-level temperament.

False positive scores could conceivably be exhibited by children with hyperthyroidism and adrenalin-producing tumors. I have not yet had any personal experience regarding the performance of children with these disorders on the steadiness tester. Diagnosing such children is generally not difficult and I would suspect that their scores would be improved after proper medical treatment.

A child's score is interpreted in the following way. After a total touch-time value is obtained, the examiner determines the child's percentile rank and/or deviation from the norm by referring to the normal and MBD tables. A 9-year-old boy, for example, obtains a total touch time of 23 sec. From Table 2.3 we note that the average boy his age obtains 10.43 ± 7.18 sec touch time. His score is 1.75 S.D. $[(23.0 - 10.43)/7.18]$ above the mean. Referring to the percentile rank table we note that he has scored worse than at least 90% of the normal group (his score is below the tenth percentile) but is at approximately the fiftieth percentile level of the MBD group. Such a score would be strongly suggestive of the presence of MBD, but not necessarily diagnostic of the disorder. The presence of other MBD manifestations would have to be demonstrated before one could conclusively make the diagnosis. An 8-year-old girl with a score of 4.1 sec has done better than over 90% of MBD children and is at about the fiftieth percentile of normals. One can reasonably conclude that she does not suffer with any of the five aforementioned neurological signs that the instrument is designed to detect. She may still have MBD, however, because she might have other MBD manifestations such as dyslexia, impaired gross motor coordination, or an auditory processing deficit. A 10-year-old boy with a score of 7 sec has done better than about 50% of normals and 70% of MBDs. Such a score is of little, if any, value in making the diagnosis, and one must rely on other criteria for diagnosis. For such a child the tension and anxiety factor must be carefully investigated to get a better understanding of the meaning of his score.

I have found the steadiness tester described in this chapter to be useful not only in diagnosing minimal brain dysfunction but in monitoring drug treatment as well. The child for whom the diagnosis has been established on the basis of many of the tests described in this book (the steadiness tester being only one) and who exhibits a score on the steadiness tester suggestive or indicative of MBD is considered a candidate for such medication. However, not all children with MBD who have high scores on the steadiness tester will necessarily respond to psycho-stimulant medication. Rather than use subjective criteria (such as parents', teachers', and therapists' observations) the steadiness tester can provide objective criteria for determining whether or not a drug is effective. The typical way in which I ascertain whether or not a child is a candidate for drug treatment is to set aside a six-hour period for medication and testing. Generally, the child is brought in at 9:00 A.M. and administered the steadiness test. Most children obtain scores similar to those they originally obtained during the diagnostic work-up. There is generally little or no improvement on practice with this instrument. At 11:00 A.M. the child is retested. By this time a three-point base line has been established. Immediately after the 11:00 A.M. recording, the child is given a test dose of psychostimulant medication. [Generally I give either 10 mg of methylphenidate (Ritalin) or 5 mg of dextroamphetamine sulfate (Dexedrine).] When the child is retested at 1:00 P.M. (two hours later), those who are sensitive to the medication will generally show an improvement (lowering) of their scores. At 3:00 P.M., the highly sensitive will often show an even further improvement (the drug has now been working over a four-hour period). Usually the improvements on the steadiness instrument correspond with the parent's description of improved behavior. Children who get worse after admininstration of the drug are either nonresponders or are receiving too high a dose of the medication. Testing on another day (a new base line need not be obtained) with a lower dose will usually settle this question. The instrument has also proved useful for adjusting dosage level once the child is being maintained on medication. Studies are presently being conducted to further evaluate the use of the steadiness tester for these purposes.

If a child's diagnostic evaluation covers a few sessions (the usual situation for this examiner), then one can get one's base line by administering the steadiness tester in each of the diagnostic sessions. If in the first diagnostic session the child's score is in the MBD range and the examiner suspects that medication will probably be recommended, then repeated scores to obtain a base line are warranted. If the initial score is borderline, then repeated scores may help the examiner to ascertain whether or not the child is hyperactive. If, however, the first score is clearly normal, then further tests with the instrument are not warranted. Generally, when I get a base line in this way, I have three or four points. Therefore, on the trial day I need only get a 9 A.M. score and can administer the medication immediately after this test is completed. This adds one more point to my base line and may shorten the trial period by two hours.

It is important for the reader to appreciate that the steadiness tester was designed to serve as only one part of the MBD diagnostic battery. It was not envisioned to be used as a simple, quick method for diagnosing hyperactivity and/or minimal brain dysfunction. It should be considered to be only one part of the MBD diagnostic battery. To use it as a simple screening device for MBD would result in some children's being diagnosed as having MBD when they do not (for example, some highly anxious and tense children), and for others the diagnosis would be missed (because although they have MBD, they do not have any of the signs that the instrument has been designed to detect).

3

Attentional Deficit
and Distractibility

For the purposes of this discussion I will use the terms attention and concentration synonymously. I will differentiate, however, between attentional impairment and distractibility. I will use the term attention to refer to the capacity to maintain involvement in a task. I will use the term distractibility to refer to the readiness with which competing stimuli can redirect attention from the primary task at hand. The two are certainly related and may vary inversely. The child who concentrates well can not usually be easily distracted. However, as will be discussed below, this is not necessarily always the case and so the differentiation can be useful.

ATTENTIONAL DEFICIT:
THE CENTRAL PROBLEM
IN MINIMAL BRAIN DYSFUNCTION?

In recent years, many workers in the field (Dykman et al., 1974; Cantwell, 1975a, 1977; Ross and Ross, 1976) have emphasized the importance of the attentional deficit in MBD. Conners (1974, 1976) held that most, if not all, of these children's poor performances on the various WISC-R subtests were the result of impaired concentration, and one need not postulate perceptual, motor, and other types of deficits to explain their difficulties. Pope (1970), using accelerometers to measure children's hyperactivity, found no difference between normal and MBD children regarding the total amount of activity each group exhibited in a fixed period. However, he found that MBD children spent less time at each activity than normals. He postulated that the hyperactivity of MBD children was specious, that it was secondary to the inability to remain fixed at a goal as long as normal children. MBD children in his study traversed more floor zones than normal children. MBD children did as well as normals, however, in performing simple short tasks. It was when performing more difficult tasks, which required prolonged concentration, that the MBD group fell down. The implication of Pope's work is that the central problem for these children is attentional and that the hyperactivity is a secondary phenomenon.

Many (Conners, 1974; Fish, 1975; Cantwell, 1975b) hold that the primary way in which psychostimulant medication helps these children is that it prolongs attention span. There is nothing "paradoxical" then in the way that these drugs act in these children. The apparent sedation is the result of the reduced activity that they produce. And the reduction of activity is the result of the improvement in concentration that such medications cause. With improved concentration there is more goal direction, less flitting from goal to goal, and hence less activity. These workers have theorized that psychostimulant medication acts similarly in both normal and MBD children. Unfortunately testing this hypothesis is very difficult because of the problem of getting parents to permit their normal children to serve as experimental subjects in studies utilizing drugs that are known to have addicting potential. Recently, Rapoport (1978) studied 14 children of colleagues, who allowed their children to receive one dose of dextroamphetamine (0.5 mg/kg). In a double-blind crossover study she found that the dextroamphetamine produced significant improvement on a variety of functions and tasks such as activity level, reaction time, continuous performance tasks, verbal learning and memory, and language performance. These are the same tasks that MBD children have been shown to improve upon after medication with psychostimulant drugs. Her work strongly supports the view that the concentration impairment is a central problem for many of these children and that psychostimulant medication acts similarly in both normal and MBD children. Peters et al. (1974) considers these children's central problem to be one of easy fatigue of attention, an impairment that is corrected by psychostimulant medication. Douglas (1972, 1974a, 1974b) has been one of the strongest supporters of this position. She has emphasized the point that the central problem is not simply one of impairment in attention, but a deficiency in the ability to *sustain* concentration. She prefers the term *vigilance* to describe this phenomenon. In addition, she has been particularly interested in understanding in greater depth the nature of the attentional deficit and the various factors that may be contributing to it.

The present emphasis on the attentional factor in MBD has become so widespread that the *Diagnostic and Statistical Manual* (DSM-III) of the American Psychiatric Association utilizes the term Attention Deficit Disorder to refer to what we presently call minimal brain dysfunction. I would prefer to keep the term MBD at this point. I consider it to be a rubric under which are subsumed a whole variety of neurological problems. There is good reason to believe that we will be able to differentiate these from one another in the future. At such time it would be appropriate to list each one of these as a separate diagnosis. At this point we seem to be dealing with a collection of symptoms with some clusters that appear to be somewhat discrete. We have children whose primary difficulties are learning, others whose central problem is attentional, others with motor coordination problems, etc. There is much overlap and we rarely find "pure" examples of one type of deficit. To choose the attentional deficit type and refer to the whole group of disorders by this name is as unreasonable as utilizing the term *hyperactivity* or *learning disability* to refer to this group of disorders. I believe also that the attentional deficit problem is primary for many, but certainly not all, children with MBD. Those who respond well to psychostimulant medication are probably in this group. Those who do not, especially those who are excited by such drugs, are probably not suffering from a primary attentional defect. These children, in my opinion, can be viewed as being "driven from within," that is, their hyperactivity is not secondary to an attentional deficit, but appears to be caused by neurological processes that seem to be running at high speed (for lack of a better description). They are like "revved up" motors that cannot be shifted into lower gear.

CLINICAL MANIFESTATIONS OF THE ATTENTIONAL DEFICIT

In every phase of development the attentional deficit interferes with the MBD child's functioning. Denhoff (1973) described how neonates who had undergone perinatal distress did not fixate as long as newborns whose births were normal. Accordingly, such infants were not as likely to learn from their environment. The first thing one must do to learn is to attend for a proper length of time to the source of information. And if there is an impairment in doing this, there will be less learning. Bowel training involves, among many other things, the ability to attend periodically to internal sensations long enough to appreciate their significance. And, if there has been an "accident" the child must be able to concentrate long enough on the resultant discomforts (cuteaneous and olfactory) to appreciate their significance. This impairment contributes to the common lateness of MBD children's bowel and bladder training, and it may also explain the MBD child's occasional wetting and soiling, after being trained, when engrossed in various activities.

The impaired ability to sustain attention is well demonstrated by the child's ability to watch TV. Television programs, especially the cartoon types traditionally enjoyed by children, involve a rapid turnover of stimuli. Accordingly, MBD children may become engrossed for hours. In addition, MBD children can attend better to *kinetic* stimuli than *static* stimuli (Peters et al., 1973; Peters, 1974). This is another reason why these children do not have trouble concentrating for long on television cartoons. Activities like reading, however, require sustained attention and this is, without question, one of the factors contributing to MBD children's reading problems. Also, reading requires active attention and work; TV watching is a passive activity requiring little if any sustained effort. It is the impairment in the ability to sustain attention, then, that explains (in part) the apparent paradox in the common comment made by parents to the teachers of MBD children: "I can't understand why you say he has a problem in concentrating. He can watch television for hours." Of course, one must not ignore the motivational element—it is much more fun to watch TV than to read most books.

In the period when the infant and toddler is learning spoken language he need not attend for long to what is being said in order to understand the kinds of simple messages imparted to children at that age level. Accordingly, early language development may not be impaired. It is later, when complex messages are imparted ("After you finish supper, go up to your room and do your homework. When you finish that you can watch TV or play games."), that the MBD child has difficulty. In play with peers the attentional deficit interferes with learning the rules of games and planning strategies. And in school MBD children learn less because they are not listening to the teacher as much as others (Forness, 1975). In conversations they do not listen long to what others are saying and so the other person soon becomes alienated.

INSTRUMENTS THAT MEASURE CONCENTRATION OBJECTIVELY

Continuous Performance Test

Probably the most sensitive and accurate test of concentration is the Continuous Performance Test (CPT). In the visual form of the test, a stream of randomized letters is flashed before the child at the rate of one every 1 to 2 seconds. In a typical task the child is instructed to press a button every time an X appears which has been preceded by an A. The child is told *not* to press the button when an X is preceded by any other letter or when an A is preceded by an X. (Of course any other combination of letters could be used.) The target sequences appear aperiodically. An auditory modification of the test is also used in which the child hears rather than views the letter sequences. The test requires sustained concentration and is very sensitive to deficiencies in this area. The greater the number of errors the more poorly the child is considered to be concentrating. However, the impulsive child is also likely to make more errors than the normal because he presses the button too quickly, rather than waiting long enough to be sure that the proper combination and sequence has indeed appeared. (As will be discussed in the next section, there is some overlap between concentration impairment and impulsivity.) Another measurement that may be taken on the CPT is reaction time. Again, the impulsive child is more likely to have a short reaction time. Lastly, impaired concentration on a psychogenic basis is also going to result in an abnormally high number of errors on the CPT, and this is an important consideration when evaluating the meaning of a child's poor performance.

Douglas (1972, 1974b) compared normal and hyperactive children's scores on the CPT for both visual and auditory stimuli (using the X preceded by an A stimulus sequence). She found that hyperactive children made significantly more errors, made more impulsive responses, and deteriorated more rapidly than normals. She considered the attentional deficit and impulsivity to explain the hyperactive children's impaired performance. Sykes et al. (1972), using the same X followed by an A target sequence, similarly found that hyperactive children made more incorrect responses and fewer correct responses than normals. Unfortunately, CPT equipment is extremely expensive (about $8,000 a unit) and so has never enjoyed widespread popularity, even among laboratory workers.

Selected Subtests of the WISC-R

The Wechsler Intelligence Scale for Children—Revised (WISC-R) (Wechsler, 1974) includes a number of subtests that will detect impairments in the ability to sustain attention. Actually, there is not one of the 12 subtests whose score would not be lowered by a child's inattentiveness, but there are a few that are particularly sensitive to this deficit. Each of these subtests, however, is not "pure" with regard to its capacity to detect concentration deficiencies. Other functions (which will be mentioned in appropriate sections) are also being measured. I mention here only the use of each of these tests with regard to its value as a measure of the ability to sustain concentration.

Digit Span

In the Digit Span subtest the examiner reads to the child a sequence of numbers that the child is asked to repeat immediately. After trial numbers are given, the child is presented with two three-digit numbers. If the child repeats both of the numerical sequences accurately, the examiner goes on to the two four-digit sequences, using different numbers. The examiner continues with longer and longer pairs of equal length (up to nine digits) until the child has missed both samples of a sequence of the same length. For each sequence of a given length, the child can receive a score of 2, 1, or 0. In the second section of the test, the child is asked to repeat verbally presented sequences in reverse order (two to eight digits in length). The two parts of the Digit Span test are referred to as Digits Forward and Digits Backward. The raw scores of each of the two parts of the subtest are added together in order to ascertain the child's scaled score. Clearly, the child must concentrate well if he is to perform adequately on this subtest.

The Digits Backward section of the subtest is an even better test of concentration than the Digits Forward. It requires the child to mentally visualize the numbers and then to scan the mentally visualized sequences. Unfortunately, Wechsler does not provide us with separate scoring data for the two parts of the subtest. Rather, the raw scores are combined to determine the scaled score. A high score on Digits Forward may so counterbalance a low score on Digits Backward that the child may appear to perform normally. The digits-backward impairment thereby gets "buried" and undetected. In order to correct this defect of the Digit Span test, I and my assistants have administered the subtest to normal children, boys and girls ages 5–16, and have presented these findings as two separate subtests. Means, standard deviations, and percentile ranks are presented so that the examiner can ascertain exactly the degree of abnormality in each of the two categories. This normative data for the Digits Forward subtest is presented in chapter 7 under auditory memory, and the data for the Digits Backward subtest is presented in chapter 8 under visual memory. However, as mentioned, both tests (especially Digits Backward) are useful for detecting concentration deficits.

Arithmetic

The Arithmetic subtest of the WISC-R is also a sensitive test of concentration. The examiner reads arithmetic questions to the child who is asked to figure out the answer without using pencil and paper. The child is required to attend well to the examiner and must concentrate on the arithmetic processes being utilized to answer the question. Some paraphrased questions from this test are shown in chapter 10 (Table 10.1) where I will be discussing this subtest in greater detail.

Coding

The Coding subtest (also known as the Digit Symbol subtest) of the WISC-R also requires the child to sustain well his concentration if he is to perform adequately. One form of the test is given to children under eight and a more difficult form to those who are eight and older. In the version for younger children, the child is shown a row of five geometric figures (star, circle, etc.) inside each of which is a simple notation (vertical line, two parallel lines, etc.). Below the model figures is a randomly sequenced array of 50 of the larger geometric forms. The child is asked to write in the center of each the notation that is shown within the geometric form in the original sample. Five practice samples are given and then the child is allowed 120 seconds to fill in as many of the remaining 45 figures as he can. Older children are shown a row of nine numbers (1–9) under each of which is a simple notation (⌐, ∨, ⊢, etc.) (a facsimile is shown in Figure 3.1). Here too the child is asked to write the appropriate notation under each of the 100 numbers that are presented in random sequence below (the first seven items are for practice). The child is given 120 seconds in which to complete as many of the remaining 93 items as he can. Younger children are given bonus credit if they get all of their answers correct. The child must concentrate well

Figure 3.1
WISC-R Coding Test B.

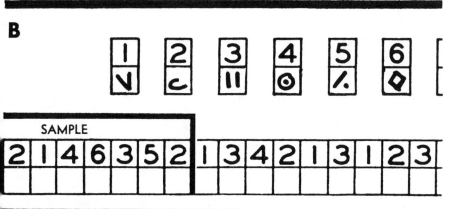

if he is to perform adequately on this test. However, the test is also sensitive to impairments in recent visual memory, visual-motor coordination, and visual discrimination. Dyspraxic children may also do poorly on the Coding subtest.

Mazes

The Mazes subtest of the WISC-R is another good test of concentration. In order to perform this test adequately, the child must focus his attention on the various pathways and follow them through to ascertain whether or not they lead into blind alleys. This test will be described further in chapter 4 in my discussion of impulsivity.

Cancellation of Rapidly Recurring Target Figures

Rudel et al. (1978) utilize a test they refer to as Cancellation of Rapidly Recurring Target Figures. Although devised as a method for differentiating dyslexics from children with other types of learning disability, it is an excellent way of detecting concentration impairment. The practice sheet (Figure 3.2) has the number 6 placed in an isolated position at the top of the page. Below is an array of 140 numbers among

Figure 3.2
Cancellation of Rapidly Recurring Target Figures

6

0	3	9	6	2	4	5	7	1	9	0	9	1	8
4	6	0	5	1	8	3	6	4	2	8	2	3	5
5	8	7	3	7	9	2	0	1	6	5	7	8	0
7	9	1	4	6	3	6	5	2	3	0	5	4	2
1	5	7	2	8	1	2	9	7	0	9	8	7	6
2	6	4	0	5	8	7	5	8	1	4	3	5	1
9	8	7	4	3	6	1	3	0	6	8	9	2	4
3	2	1	9	7	4	0	2	4	3	7	4	6	9
6	9	8	2	4	8	9	4	5	1	6	5	7	0
8	0	3	1	5	0	3	1	7	6	9	2	0	3

Reprinted with the permission of Rita Rudel, Ph.D., Martha Denckla, M.D. and Melinda Broman, Ph.D.

which are randomly placed the number 6. The child is instructed to draw a line through all 6s, but to leave all other numbers alone. If he demonstrates the ability to understand the instructions and to execute them with some degree of accuracy, then he is given the two test sections.

In the first (Figure 3.3), the model figure is a diamond and the diamond figure is randomly placed below among an array of 140 other geometric forms. Again the child is instructed to place a line through the diamonds only, and to leave all nondiamond figures alone. The total amount of time the child takes and the number of errors, both omissions (failing to place a line through a diamond) and commissions (placing a line through a nondiamond), are recorded. The second test, the more

Figure 3.3
Cancellation of Rapidly Recurring Target Figures.

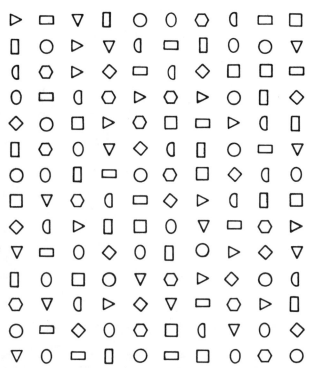

Reprinted with the permission of Rita Rudel, Ph.D., Martha Denckla, M.D., and Melinda Broman, Ph.D.

difficult one, uses as the model figure the number sequence 592 (Figure 3.4). In the array of 140 three-digit numbers below, all begin with a 5. The second digit is either a 6 or a 9. And the third can be a 1, 2, 3, 4, 5, 8 or 9. Again the child is instructed to place a line through the 592 sequence *only*. The time it takes the child to complete the task is recorded as well as the total number of errors. Means and standard deviations are provided (Table 3.1) enabling the examiner to compare the child with others his age. Although the test measures visual discrimination, visual sequential memory, and impulsivity, it is described here because of its value as an objective test of concentration capacity. Some of the optometric problems to be described in chapter 8 may interfere with a child's performance on these tests, especially the 592 test. Accordingly, the examiner must be certain that such difficulties do not exist before administering the test of Rapidly Recurring Target Figures. In chapter 8 I will discuss this test further.

Figure 3.4
Cancellation of Rapidly Recurring Target Figures

592

569	562	598	561	591	564	563	591	569	561
564	561	592	599	562	594	591	562	598	592
599	593	563	564	591	598	562	564	569	599
563	599	594	569	561	591	592	599	592	564
561	564	591	562	599	599	561	569	598	594
594	592	563	569	594	564	594	599	561	563
569	562	569	599	598	563	591	564	599	592
563	592	561	563	591	561	569	598	562	569
562	591	594	564	592	563	599	592	599	591
598	561	592	599	562	594	564	562	563	598
564	563	599	598	594	569	592	561	599	562
598	592	569	591	564	562	594	598	594	591
561	563	564	562	592	598	563	562	592	564
569	591	598	594	561	569	591	594	561	563

Reprinted with the permission of Rita Rudel, Ph.D., Martha Denckla, M.D., and Melinda Broman, Ph.D.

Table 3.1

Cancellation of Rapidly Recurring Target Figures—Normative Data

| | | **Diamond** | | |
| | | Total Errors | | Time |
Age	Mean	S.D. [rounded off]	Mean	S.D.
4-5	12	(4)	—	—
6-7	5	(3)	103.43	(46.30)
8-9	4	(3)	66.26	(21.63)
10-11	3	(3)	70.10	(24.55)
12-13	2	(3)	40.90	(8.88)

| | | **592** | | |
| | | Total Errors | | Time |
Age	Mean	S.D. [rounded off]	Mean	S.D.
4-5	13	(4)	—	—
6-7	6	(3)	200.76	(81.51)
8-9	2	(2)	116.00	(33.71)
10-11	2	(2)	90.70	(24.66)
12-13	2	(2)	67.13	(15.76)

Reprinted with the permission of Rita Rudel, Ph.D., Martha Denckla, M.D., and Melinda Broman, Ph.D.

The Visual Closure Subtest of the ITPA

Although the Visual Closure subtest of The Illinois Test of Psycholinguistic Abilities (Kirk et al., 1968) tests short-term visual memory and visual gestalt, I consider it a good test for concentration. A picture of three dogs alone is first used as a sample. The examiner explains to the child that he is to find as many dogs as he can in the adjacent complex array in which parts of dogs can be seen if one carefully scans the scene. "Some of them are hiding." "Do you see this one?" "Do you see this dog's tail?" With each of the actual test items—fish (Figure 3.5), shoes, bottles, hammers and saws—the child is told,"I want to see how quickly you can find all the _____ in here," "Put your finger right on each one you can find." During the 30-sec period the examiner marks each spot where the child has correctly identified the partially hidden figure. The child is given one point for every item correctly identified. Raw scores can be converted to age-equivalents. For example, a raw score of 18 is the mean for a 5-year-10-month-old child. The raw score can be converted to a scaled score by referring to the appropriate chart for the child's age. For example, a 6½-year-old child gets a raw score of 31. This corresponds to a scaled score of 49. As is true for all of the subtests of the ITPA, the mean scaled score is 36 with a standard deviation of 6. Accordingly, this child's score is over 2 standard deviations above the mean. The likelihood of there being a problem in any of the areas that the test assesses is very small.

Figure 3.5
Visual Closure Subtest of the ITPA.

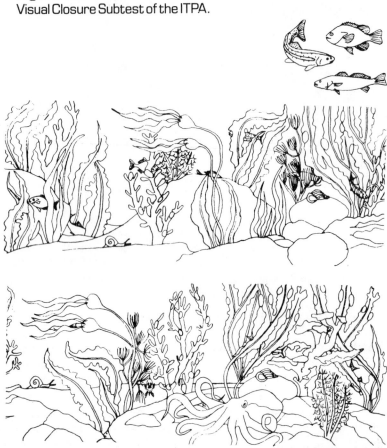

The Gardner Steadiness Tester

In chapter 2 I described the steadiness tester as a useful instrument for detecting hyperactivity, concentration impairment, motor impersistence, resting tremors, and choreiform movements. The presence of resting tremors and choreiform movements can usually be determined by closely observing the fingers of the child's outstretched hands. Tests of motor persistence will be described in chapter 6. Actually the last three symptoms (motor impersistence, resting tremors, and choreiform movements), in my experience, are relatively uncommon in MBD children. Accordingly, for all practical purposes the steadiness tester detects hyperactivity and/or attentional deficit. If a child does well on most, if not all, of the aforementioned tests of concentration, then one can assume that a child's poor score on the steadiness tester is the result of hyperactivity, of the "driven from within" type. If he does poorly, then it is probable that concentration impairment is contributing to the steadiness problem. Such children are among the more common when hyperactivity is present and are in the group that is more likely to respond to psychostimulant medication.

SOME FINAL COMMENTS ABOUT CONCENTRATION

If it is true that concentration impairment is a central problem for many, if not most, children with MBD, then we are in serious need of normative data on attentional capacity. Many of the instruments and tests described (such as the Digit Span, Coding, and the steadiness tester) also measure other functions to a significant degree. The Continuous Performance Test is probably the "purest" test of concentration, but it too measures other functions (such as visual memory and impulsivity). Hopefully, normative data on this test will soon be collected so that we can more profitably use this valuable instrument. In addition, a lower-priced version would also enable more examiners to utilize it.

Tension and anxiety can also impair concentration to a significant degree. Accordingly, one must always consider this factor when deciding whether a child has an attentional impairment. As mentioned, it is the author's belief that some of the normal children who obtained high scores on the steadiness tester did so because of anxiety rather than from basic neurological factors. This has been confirmed by pilot studies conducted by my staff in which children with no evidence for MBD, but with definite psychogenic symptoms such as phobias, compulsions, and generalized tension, obtained scores in the high normal range. I would be most hesitant to place the MBD label on a child whose only manifestation of the disorder was concentration impairment. Rather, I would consider anxiety and tension to be the more likely causes of the concentration deficit and look for other signs and symptoms of psychogenic disturbance.

One cannot consider attentional capacity without taking into consideration the attractiveness of the stimulus and the motivation of the child to attend to it. It is certainly true that one reason why MBD children concentrate better on television than on reading is that the former requires mainly short-term attention to rapidly changing stimuli, whereas the latter requires sustained attention. However, it is also a fact that television viewing is a far more attractive activity (if it can be called that) than learning to read or do arithmetic. Jansky and de Hirsch (1972) go so far as to state that "one can hardly discuss attention without taking into account motivation."

Denckla (1976) points out that one must also take into consideration the particular deficit of the MBD child when one is talking about attentional deficit. For example, the dyslexic child may be able to concentrate well on sports, art, woodwork, science experiments, and arithmetic because his impairment does not interfere with his functioning in these areas. However, he may concentrate poorly when the teacher reads a story or when he is asked to read himself because of difficulties in performing these functions. Therefore, it is not enough to say that the MBD child has trouble concentrating. It is necessary to specify in which particular area the child's attentional deficit exhibits itself. Most examiners today view the attentional deficit as a central one and consider it to manifest itself in many areas. If Denckla is correct, then such a view would be an oversimplification of the problem.

Lastly, we must consider the child's basic temperamental pattern when considering whether there is an attentional deficit. Among the temperamental patterns described by Thomas et al. (1963) are *decreased attention span* and *distractibility*. Children so diagnosed would have no signs of MBD or psychogenic difficulty. Their attentional deficit would then be considered a normal human variation.

DISTRACTIBILITY

As mentioned, concentration capacity and distractibility are best viewed as two separate phenomena. In their classic works *Psychopathology and Education of the Brain-Injured Child,* Strauss and Lehtinen (1947) and Strauss and Kephart (1955) describe distractibility to be the central problem of children with MBD. These children's hyperactivity was viewed as secondary to the excessive movements caused by their being drawn to every competing stimulus. In accordance with this theory, they suggested that classrooms reduce as much as possible stimuli that could potentially distract children from the important tasks at hand. Accordingly, they recommended that classrooms be free of distracting stimuli such as pictures. They suggested that teachers wear plain clothing and refrain from wearing attractive jewelry. They recommended that the walls of the classroom be painted in soft, flat tones and that the windows of the classroom be so covered that the children would not be able to look outside. As far as possible, they suggested that auditory stimulation also be reduced. By having very few children in a classroom

and placing the most distractible behind a screen (without the implication of punishment) they hoped to further reduce distracting stimulation.

Cruickshank et al. (1961) tried to determine whether the Strauss
et al. stimulus reduction approach did indeed improve children's learning. In a well-controlled experiment in which children studied in cubicles
in order to maximally reduce distracting stimuli, they did not find any
significant difference between educationally retarded and normal
children in their improvement on a variety of psychological tests after
such a program. Similarly, Rost and Charles (1967) were not able to
find any specific educational benefit derived from children's using
cubicles. Jenkins, Gorrafa, and Griffiths (1972) and Scott (1970) concluded
from their studies that cubicles helped increase a child's productivity.
Others hold that depriving the MBD child of extraneous stimuli may
increase hyperactivity (W. I. Gardner, et al., 1959; Cromwell, et al.,
1963; Turnure, 1970, 1971; Dykman, et al., 1971; Satterfield and Dawson,
1971). These investigators believe that extraneous stimulation is necessary for optimum performance and that the MBD child may need
more, not less, environmental stimulation than normals. They hold that
to deprive the MBD child of such stimulation may reduce his academic
performance. Leuba (1955) has introduced the concept of *optimal stimulation.* He holds that each individual needs a certain level of extraneous
stimulation for optimal functioning. If there is too little external stimulation then the individual will attempt to create such stimulation by
methods such as increasing motor activity. If such stimulation is too
high the individual will attempt to reduce it by withdrawal or immobility.

Douglas (1974b, 1975) compared normal and hyperkinetic children's
performance on the Continuous Performance Test regarding their responses to distracting stimuli. While being given the test, distracting
auditory stimuli were introduced. She found no significant difference
between the two groups. She not only believes that distractibility is not
a symptom of MBD but goes further and raises the possibility that if
one deprives MBD children of a significant amount of external stimulation
they may become more restless and hyperactive.

Studies such as these shed much doubt on the original Strauss et
al. concept that distractibility is a fundamental symptom of MBD. In
fact, they make one wonder whether distractibility is a symptom of
MBD at all. Therefore, considering the many questions that have been
raised on this issue, I believe that the most judicious position to take at
this time is to withhold using distractibility as a criterion for making
the diagnosis of MBD. Therefore, I do not include specific distractibility
tests in my battery at this time.

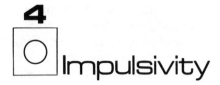

4
Impulsivity

Impulsivity refers to the tendency to act without forethought. An impulsive act is one that is performed without significant deliberation. Without advance reflection and consideration of consequences. acts are performed that may be socially alienating or that may compromise in other ways the individual's capacity to relate and adapt to others. Impulsivity is a common manifestation of MBD. Most workers in the field consider it to be one of the most common manifestations of the disorder. Douglas (1972, 1974a, 1974b) holds that impulsivity along with the attentional impairment are the central problems in MBD, and that the other manifestations are derivatives of these deficits.

CLINICAL MANIFESTATIONS
OF IMPULSIVITY

Although some of the clinical manifestations of impulsivity are similar to those of hyperactivity, there is a distinct difference between the two types of symptoms. In impulsivity there is the element of the unexpected. The behavior often occurs suddenly, without warning. Hyperactivity is more likely to be ongoing with ups and downs; impulsivity comes in dramatic episodes. Eisenberg (1973) refers to this distinction in his comment about the MBD child: "The youngster has a 'motor' but no 'governor.'" Kinsbourne (1975) similarly describes the mechanism in this way: "They are the 'fools who rush in' where introverted 'angels fear to tread.'" Although the child may be able to exert some degree of conscious control, such self-monitoring is difficult for MBD children. It is common for many of these impulsive children to suffer significant guilt after they have quieted down enough to observe the consequences of their impulsivity (Pontius, 1973).

It is probably in the classroom, more than anywhere else, that the MBD child's impulsivity causes him trouble. The classroom is generally a highly structured situation, and even those referred to as "open" or "free" require a significant degree of self-discipline on the child's part if he is to function adequately. Academic performance is compromised because they do not take the time to consider the various alternative solutions to a problem. They make many errors, in areas of proven competence, because they so quickly jump to conclusions. This is certainly one of the contributing factors to these children's learning disability. They cannot resist the desire for short, quick solutions to a problem, and this tendency may play a role in their cheating on examinations (Douglas, 1974a). One of the most common problems that MBD children have in the classroom is blurting out their answers (more often wrong than right). Holding their hands raised while waiting for the teacher to call upon them is something that is extremely difficult for these children to do. They thereby suffer the irritation of their teachers and alienation of their classmates. Although often among the least knowledgeable in the class, they are among those who most frequently raise their hands, with significantly more of the associated movements and vocalizations designed to attract the teacher's attention. They are quick to jump out of their seats and are among the most inveterate jokers and pranksters.

Of course, psychogenic factors are also operative in classroom impulsivity. These children's desire for peer recognition and respect is especially strong because of their frequent frustration in gaining such positive feedback. By frequently offering answers they hope to get a few right. They fail to realize, however, that their higher frequency of incorrect responses just brings about even further alienation. The child who blurts out answers as a manifestation of purely psychogenic problems will generally have an angry, smug, or defiant attitude while doing so. There is a calmness and deliberate quality to such responses that the impulsive MBD child does not possess.

At home and in the child's neighborhood the impulsivity problem will also cause difficulty. It is not uncommon for a young MBD child to suddenly break away from a parent and dart into the street, totally oblivious to the dangers of traffic. Jumping out of first and second story windows and off low roofs is a common occurrence for such children. They may suddenly jump into swimming pools even though they cannot swim. With peers their impulsivity may cause significant interpersonal problems. Not being able to tolerate delay, they find it difficult to wait their turns in games. They quickly gain for themselves the epithet of "sore loser" because they so frequently react with violent outbursts if they do not end up winner. They interrupt freqently during conversations, so much so that the other person doesn't feel that he or she is being listened to. Interrupting, in my experience, is one of the hallmarks of the impulsivity problem in MBD children. They do not censor much of what they are saying, and so they often make tactless and socially alienating comments. Dealing with bullies may be particularly difficult for MBD children. They can neither ignore taunts nor suppress anger or tears. They cannot react with calm and restraint and "make believe" that they are not being bothered. They thereby invite further tormenting as they gain for themselves the reputation of being perfect prey for scapegoaters. Lastly, when their impulsive demands are not satisfied, they reiterate them so often that those around remove themselves if they can in order to avoid continuously being plagued.

ETIOLOGICAL CONSIDERATIONS

The "catastrophic reaction" described by Goldstein (1952) is probably related to the impulsivity problem of children with MBD. Although Goldstein's work was primarily with brain-damaged adults, others such as Strauss and Lehtinen (1947) used the term to refer to similar outbursts in brain-injured children. These outbursts of anger and woeful frustration often appear without known cause. However, on careful inquiry or examination, one will usually find some precipitating frustration (Stone, 1959). Gainotti (1972) found that adult patients with left-hemisphere lesions were more likely than those with right-hemisphere lesions to exhibit outbursts of rage, cursing, crying, and tension. Whether these findings are applicable to MBD children remains to be seen. It is certainly the case that some MBD children are much more impulsive than others, but I know of no studies in which a correlation is described between impulsivity and left-hemisphere impairment in these children.

Douglas (1974a) considers a strong interrelationship to exist between impulsivity and impaired ability to sustain attention. She also relates these children's impulsivity to their cognitive style. By cognitive style she refers to the *way* in which the individual approaches a task. Problem solving *strategies* are separate from cognition and intelligence.

She views these children as having *impulsive* rather than *reflective* cognitive styles. Elsewhere (1975) she states: "They tend to react with the first idea that occurs to them or to those aspects of a situation which are the most obvious or compelling."

Ross and Ross (1976) describe studies that suggest that the MBD child has a narrower *response range* than normal children. On the one hand, they react too fast when a slow reaction is warranted. For example, they do not wait to be called upon in the classroom. On the other hand, they react too slowly when a rapid reaction is called for. For example, in a race they do not start rapidly enough and do not run as fast as they are physically capable of running. The normal child has a wider range of response rates. However, they view average children to have a mean response rate that is slower than that of children with MBD. In other words, although MBD children have a wider response rate range, they generally react more rapidly than normal children.

It is my opinion that one factor in MBD children's impulsivity is their impaired ability to appreciate future consequences of their acts. Time appreciation is often impaired in these children. They live much more for the present and often even behave as if there were no future. This "mañana" philosophy of life, in which they take the attitude that the future will somehow take care of itself, may make them less concerned with the consequences of their impulsive acts. So they indulge themselves in their interrupting, shouting out, and pushing ahead in line because they do not anticipate the consequences of such behavior. Another factor that I believe contributes to these children's impulsivity is their impairment in projecting themselves into another person's situation. This capacity is central to what we refer to as intimacy, empathy, and sympathy. Without this capacity one is seriously impaired in developing meaningful relationships. This is what the ancient Golden Rule ("Do unto others as you would have them do unto you") is all about. When one is incapable of appreciating what others want and need, of surmising what others are thinking and feeling, one is not going to have many friends. Deficiency in this area probably has both neurological and psychological components.

Piaget and Inhelder (1948), in a series of ingenious studies, have described the normal development of children's capacity to view a situation from a point outside of themselves. The child is shown a model scene of three mountains, each of which is different from the others. They are of different heights and colors and have other distinguishing characteristics (one has a house, another a red cross on the top, and the third an incecap). The mountains are set on a board one meter square and the child is asked to construct from shaped cardboard the view that would be seen by a 2–3 cm figurine from four different positions, namely, the middle point on each of the four edges of the board. In another phase of the study the child is shown 10 pictures and asked to select those that correspond to the views the man would have from various positions. Piaget and Inhelder found that up to about 8 years of age the child considers the figurine to have the same view that he has in reality, regardless of where the figurine is set. Ages 8–9 represents a transition stage for the development of the capacity to make correct discriminations. After 9, and especially by 10, children are able to ascertain the scene visualized from the various points of view of the figurine. Benton (1968), in his studies of the development of right-left discrimination, has found that children are usually able to point out various parts of their own body ("Touch your left eye with your right hand") by age 9. However, the capacity to ascertain right and left on another person ("Point to my right eye") does not appear until 11 and the ability to consider simultaneously one's own and an outsider's orientation ("Put your right hand on my left ear") does not occur until 12. Although these studies pertain to a concrete capacity (Piaget's is part of a study of geometric perspective), it is reasonable to consider the findings relevant to the child's capacity to appreciate the more complex phenomenon of another person's thoughts and feelings. It may be that children with MBD are defective in their ability to view a situation from another person's vantage point because of lags in the development of cerebral centers involved in this capacity. However, psychological factors related to immaturity and egocentricity are probably also operative.

MBD children do not seem to appreciate others' reactions to their picking their noses, drooling, scratching their genitalia, and interrupting. The inability to project oneself into another's situation may play a role in the cruelty to animals often seen in MBD children (Gardner, 1973b). Parents will often complain that the MBD child hurts his dog unmercifully, to the point where the animal flees the child whenever possible. Peers cannot but be alienated by such insensitivity, especially because animals play such an important role in the lives of many children. MBD children may not feel the need to say anything when they don't wish to answer a question. They may sit silently, without any change in facial expression, not recognizing that the questioner is waiting for a response. They do not feel the need to compliment others because they fail to appreciate how good such statements make the other person feel. When they hit other children they are surprised that the recipient of their blows reacts with anger and cannot understand why those who observe such bullying are also alienated (Gardner, 1975a). Goldstein (1952), in his studies of adults with brain damage, describes how these patients do not appear to understand situations not directly related to themselves. When they hear a story about events occurring to someone else, and the story is not at all relevant to themselves, they neither understand nor show interest in the story. When, however, the story is about a person whose situation is very similar to their own, such patients may be able to understand. Such inability, in my opinion, plays a role in these children's impulsivity. Were they to be more appreciative of how others were reacting to their impulsivity, they would be more likely to inhibit themselves.

Cultural factors also play a role in these children's impulsivity. Socieites in which meditation, reflection, and deep concern for the social consequences of one's behavior are important are less likely to have impulsive children. Children of oriental cultures, in my experience, exhibit such qualities, and even when they suffer with MBD they are less likely to be hyperactive and impulsive. Perhaps future studies will be able to either confirm or refute this observation. Jansky and de Hirsch (1972) describe how black children raised in ghettos are reared in an environment in which quick action and instant gratification are the norm. Accordingly, such children, they believe, are more likely to exhibit impulsivity as a manifestation of their MBD.

It is apparent, then, from the foregoing discussion that although impulsivity in MBD children probably has a neurological basis, there are many ways in which psychological factors can contribute to this symptom. In addition to those already referred to, one must consider parental toleration and even indulgence of the symptom. Some parents ignore some of the impulsive behavior and act as if it were not even occurring. Sometimes the child has an impulsive parent as a model. Even though the parent may not have MBD (although he or she may) the parent's impulsivity serves to increase that which the MBD child has on a neurological basis. Lastly, anxiety may increase impulsivity. Tension makes all of us "edgy" and more likely to "explode," and this is particularly true of the MBD child.

INSTRUMENTS THAT MEASURE
IMPULSIVITY OBJECTIVELY

Continuous Performance Test

The Continuous Performance Test measures impulsivity as well as concentration. The impulsive child tends to press the button too quickly, before he is sure that the correct letter combinations have appeared. Douglas (1974a) has demonstrated that MBD children make more errors and have shorter reaction times than normals when utilizing this device. As mentioned, the instrument is so expensive that it cannot be considered of value for all but the wealthiest practitioners. Accordingly, in its present form it is not likely that it will enjoy widespread use.

Mazes Subtest of the WISC-R

The Mazes subtest of the WISC-R is very sensitive to impulsivity. The child is shown a typical maze drawing with a picture of a boy in the middle. The child is asked to trace with a pencil a path that would enable the boy to "get out to the street" without getting "stuck by the blind road." The mazes presented to the child become ever more complex. The number of errors are recorded and there is a time limit for the completion of each maze. Raw scores are converted to scaled scores and, if desired, to age-equivalents. The impulsive child will quickly maneuver into blind alleys and either retract or cross barriers in order to try alternative pathways. The lack of planning and forethought is readily revealed by this instrument. As mentioned in chapter 3, the test is also sensitive to attentional impairments. Although the child with a visual-motor-coordination problem may have difficulty keeping his pencil line within a particular pathway, this impairment does not necessarily cause the child to get a low score. There is no penalty for mildly crooked lines. The penalties are for entering blind alleys, not for poor penmanship.

Matching Familiar Figures Test

The Matching Familiar Figures Test (MFFT) (Kagan, 1964) can be useful in detecting impulsivity. Whereas the CPT and the Mazes subtest of the WISC-R were not designed primarily to serve as tests for impulsivity, the MFFT was specifically originated for this purpose. The test consists of 12 items. Each item contains a standard picture of an object readily recognizable to most children (boat, scissors, telephone) and 4, 6, or 8 similar pictures, only one of which exactly matches the standard. The child is simply asked to point to that figure among the facsimiles that matches the standard (Figure 4.1). If the child errs, he is given another chance, but the total number of errors is recorded. In addition, the time it takes the child between the presentation of the item and the completion of his responses is also recorded.

Messer (1976) has collected normative data on the MFFT. In collaboration with Kagan, they have defined four subgroups of respondants. *Impulsives* make many errors and have short reaction times. *Reflectives* make few errors but have long reaction times. The *fast-accurate* subjects are both quick to react and make few errors. (These are generally the brightest.) And the *slow-inaccurate* group is slow to respond and

Figure 4.1
Matching Familiar Figures Test.

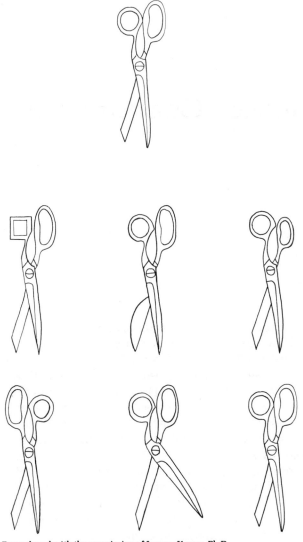

still makes many errors. (These are generally the less intelligent subjects.) My experience with the test has been that on occasion it does prove useful in detecting impulsivity. However, some patients do not fit neatly into any one of the four groups, and in such cases the results are not of much value. The test is also a useful measure of visual discrimination because the items are often very similar to one another.

5

☐ Motor Coordination

Motor coordination is generally divided into two categories: fine and gross. However, many functions subsumed under one of these two subgroups are combinations of both. For example, ball throwing is generally considered to be a gross motor function. However, finger movements (a fine motor function) are also involved in this maneuver. Placing pegs in holes is usually considered to be a fine motor function. However, wrist and arm movements also determine the subject's performance in such tasks. Accordingly, I recognize that my differentiation between the two groups may not at times be fully warranted. The tradition, however, is deep seated and does have merit. In this discussion, therefore, I will maintain the differentiation, but recognize that some of the tasks that I will be describing under fine motor coordination may have a minor gross motor component. Likewise, some discussed under gross motor may have a fine motor component.

Subjectivity in defining motor-coordination problems has been widespread, especially in the field of medicine. The tradition has been to rely on "clinical observation," and the older and more experienced physicians enjoy the greatest credibility in this area. Observations rather than direct measurements have been the tradition. The examiner observes the patient's gait and describes in general what he considers to be the coordination deficits. The examiner "plays catch" with the child to determine whether he throws a ball well. Handwriting is examined to see if it is "poor" or "uncoordinated." Objective measurements are not even considered by many examiners because the view is that one can determine such deficits with a "sharp eye" and accumulated experience.

The phenomenon is well demonstrated in the following vignette. Although not specifically true, it epitomizes a commonplace interchange between physicians. A senior pediatric neurologist is examining a 5-year-old boy in front of a resident in child neurology. The boy is asked to oppose the tip of his thumb to the tips of each of the other four fingers, in succession, as rapidly as he can. As the child attempts to perform this maneuver, he is observed to execute the task somewhat slowly (as compared to the adult) and to frequently miss proper contact between fingers so that he has to repeat his attempts before going on to the next finger (again, with an error frequency that appears to be higher than what one would expect of an adult). The senior man then states to the resident: "This boy demonstrates a fine-motor-coordination problem. Notice how slowly he moved his fingers and how frequently he missed making contact so that he had to go back and repeat a maneuver quite frequently." To this the junior man responds: "All 5-year-olds do this slowly and make mistakes. How do you know that this boy's error range is pathological? How do you know the point at which the normal functioning ends and the pathological begins?" To which the senior man responds: "I've been doing child neurology for 35 years and the number of children I've seen are too numerous to count. I can tell you that this degree of slowness and error frequency is definitely abnormal."

Now there are two possibilities here: the older man is right or the older man is wrong. It may be that over the years he has accumulated enough knowledge about normal functioning for this task that he can differentiate the normal from the pathological. But even if this is so, how does he teach the younger man these differentiating criteria? If they are so subtle that they cannot be directly taught, must the young man himself have 35 years of experience before he can speak with authority about this function? If this is the case, then patients would probably be wise to subscribe to the dictum: "Never trust a pediatric neurologist under the age of 70." Or the older man may be wrong. His line of demarcation between normal and abnormal is erroneous and he has been making wrong diagnoses for 35 years. Even if it were possible to teach these criteria to others, he would be imparting incorrect information. The solution to the problem lies, of course, in collecting and utilizing objective criteria. But even when this is done, the tests so devised may not be valid. Take, for example, the Lincoln-Oseretsky Motor Development Scale (Sloan, 1955) which includes a subtest in which the child's ability to catch a ball is allegedly measured. In this test, the examiner throws tennis balls (five trials for each hand) to the patient, and the number of completed catches is recorded. The test is based on the assumption that the examiner has perfect coordination and that each of his or her throws traverses the exact same arc and ends in the exact same place. I think that the only thing one can conclude when a child exhibits a low score on this subtest is that either he or the examiner (or both of them) have poor coordination with regard to this function.

FINE MOTOR COORDINATION

Hand Tally Counter

Knights and Moule (1967) utilize a standard hand tally counter mounted on a board (Figure 5.1) to measure finger- and foot-tapping coordination. The counter they use is available from the Lafayette Instrument Company of Lafayette, Indiana (catalog no. 56016). The counter requires 1/4 in. depression of the lever to rotate the read-out to the next digit, and a static weight of 400 gm is necessary to fully depress the lever. The counter is so mounted on the board that the lever is 1¾ in. above the board. The authors recommend a 6 in. × 10 in. board. This dimension is fine for use on tests of finger coordination. However, my experience has been that a larger board would have been preferable when using the device to measure foot-tapping speed, because this smaller board does not provide an optimally stable base for testing that

Figure 5.1
Hand Tally Counter.

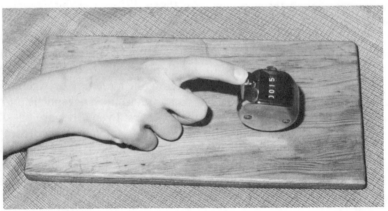

function. (The use of this unit for measuring foot-tapping speed will be described in the section on gross motor coordination.)

The subject is instructed to rest his wrist on the board and to depress the lever on the tally counter with his index finger as rapidly as he can after the examiner tells him to start. He is advised to try to keep the other fingers motionless while executing the task. It has been this examiner's experience that most children cannot comply with this part of the instructions and they almost automatically bring the other fingers into play while the index finger is moving. Such "associated movements" (to be discussed in detail in chapter 6) are especially common in children with MBD. Both the dominant and the nondominant hands are tested. Four 10-sec trials are given to each hand, with the hands being alternated between trials. In other words, the dominant hand is tested for 10 sec, then the nondominant, then the dominant again, etc., until each hand has been tested four times. The mean of the best three of the four 10-sec trials is used as the child's score. Normative data for this test is shown in Table 5.1. Although the average number of subjects in each of the 10 age groups is 17, the author has found the data useful and his experience suggests the test to be valid and reliable.

Table 5.1

Means and Standard Deviations for Finger Tapping for Each Chronological Age

| | | Chronological Age in Years | | | | | | | | | |
		5.7	6.5	7.5	8.5	9.5	10.4	11.5	12.5	13.5	14.4
Dominant Hand	Mean	22.6	25.8	26.6	29.3	31.8	34.8	38.5	39.7	43.2	45.3
	S.D.	3.0	3.4	3.8	3.6	4.4	5.3	4.9	5.3	4.5	4.5
Nondominant Hand	Mean	21.5	22.6	24.4	27.3	29.2	32.6	35.5	36.6	38.9	40.8
	S.D.	4.9	2.8	2.8	3.1	3.7	5.2	5.4	5.4	5.8	4.5
		10	12	27	22	19	17	25	11	16	10

Reprinted with permission of author and publisher from: Knights, Robert M., and Moule, Allan D. Normative and Reliability Data on Finger and Foot Tapping in Children. PERCEPTUAL AND MOTOR SKILLS, 1967, 25, 717–720.

Purdue Pegboard

The Purdue Pegboard (Lafayette Instrument Company, catalog no. 32020) provides an excellent test of fine motor coordination. The board (Figure 5.2) consists of two parallel rows of 25 holes in each row. Pins, collars, and washers are located in four cups at the top of the board. Pins are placed at the extreme right-hand and left-hand cups. Collars and washers occupy the two middle cups. The subject is asked which hand he prefers to use first. For example, if the child indicates that he prefers to use the right hand, he is instructed to practice taking pegs from the right-hand cup and placing them as rapidly as he can in the right row, from top to bottom. When the child demonstrates under-

Figure 5.2
Purdue Pegboard.

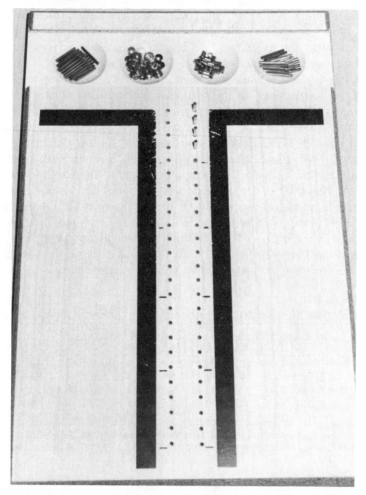

standing, he is told that when the examiner says "begin" he is to try to place as many pegs as he can in the right column of holes during the allotted time. He is instructed to take only one pin at a time and that if he drops a pin he should not pick it up, but go back to the cup for another. (When I have used the test, I started all over again if the child takes two pins at the same time.) A stopwatch is used and the total number of pegs the child places in the holes during the 30-sec trial period is recorded. The pegs are allowed to remain in the holes and the same procedure is repeated with the nonpreferred hand. Again, the trial period is 30 sec. The pins are then removed and the test is repeated with the child using both hands simultaneously. Again, the trial period is 30 sec.

The pegs are then removed in preparation for the fourth part of the test. Here the child is asked to form "assemblies" consisting of a peg, a washer, a collar, and another washer (Figure 5.3). The examiner demonstrates to the child that the best way to do this is to alternate hands so that, for example, a peg is inserted with the right hand while a washer is being picked up with the left. While this washer is being placed on the peg, the right hand is picking up a collar. While this collar is being placed on the peg, the left hand is picking up the second washer. While the second washer is being placed on the peg, the right hand is picking up a second peg—to start the whole process all over again. Only one column is used and the trial period is one minute. Although the examiner demonstrates the continuous alternating movements as the optimum way to do the task, and although the child may be encouraged to use this system during the trial period, it has been my experience that most children (especially young ones) cannot utilize such smooth integration and usually accomplish the task in a more haphazard way. They are permitted to do so even though this lessens their efficiency and reduces their score. The total score is the total number of items (pegs plus washers plus collars) assembled in the allotted time. Each unit is scored as 4 points and partial units are also calculated. The assembly shown in Figure 5.3 would be scored 15 points (The three completed assemblies of 4 points each are scored 12 points. And the partially completed assembly is scored 3 points, bringing the total to 15 points).

Figure 5.3
Purdue Pegboard Assemblies.

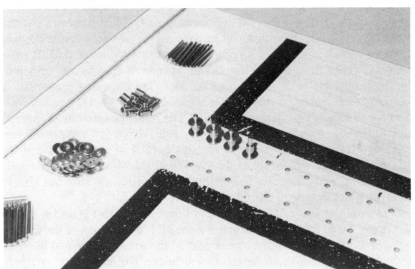

Unfortunately, the original pegboard was standardized for factory workers in a wide variety of industrial jobs: general factory workers, production workers, electronics production workers, maintenance and service employees, sewing machine operators, etc. The normative data on these subjects (provided in the Lafayette Instrument Co. manual) is not broken down by age under the assumption that this would not be a significant variable among adults over the age range employed in factories. Presumably, the youngest subjects utilized in the collection of this data were 17 or 18. Accordingly, this potentially useful test of fine motor coordination has not been utilized optimally in diagnosing children's coordination deficits. Many examiners, recognizing its value, have used it, but they base their conclusions on their subjective accumulated experience.

Costa et al. (1964) did collect data on Purdue Pegboard performance on 183 normal children from ages 6-15. Normative data is presented for the 160 right-handed children, and the authors claim that the scores for the 23 left-handed children is comparable at each age level. (Considering an average of 2-3 left-handed children at each of the 10 levels, this statement is not too convincing.) For the right-handed group of 160 children at 10 age levels, the average number of children at each level is 16. The number of children at the 14-year level is 6 and at the 15-year level is 1. Such small numbers of subjects cannot provide examiners with great confidence in the data. Unfortunately, this study did not include the assembly section of the test which, in my opinion, is the one that is most sensitive to fine motor coordination deficits. This more complex task is the one that is more likely to detect such defects.

In order to provide more extensive normative data my associates and I collected performance data on 1334 normal school children (663 boys and 671 girls, ages 5-16) in Bergen County, New Jersey (a suburb of New York City). Only children in regular classes were utilized, and any who were suspected of having any signs or symptoms of MBD were excluded from the study. The means, standard deviations, and percentile ranks, for each of the four subtests for boys are presented in Tables 5.2-5.6. Similar data for girls are in Tables 5.7-5.11. Age brackets are broken down into half-year levels. The average number of boys at each half-year level is 30.1 and for girls 30.5. When full-year levels are considered, the average number of boys is 60.2 at each level and for girls 61.0 in each age bracket. I have found this data to be extremely useful not only in detecting fine-motor-coordination deficits but also in describing the degree of deficit objectively.

In another study, 145 MBD boys (ages 5-0 to 15-11) and 67 MBD girls (ages 5-0 to 13-11) were administered all four sections of the Purdue Pegboard. The MBD children were part of the group described in chapter 2 who provided data for the steadiness tester. The means and standard

Table 5.2

urdue Pegboard: Means and Standard Deviations for Boys

Age	N	Preferred Hand		Nonpreferred Hand		Both Hands		Assembly	
		Mean	S.D.	Mean	S.D.	Mean	S.D.	Mean	S.D.
-0 to 5-5	30	9.33	1.81	8.40	1.33	6.73	1.17	14.10	3.29
-6 to 5-11	30	9.93	1.51	8.83	1.95	6.97	1.54	15.57	3.56
-0 to 6-5	30	9.77	1.57	9.13	1.83	7.30	1.53	15.93	2.94
-6 to 6-11	30	11.57	1.45	10.17	2.17	8.23	1.77	19.20	3.84
-0 to 7-5	30	11.67	1.67	11.00	1.70	8.77	1.41	19.23	4.95
-6 to 7-11	30	12.07	1.95	11.23	1.68	9.57	1.59	20.40	4.10
-0 to 8-5	30	12.70	1.60	12.17	1.51	9.83	1.51	23.20	3.80
-6 to 8-11	30	13.90	2.19	12.57	1.85	10.90	1.73	24.47	5.35
-0 to 9-5	30	13.33	1.60	12.43	1.59	10.50	1.48	24.57	3.75
-6 to 9-11	30	13.87	1.91	12.87	2.05	11.33	1.65	27.37	4.55
-0 to 10-5	30	14.03	1.88	12.87	1.72	10.93	1.84	26.37	6.15
-6 to 10-11	30	14.73	1.51	13.90	1.84	11.77	1.65	28.17	5.38
-0 to 11-5	30	14.93	1.86	14.00	1.98	11.30	1.68	29.53	6.19
-6 to 11-11	30	14.83	1.60	13.93	1.60	12.27	1.41	31.33	5.19
-0 to 12-5	30	14.83	1.78	13.67	2.02	11.67	1.52	31.13	5.78
-6 to 12-11	30	15.37	2.81	14.00	2.38	11.87	1.87	30.13	6.08
-0 to 13-5	40	15.15	1.92	13.90	2.00	11.85	1.58	33.73	5.00
-6 to 13-11	30	14.87	1.72	14.10	1.47	11.53	1.80	34.57	5.88
-0 to 14-5	30	15.67	1.47	14.40	1.57	12.03	1.67	33.97	6.58
-6 to 14-11	30	14.70	1.49	14.33	1.65	12.20	1.61	31.37	7.24
-0 to 15-5	30	15.57	1.59	14.87	1.50	12.57	1.48	32.20	6.21
-6 to 15-11	23	15.09	1.50	14.30	1.61	12.65	1.30	33.04	6.24
	663								

Table 5.3

urdue Pegboard: Percentiles for Boys Using Preferred Hand

Age	N	10	20	30	40	50	60	70	80	90
-0 to 5-5	30	7.0	8.0	8.0	9.0	9.0	10.0	10.0	11.0	11.0
-6 to 5-11	30	8.0	9.0	9.0	10.0	10.0	10.0	11.0	11.8	12.0
-0 to 6-5	30	7.1	9.0	9.0	9.0	9.5	10.0	11.0	11.0	11.9
-6 to 6-11	30	9.1	10.2	11.0	11.0	12.0	12.0	12.0	13.0	13.0
-0 to 7-5	30	9.1	10.2	11.0	11.4	12.0	12.0	12.7	13.0	13.9
-6 to 7-11	30	9.0	10.0	11.0	12.0	12.0	12.6	13.0	14.0	14.0
-0 to 8-5	30	11.0	12.0	12.0	12.0	13.0	13.0	14.0	14.0	14.0
-6 to 8-11	30	11.1	12.0	12.3	13.0	14.0	15.0	15.0	16.0	17.0
-0 to 9-5	30	11.0	12.0	12.0	13.0	13.0	14.0	15.0	15.0	15.0
-6 to 9-11	30	12.0	12.0	13.0	13.0	14.0	14.6	15.0	15.0	15.9
-0 to 10-5	30	11.1	12.2	13.0	14.0	14.0	15.0	15.0	15.8	16.9
-6 to 10-11	30	13.0	13.2	14.0	14.0	15.0	15.0	15.0	16.0	17.0
-0 to 11-5	30	13.0	13.0	13.0	14.0	14.5	16.0	16.0	16.8	17.0
-6 to 11-11	30	13.0	14.0	14.0	14.0	15.0	15.0	15.0	16.8	17.0
-0 to 12-5	30	13.0	13.0	14.0	14.0	14.5	15.0	15.7	16.0	17.9
-6 to 12-11	30	13.0	13.2	15.0	15.0	15.0	15.0	16.0	17.0	18.9
-0 to 13-5	40	12.1	14.0	14.0	15.0	15.0	15.0	16.0	16.8	18.0
-6 to 13-11	30	13.0	13.0	14.0	14.4	15.0	15.0	16.0	16.0	17.0
-0 to 14-5	30	14.0	14.0	14.3	15.0	16.0	16.0	17.0	17.0	17.9
-6 to 14-11	30	13.0	13.0	14.0	14.4	15.0	15.0	15.0	16.0	16.9
-0 to 15-5	30	14.0	14.0	14.0	15.0	15.5	16.0	16.7	17.0	18.0
-6 to 15-11	23	13.0	14.0	14.0	15.0	15.0	15.0	16.0	17.0	17.0
	663									

Table 5.4

Purdue Pegboard: Percentiles for Boys Using Nonpreferred Hand

Age	N	10	20	30	40	50	60	70	80	90
5-0 to 5-5	30	6.1	7.0	8.0	8.0	8.5	9.0	9.0	9.0	10.
5-6 to 5-11	30	6.1	8.0	8.0	8.0	9.0	9.6	10.0	10.0	11.
6-0 to 6-5	30	6.0	8.0	9.0	9.0	9.0	10.0	10.0	10.0	12.
6-6 to 6-11	30	7.1	8.2	9.0	10.0	10.5	11.0	11.7	12.0	13.
7-0 to 7-5	30	9.0	10.0	10.0	11.0	11.0	11.0	12.0	12.0	12.
7-6 to 7-11	30	9.1	10.0	10.0	11.0	11.0	11.0	12.0	13.0	13.
8-0 to 8-5	30	10.0	11.0	11.0	12.0	12.5	13.0	13.0	13.0	14.
8-6 to 8-11	30	10.1	11.0	11.0	12.0	12.0	13.0	13.7	14.0	15.
9-0 to 9-5	30	10.0	11.0	11.3	12.0	13.0	13.0	13.7	14.0	14.
9-6 to 9-11	30	10.0	11.2	12.0	12.0	12.0	13.0	14.0	15.0	16.
10-0 to 10-5	30	10.1	12.0	12.0	13.0	13.0	13.6	14.0	14.0	15.
10-6 to 10-11	30	11.0	12.2	13.0	13.0	14.0	14.0	15.0	15.8	17.
11-0 to 11-5	30	12.0	13.0	13.0	13.0	13.5	14.0	15.0	15.8	16.
11-6 to 11-11	30	11.1	13.0	13.0	14.0	14.0	14.0	15.0	15.0	16.
12-0 to 12-5	30	12.0	13.0	13.0	13.0	14.0	14.0	15.0	15.0	16.
12-6 to 12-11	30	11.0	12.2	13.0	13.4	14.0	14.0	15.0	16.0	16.
13-0 to 13-5	40	11.0	11.2	13.0	14.0	14.0	15.0	15.0	16.0	16.
13-6 to 13-11	30	12.0	13.0	13.0	14.0	14.0	14.0	15.0	15.8	16.
14-0 to 14-5	30	12.1	13.0	14.0	14.0	14.5	15.0	15.7	16.0	16.
14-6 to 14-11	30	11.2	13.2	14.0	14.0	14.5	15.0	15.0	15.8	16.
15-0 to 15-5	30	13.0	14.0	14.3	15.0	15.0	15.0	16.0	16.0	16.
15-6 to 15-11	23	12.0	13.0	13.0	14.0	15.0	15.0	15.0	16.0	16.
	663									

Table 5.5

Purdue Pegboard: Percentile for Boys Using Both Hands

Age	N	10	20	30	40	50	60	70	80	90
5-0 to 5-5	30	5.1	6.0	6.0	6.0	7.0	7.0	7.0	8.0	8.
5-6 to 5-11	30	5.0	6.0	6.0	6.4	7.0	7.0	8.0	8.0	9.
6-0 to 6-5	30	5.0	6.0	6.3	7.0	7.0	7.6	8.0	9.0	9.
6-6 to 6-11	30	6.0	7.0	8.0	8.0	8.0	8.6	9.0	9.0	10.
7-0 to 7-5	30	7.0	8.0	8.0	8.0	8.0	9.0	10.0	10.0	10.
7-6 to 7-11	30	8.0	8.0	8.0	9.0	9.5	10.0	10.7	11.0	12.
8-0 to 8-5	30	8.0	8.0	9.0	9.0	10.0	10.0	11.0	11.0	12.
8-6 to 8-11	30	9.0	9.2	10.0	10.0	11.0	11.0	12.0	12.8	13.
9-0 to 9-5	30	8.1	9.0	10.0	10.0	10.0	11.0	11.0	12.0	12.
9-6 to 9-11	30	9.1	10.0	10.0	11.0	11.0	11.6	12.0	13.0	13.
10-0 to 10-5	30	9.0	9.0	10.0	10.4	11.0	11.0	11.0	12.8	13.
10-6 to 10-11	30	10.0	10.2	11.0	11.0	12.0	12.0	12.0	13.0	14.
11-0 to 11-5	30	9.0	10.0	10.3	11.0	11.0	12.0	12.7	13.0	13.
11-6 to 11-11	30	11.0	11.0	12.0	12.0	12.0	13.0	13.0	13.8	14.
12-0 to 12-5	30	9.1	11.0	11.0	11.0	12.0	12.0	12.0	12.8	14.
12-6 to 12-11	30	9.1	10.2	11.0	12.0	12.0	12.6	13.0	13.8	14.
13-0 to 13-5	40	9.1	11.0	11.0	11.4	12.0	12.0	13.0	13.0	14.
13-6 to 13-11	30	9.1	10.0	11.0	11.0	11.0	12.0	12.0	13.0	14.
14-0 to 14-5	30	10.1	11.0	11.0	11.0	12.0	12.0	13.0	14.0	14.
14-6 to 14-11	30	10.0	11.0	11.0	12.0	12.0	12.0	13.0	14.0	15.
15-0 to 15-5	30	10.1	11.0	12.0	12.0	13.0	13.0	13.0	14.0	14.
15-6 to 15-11	23	11.0	11.8	12.0	12.0	13.0	13.0	13.0	14.0	14.
	663									

Table 5.6

ırdue Pegboard: Assembly Percentiles for Boys

Age	N	10	20	30	40	50	60	70	80	90
-0 to 5-5	30	10.0	11.2	12.0	13.0	14.0	14.6	16.0	16.0	17.9
-6 to 5-11	30	10.1	12.2	14.0	15.0	16.0	16.0	17.7	18.0	20.9
-0 to 6-5	30	12.1	14.0	15.0	15.0	16.0	16.0	17.0	19.0	20.0
-6 to 6-11	30	14.0	16.2	18.0	18.0	19.5	20.6	22.0	22.8	24.0
-0 to 7-5	30	12.1	16.0	17.3	18.4	19.0	20.6	21.7	23.0	26.7
-6 to 7-11	30	16.0	17.2	18.3	19.4	21.0	22.0	22.7	24.0	25.0
-0 to 8-5	30	19.0	20.2	21.0	22.4	23.5	24.0	24.0	26.8	28.9
-6 to 8-11	30	18.0	20.0	20.3	23.4	24.0	25.0	27.1	30.0	32.0
-0 to 9-5	30	20.0	21.2	23.0	24.0	24.0	26.0	26.0	27.0	28.0
-6 to 9-11	30	21.1	24.0	24.3	25.4	26.0	29.2	30.7	31.8	32.0
-0 to 10-5	30	19.1	20.2	24.0	25.0	26.0	26.0	28.7	30.0	35.7
-6 to 10-11	30	22.0	24.0	25.3	28.4	29.0	30.0	30.0	31.0	33.8
-0 to 11-5	30	22.0	22.2	26.0	27.4	28.0	31.0	32.0	34.6	39.9
-6 to 11-11	30	25.1	27.0	28.6	30.0	31.0	32.6	33.7	35.0	39.0
-0 to 12-5	30	25.0	26.0	27.0	29.0	29.0	32.6	35.4	36.0	40.9
-6 to 12-11	30	23.1	25.4	28.0	29.0	30.5	32.2	34.0	35.8	37.0
-0 to 13-5	40	27.0	30.0	31.0	32.0	34.0	34.8	36.0	37.0	40.9
-6 to 13-11	30	27.1	30.0	30.0	33.0	34.5	35.6	36.7	39.8	43.8
-0 to 14-5	30	26.1	29.2	31.0	32.0	34.0	36.0	38.7	40.0	41.0
-6 to 14-11	30	23.0	25.2	26.3	29.0	30.5	32.0	34.7	35.8	45.4
-0 to 15-5	30	24.0	26.0	28.0	31.4	33.5	35.6	36.0	37.8	39.9
-6 to 15-11	23	24.4	26.8	29.4	32.0	33.0	34.4	35.8	39.0	42.0
	663									

Table 5.7

ırdue Pegboard: Means and Standard Deviations for Girls

Age	N	Preferred Hand		Nonpreferred Hand		Both Hands		Assembly	
		Mean	S.D.	Mean	S.D.	Mean	S.D.	Mean	S.D.
ı-0 to 5-5	30	10.00	1.53	8.50	1.36	6.97	1.25	14.70	2.55
ı-6 to 5-11	30	9.30	1.73	9.13	1.59	6.77	1.28	14.37	4.02
ı-0 to 6-5	30	11.43	1.33	10.23	1.52	8.53	1.46	18.03	3.54
ı-6 to 6-11	30	11.87	1.68	10.47	1.38	8.67	1.79	20.63	4.27
'-0 to 7-5	30	12.03	1.65	10.47	2.08	8.83	1.80	19.77	4.49
'-6 to 7-11	30	12.47	1.53	11.50	1.80	9.50	1.70	20.20	4.61
ı-0 to 8-5	30	13.07	1.78	12.03	1.40	10.10	1.81	21.93	4.31
ı-6 to 8-11	30	13.77	1.63	12.30	1.26	10.43	1.59	24.50	5.83
)-0 to 9-5	30	13.37	1.79	11.83	2.12	9.83	1.62	24.97	6.81
)-6 to 9-11	30	14.40	1.52	13.03	1.67	11.60	1.65	29.07	6.01
)-0 to 10-5	30	15.13	1.48	13.20	1.35	11.33	1.42	27.90	5.10
)-6 to 10-11	30	15.47	1.59	13.63	1.33	12.27	1.46	31.70	6.02
ı-0 to 11-5	30	14.90	1.79	14.00	2.00	11.67	1.63	32.77	5.50
ı-6 to 11-11	30	15.70	1.84	13.83	1.88	12.00	1.82	33.47	7.24
2-0 to 12-5	30	15.57	1.65	14.20	1.73	12.00	1.23	34.57	5.20
2-6 to 12-11	30	15.40	1.96	14.07	1.66	12.03	1.65	34.70	7.52
3-0 to 13-5	40	15.55	1.69	14.15	1.64	12.03	1.44	34.85	5.57
3-6 to 13-11	32	15.38	1.58	14.09	1.44	12.13	1.31	37.40	5.34
ı-0 to 14-5	30	16.33	1.73	14.93	1.78	12.63	1.61	36.43	6.76
ı-6 to 14-11	30	16.03	1.77	14.83	1.66	12.40	1.94	34.17	6.62
5-0 to 15-5	28	16.68	1.49	14.89	1.40	12.89	1.64	36.89	7.75
5-6 to 15-11	31	16.42	1.84	15.29	2.04	12.77	1.45	37.35	8.24
	671								

Table 5.8
Purdue Pegboard: Percentiles for Girls Using Preferred Hand

Age	N	10	20	30	40	50	60	70	80	9
5-0 to 5-5	30	8.0	8.2	9.3	10.0	10.0	10.6	11.0	11.0	12
5-6 to 5-11	30	7.0	8.0	8.0	9.0	9.5	10.0	11.0	11.0	11
6-0 to 6-5	30	9.1	10.2	11.0	11.0	11.5	12.0	12.0	12.0	13
6-6 to 6-11	30	10.1	11.0	11.0	11.0	11.0	12.0	13.0	14.0	14
7-0 to 7-5	30	10.0	11.0	11.0	12.0	12.0	12.6	13.0	13.0	14
7-6 to 7-11	30	10.1	11.0	12.0	12.0	13.0	13.0	13.0	14.0	14
8-0 to 8-5	30	11.0	12.0	12.0	12.4	13.0	13.0	14.0	14.8	15
8-6 to 8-11	30	12.0	12.0	13.0	13.0	14.0	14.0	14.7	15.0	16
9-0 to 9-5	30	10.1	12.0	13.0	13.0	13.0	14.0	14.0	15.0	16
9-6 to 9-11	30	12.0	13.0	14.0	14.0	14.0	15.0	15.0	16.0	16
10-0 to 10-5	30	13.0	14.0	14.0	15.0	15.0	15.0	16.0	16.0	17
10-6 to 10-11	30	13.1	14.0	14.3	15.0	15.5	16.0	16.0	16.8	17
11-0 to 11-5	30	12.0	13.2	14.0	15.0	15.0	15.0	15.7	16.8	17
11-6 to 11-11	30	14.0	14.0	15.0	15.0	16.0	16.0	17.0	17.0	18
12-0 to 12-5	30	14.0	14.0	14.0	15.0	15.0	16.0	17.0	17.0	17
12-6 to 12-11	30	12.1	13.2	15.0	15.0	16.0	16.0	16.0	17.0	18
13-0 to 13-5	40	14.0	14.0	15.0	15.0	16.0	16.0	16.0	17.0	18
13-6 to 13-11	32	13.3	14.0	14.0	15.0	15.0	15.0	16.0	17.0	18
14-0 to 14-5	30	14.1	15.0	15.0	16.0	16.0	16.0	17.0	17.8	19
14-6 to 14-11	30	14.0	14.0	15.0	15.0	16.0	16.6	17.0	17.0	18
15-0 to 15-5	28	15.0	15.0	16.0	16.0	17.0	17.0	18.0	18.0	19
15-6 to 15-11	31	14.0	15.0	15.6	16.0	16.0	17.0	17.4	18.0	19
	671									

Table 5.9
Purdue Pegboard: Percentiles for Girls Using the Nonpreferred Hand

Age	N	10	20	30	40	50	60	70	80	9
5-0 to 5-5	30	7.0	7.0	8.0	8.0	9.0	9.0	9.0	10.0	10
5-6 to 5-11	30	7.0	7.2	8.0	8.4	9.0	10.0	10.0	11.0	11
6-0 to 6-5	30	8.0	8.2	9.3	10.0	10.0	11.0	11.0	11.8	12.
6-6 to 6-11	30	9.0	9.2	10.0	10.0	10.0	11.0	11.0	12.0	12
7-0 to 7-5	30	8.0	9.0	10.0	10.0	11.0	11.0	11.0	12.0	13
7-6 to 7-11	30	9.0	10.0	10.3	11.0	11.0	12.0	13.0	13.0	14.
8-0 to 8-5	30	10.0	11.0	11.0	12.0	12.0	12.0	12.7	13.0	14.
8-6 to 8-11	30	11.0	11.0	12.0	12.0	12.0	12.6	13.0	13.8	14.
9-0 to 9-5	30	9.0	10.0	11.0	11.0	11.5	12.6	13.0	14.0	14.
9-6 to 9-11	30	11.0	11.0	12.0	12.0	13.0	13.6	14.0	14.8	15
10-0 to 10-5	30	11.0	12.0	13.0	13.0	13.0	13.6	14.0	14.8	15.
10-6 to 10-11	30	11.2	13.0	13.0	13.4	14.0	14.0	14.0	14.8	15.
11-0 to 11-5	30	10.2	12.4	14.0	14.0	14.0	15.0	15.0	15.0	16.
11-6 to 11-11	30	11.0	12.0	13.0	14.0	14.0	14.0	15.0	15.0	16.
12-0 to 12-5	30	12.0	13.0	13.3	14.0	14.0	14.0	15.0	16.0	16.
12-6 to 12-11	30	12.0	13.0	13.0	13.0	14.0	15.0	15.0	15.0	16.
13-0 to 13-5	40	12.1	13.0	13.0	13.4	14.0	14.0	15.0	16.0	16.
13-6 to 13-11	32	12.0	13.0	14.0	14.0	14.0	15.0	15.0	15.0	16.
14-0 to 14-5	30	13.0	13.0	14.0	15.0	15.0	15.0	15.7	16.0	17.
14-6 to 14-11	30	13.0	13.2	14.0	14.0	15.0	15.0	16.0	16.8	17.
15-0 to 15-5	28	12.9	14.0	14.0	14.6	15.0	15.4	16.0	16.0	17.
15-6 to 15-11	31	13.0	13.0	14.0	14.0	15.0	16.0	16.4	17.6	18.
	671									

Table 5.10

Purdue Pegboard: Percentiles for Girls Using Both Hands

Age	N	10	20	30	40	50	60	70	80	90
5-0 to 5-5	30	5.0	6.0	6.0	7.0	7.0	7.6	8.0	8.0	8.0
5-6 to 5-11	30	5.0	6.0	6.0	6.4	7.0	7.0	7.7	8.0	8.0
6-0 to 6-5	30	6.1	7.2	8.0	8.0	9.0	9.0	9.0	10.0	10.0
6-6 to 6-11	30	6.1	8.0	8.0	8.0	8.0	8.6	9.7	10.0	12.0
7-0 to 7-5	30	6.0	7.2	8.0	9.0	9.0	9.0	10.0	10.8	11.0
7-6 to 7-11	30	7.0	8.0	9.0	9.0	9.5	10.0	10.7	11.0	11.0
8-0 to 8-5	30	8.0	8.2	9.0	10.0	10.0	11.0	11.0	11.0	12.0
8-6 to 8-11	30	8.0	9.0	10.0	10.0	10.5	11.0	11.0	12.0	12.9
9-0 to 9-5	30	8.0	8.0	9.0	9.4	10.0	10.0	11.0	11.0	12.0
9-6 to 9-11	30	9.0	10.0	11.0	12.0	12.0	12.0	13.0	13.0	13.0
10-0 to 10-5	30	10.0	10.0	11.0	11.0	11.0	11.6	12.0	12.0	13.0
10-6 to 10-11	30	11.0	11.0	11.3	12.0	12.0	12.0	13.0	13.8	14.9
11-0 to 11-5	30	9.1	10.0	11.0	11.4	12.0	12.0	12.7	13.0	13.0
11-6 to 11-11	30	9.1	10.2	11.0	11.0	13.0	13.0	13.0	14.0	14.0
12-0 to 12-5	30	10.0	11.0	12.0	12.0	12.0	12.0	12.0	13.0	14.0
12-6 to 12-11	30	10.0	10.2	11.0	12.0	12.0	12.0	13.0	13.8	14.0
13-0 to 13-5	40	10.0	11.0	11.0	12.0	12.0	12.0	13.0	13.0	14.0
13-6 to 13-11	32	10.3	11.0	11.9	12.0	12.0	12.0	13.0	13.0	13.7
14-0 to 14-5	30	11.0	11.0	12.0	12.0	12.0	13.0	13.0	14.8	15.0
14-6 to 14-11	30	9.1	11.0	11.3	12.0	12.0	13.0	13.7	14.0	15.0
15-0 to 15-5	28	11.0	11.0	12.0	12.0	13.0	13.0	14.0	14.0	16.0
15-6 to 15-11	31	11.0	11.0	12.0	13.0	13.0	13.0	13.4	14.0	14.0
	671									

Table 5.11

Purdue Pegboard: Percentiles for Girls

Age	N	10	20	30	40	50	60	70	80	90
5-0 to 5-5	30	11.1	13.0	13.0	14.0	15.0	15.6	16.0	17.0	18.0
5-6 to 5-11	30	9.0	11.0	12.3	13.4	14.0	15.6	16.0	17.0	20.0
6-0 to 6-5	30	14.0	16.0	16.0	16.0	17.0	18.0	20.0	22.0	23.9
6-6 to 6-11	30	16.0	17.0	18.0	19.0	20.0	21.0	22.7	25.6	27.8
7-0 to 7-5	30	14.0	15.2	17.0	18.0	19.5	21.6	22.0	24.0	24.9
7-6 to 7-11	30	14.0	16.0	17.0	18.4	19.5	21.6	23.4	25.8	26.9
8-0 to 8-5	30	16.0	17.0	20.0	21.0	22.0	23.0	23.0	24.8	28.9
8-6 to 8-11	30	18.0	19.2	20.3	21.4	23.0	24.6	27.4	31.8	32.0
9-0 to 9-5	30	18.0	19.0	20.3	22.0	23.5	26.0	29.0	31.8	36.0
9-6 to 9-11	30	22.1	23.2	26.0	27.0	28.0	31.0	32.0	34.8	37.9
10-0 to 10-5	30	20.3	23.2	26.0	27.0	28.0	29.0	29.7	30.8	35.8
10-6 to 10-11	30	24.1	27.0	28.3	29.4	30.5	31.6	35.7	37.8	39.8
11-0 to 11-5	30	25.1	28.0	29.3	31.4	32.5	34.0	35.7	37.0	40.9
11-6 to 11-11	30	22.2	25.4	28.3	31.0	34.5	37.0	39.0	40.0	41.0
12-0 to 12-5	30	28.0	31.0	32.0	34.0	34.0	34.6	36.7	39.0	43.6
12-6 to 12-11	30	24.0	28.0	30.3	32.8	35.0	36.0	38.7	41.7	45.7
13-0 to 13-5	40	27.0	31.2	32.3	33.4	35.0	37.6	38.0	39.0	41.9
13-6 to 13-11	32	29.5	33.0	34.9	36.4	38.0	38.0	40.0	42.0	44.1
14-0 to 14-5	30	25.3	30.2	34.0	34.0	36.0	38.0	40.7	43.0	45.9
14-6 to 14-11	30	27.1	28.2	30.3	32.0	33.0	35.2	37.7	40.8	44.9
15-0 to 15-5	28	28.7	29.8	31.7	33.6	35.5	38.4	41.3	43.2	50.2
15-6 to 15-11	31	23.2	29.4	33.0	36.8	39.0	40.0	41.0	43.0	47.8
	671									

deviations of each one-year age level are shown in the columns on the right of Tables 5.12–5.15 (under MBD Boys and MBD Girls). T-test comparisons of normals and MBDs at each one-year age level revealed that the differences between the two groups were significant at the $p < .001$ level for 62 of the 76 comparisons. The differences were significant at the $p < .01$ level for 12 of the 76 age-level comparisons. Between only 2 of the 76 age levels studied were there no significant differences. It is reasonable to conclude then that MBD children do significantly more poorly than normals on the Purdue Pegboard, and this confirms the general clinical impression that as a group they are more likely to exhibit fine-motor-coordination impairments.

Table 5.12

Purdue Pegboard: Preferred Hand. Significance of t-Test Group Comparisons for Normals and MBDs

Age	Normal Boys			MBD Boys			p
	N	Mean	S.D.	N	Mean	S.D.	
5-0 to 5-11	60	9.63	1.68	7	5.71	2.98	< .001
6-0 to 6-11	60	10.67	1.75	21	8.10	3.16	< .001
7-0 to 7-11	60	11.87	1.81	22	8.45	2.46	< .001
8-0 to 8-11	60	13.30	1.99	17	10.06	2.97	< .001
9-0 to 9-11	60	13.60	1.77	13	11.69	2.78	< .01
10-0 to 10-11	60	14.38	1.73	16	12.25	1.88	< .001
11-0 to 11-11	60	14.88	1.72	20	11.65	2.81	< .001
12-0 to 12-11	60	15.10	2.35	15	12.53	2.17	< .001
13-0 to 13-11	70	15.03	1.83	10	13.90	2.28	NS[a]
14-0 to 14-11	60	15.18	1.55	4	11.75	3.30	< .001
15-0 to 15-11	53	15.35	1.55				
	663			145			

Age	Normal Girls			MBD Girls			p
	N	Mean	S.D.	N	Mean	S.D.	
5-0 to 5-11	60	9.65	1.66	4	6.75	2.22	< .01
6-0 to 6-11	60	11.65	1.52	10	6.90	3.45	< .001
7-0 to 7-11	60	12.25	1.59	12	8.58	3.12	< .001
8-0 to 8-11	60	13.42	1.73	10	9.60	3.13	< .001
9-0 to 9-11	60	13.88	1.73	5	10.40	2.70	< .001
10-0 to 10-11	60	15.30	1.53	4	9.75	3.40	< .001
11-0 to 11-11	60	15.30	1.84	13	10.77	2.95	< .001
12-0 to 12-11	60	15.48	1.80	5	9.20	2.39	< .001
13-0 to 13-11	72	15.47	1.64	4	11.50	3.00	< .001
14-0 to 14-11	60	16.18	1.74				
15-0 to 15-11	59	16.54	1.67				
	671			67			

[a] NS, Not Significant

Table 5.13

Purdue Pegboard: Nonpreferred Hand. Significance of t-Test Group Comparisons for Normals and MBDs

Age	Normal Boys N	Mean	S.D.	MBD Boys N	Mean	S.D.	p
5-0 to 5-11	60	8.62	1.67	7	5.57	3.87	$<.001$
6-0 to 6-11	60	9.65	2.06	21	7.52	3.49	$<.01$
7-0 to 7-11	60	11.12	1.68	22	8.14	2.21	$<.001$
8-0 to 8-11	60	12.37	1.69	17	9.47	2.27	$<.001$
9-0 to 9-11	60	12.65	1.83	13	10.62	2.36	$<.01$
10-0 to 10-11	60	13.38	1.84	16	11.13	2.63	$<.001$
11-0 to 11-11	60	13.97	1.78	20	11.10	2.29	$<.001$
12-0 to 12-11	60	13.83	2.20	15	10.93	2.05	$<.001$
13-0 to 13-11	70	13.99	1.78	10	11.50	2.07	$<.001$
14-0 to 14-11	60	14.20	2.16	4	10.00	2.31	$<.001$
15-0 to 15-11	53	14.62	1.56				
	663			145			

Age	Normal Girls N	Mean	S.D.	MBD Girls N	Mean	S.D.	p
5-0 to 5-11	60	8.82	1.50	4	2.50	2.38	$<.001$
6-0 to 6-11	60	10.35	1.45	9	6.00	2.74	$<.001$
7-0 to 7-11	60	10.98	2.00	11	9.09	2.81	$<.01$
8-0 to 8-11	60	12.17	1.33	9	7.33	2.00	$<.001$
9-0 to 9-11	60	12.43	1.99	5	9.60	3.05	$<.01$
10-0 to 10-11	60	13.42	1.34	4	10.50	2.52	$<.001$
11-0 to 11-11	60	13.92	1.92	13	9.69	2.59	$<.001$
12-0 to 12-11	60	14.13	1.68	5	8.20	1.48	$<.001$
13-0 to 13-11	72	14.13	1.55	4	10.00	3.37	$<.001$
14-0 to 14-11	60	14.88	1.71				
15-0 to 15-11	59	15.12	1.77				
	671			64			

Table 5.14

Purdue Pegboard: Both Hands. Significance of t-Test Group Comparisons for Normals and MBDs

Age	Normal Boys N	Mean	S.D.	MBD Boys N	Mean	S.D.	p
5-0 to 5-11	60	6.85	1.36	5	4.20	3.03	$<.001$
6-0 to 6-11	60	7.77	1.71	18	6.61	2.40	NS[a]
7-0 to 7-11	60	9.17	1.54	21	6.14	2.03	$<.001$
8-0 to 8-11	60	10.37	1.70	17	7.41	2.09	$<.001$
9-0 to 9-11	60	10.92	1.61	13	8.15	2.82	$<.001$
10-0 to 10-11	60	11.35	1.78	16	8.75	2.41	$<.001$
11-0 to 11-11	60	11.78	1.62	20	9.30	2.74	$<.001$
12-0 to 12-11	60	11.77	1.69	15	9.13	1.77	$<.001$
13-0 to 13-11	70	11.70	1.67	10	9.50	2.37	$<.001$
14-0 to 14-11	60	12.12	1.63	4	9.25	1.71	$<.01$
15-0 to 15-11	53	12.60	1.39				
	663			139			

Table 5.14 [Continued]

Age	Normal Girls N	Mean	S.D.	MBD Girls N	Mean	S.D.	p
5-0 to 5-11	60	6.87	1.26	3	2.67	1.53	< .001
6-0 to 6-11	60	8.60	1.62	9	3.44	1.94	< .001
7-0 to 7-11	60	9.17	1.77	10	6.50	1.90	< .001
8-0 to 8-11	60	10.27	1.70	9	6.11	2.32	< .001
9-0 to 9-11	60	10.72	1.85	5	7.40	2.88	< .001
10-0 to 10-11	60	11.80	1.50	4	7.00	2.83	< .001
11-0 to 11-11	60	11.83	1.72	13	7.77	3.09	< .001
12-0 to 12-11	60	12.02	1.44	5	6.80	1.48	< .001
13-0 to 13-11	72	12.07	1.38	4	8.00	2.94	< .001
14-0 to 14-11	60	12.52	1.77				
15-0 to 15-11	59	12.83	1.53				
	671			62			

^{a} NS—Not Significant

Table 5.15

Purdue Pegboard: Assembly. Significance of *t*- Test Group Comparisons for Normals and MBDs

Age	Normal Boys N	Mean	S.D.	MBD Boys N	Mean	S.D.	p
5-0 to 5-11	60	14.83	3.48	5	10.60	6.23	< .01
6-0 to 6-11	60	17.57	3.77	16	12.13	4.86	< .001
7-0 to 7-11	60	19.80	4.54	20	12.15	3.76	< .001
8-0 to 8-11	60	23.83	4.64	17	16.94	4.55	< .001
9-0 to 9-11	60	25.97	4.37	13	19.38	5.74	< .001
10-0 to 10-11	60	27.27	5.80	16	22.75	6.37	< .01
11-0 to 11-11	60	30.43	5.74	20	22.50	6.54	< .001
12-0 to 12-11	60	30.63	5.90	15	21.93	6.03	< .001
13-0 to 13-11	70	34.09	5.37	10	25.60	5.10	< .001
14-0 to 14-11	60	32.67	6.99	4	21.25	5.56	< .01
15-0 to 15-11	53	32.56	6.17				
	663			136			

Age	Normal Girls N	Mean	S.D.	MBD Girls N	Mean	S.D.	p
5-0 to 5-11	60	14.53	3.34	3	7.33	1.15	< .001
6-0 to 6-11	60	19.33	4.10	9	8.22	3.11	< .001
7-0 to 7-11	60	19.98	4.52	10	12.10	4.23	< .001
8-0 to 8-11	60	23.22	5.24	7	14.86	1.86	< .001
9-0 to 9-11	60	27.02	6.69	5	18.40	7.70	< .01
10-0 to 10-11	60	29.80	5.85	4	19.25	9.03	< .01
11-0 to 11-11	60	33.12	6.38	13	18.08	8.25	< .001
12-0 to 12-11	60	34.63	6.41	5	18.80	3.42	< .001
13-0 to 13-11	72	35.99	5.58	4	20.75	8.42	< .001
14-0 to 14-11	60	35.30	6.73				
15-0 to 15-11	59	37.13	7.95				
	671			60			

Clinically, the data presented in Tables 5.12–5.15 could be used in this way. A 7-year-old boy, for example, obtains the following scores on the pegboard test: preferred hand 11, nonpreferred hand 10, both hands 9, and assembly 19. Referring to the tables, we see that his scores are below the means for *normal* boys his age, but well within 1 standard deviation difference. However, his scores are generally 1–2 standard deviations above the means for *MBD* boys. One can conclude that this patient's motor coordination on this test is in the normal range.

The Eye-Motor Coordination Subtest (I) of the Development Test of Visual Perception

The Eye-Motor Coordination subtest of Frostig's Test of Visual Perception (Frostig, 1961) is a useful instrument for measuring fine motor coordination. In the section of this subtest shown in Figure 5.4, the subject is first asked to connect the mouse on the left of the top path

Figure 5.4
Eye-Motor Coordination Subtest (I) of the Development Test of Visual Perception

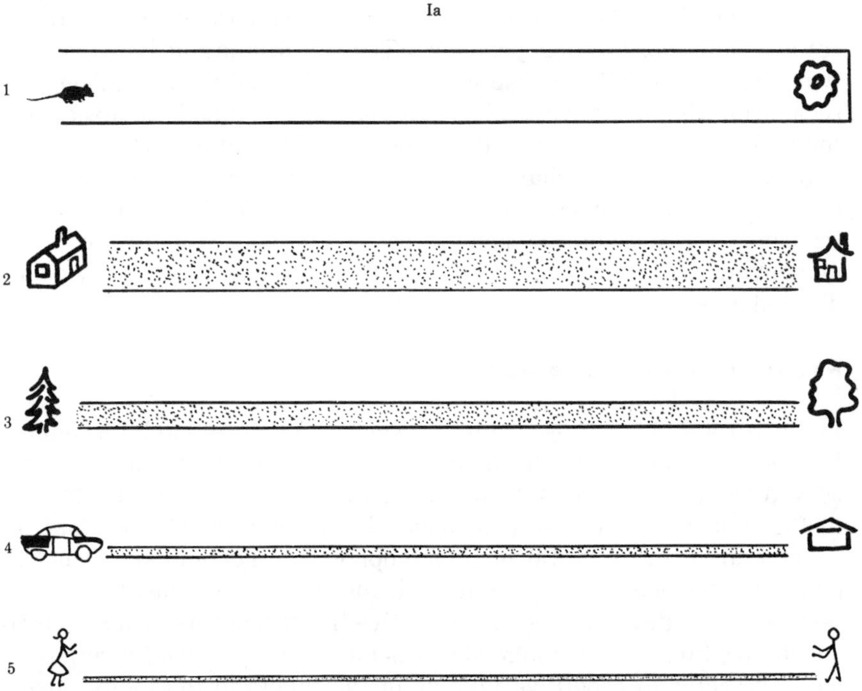

Reproduced by special permission from the Developmental Test of Visual Perception by Marianne Frostig, Ph.D. Copyright, 1961. Published by Consulting Psychologists Press, Inc.

with the cheese on the right. The child is encouraged to draw his line as straight as possible, without going outside of the path or even touching the sides. Next, he is asked to connect the two houses in the same way. Similar instructions are provided for the other tasks on this page as well as others in the subtest. The child is given 2 points if his line makes no contact at all with the sides of the path, 1 point if side contact is made but the line does not loop outside of the path edge, and no points if the line goes outside of the path edge. Raw scores are converted into age-equivalents and scaled scores for each subtest. A scaled score of 10 is average. Although all five subtests together are used to determine the child's "perceptual quotient," one can use each individual subtest to compare objectively the child's score with that which is normal for his age. Unfortunately, the upper age limit for which the test is standardized is 7 years, 11 months. Normative data on older children would have proved useful. On occasion, however, I have tested older children (especially those whom I strongly suspected to have a fine-motor-coordination problem) and expressed such findings in the following way: "Although John is 8 years 6 months old, his score on subtest I is comparable to the average child of 7 years 3 months, suggesting the presence of a fine-motor-coordination problem.

This test is also very sensitive to the presence of dyspraxia. There are some children who cannot draw the lines straight because of dyspraxic rather than coordination problems. The differentiation between the two may be difficult because in both cases the child's hand does not seem to do what he desires and he may recognize that he is not executing the task correctly. The Manual Expression subtest of the ITPA, which I will discuss in detail in chapter 9, can be useful in helping the examiner discriminate between coordination and dyspraxic deficits. In the ITPA instrument, if the child demonstrates that he can execute the basic maneuvers, he is given full credit. No points are lost for poorly coordinated imitation of the tasks.

Finger-Thumb Opposition

In the introduction to this section I described a theoretical interchange between a senior pediatric neurologist and a resident. The vignette served to illustrate the subjectivity of criteria for making diagnoses of fine-motor-coordination problems. The example given was that of speed and accuracy of finger-thumb opposition. Fortunately, Denckla (1973, 1974) has provided us with such normative data. She utilizes two tests of finger dexterity: one of repetitive finger movements and one of successive finger movements. She uses the term *repetitive finger movements* to refer to repetitive tapping of the thumb to the index finger only. She uses the term *successive finger movements* to refer to the serial tapping of the thumb to each of the other four fingers, that is, the thumb to the index finger first, then to the middle finger, then to the ring finger, and lastly to the fifth finger. Her instructions are a little complicated but serve to ensure standardization of the task.

Twenty Repetitive Finger Movements

The child is first asked to perform 20 repetitive finger movements (thumb to index finger only) with the preferred hand (usually the right). It is generally helpful for the examiner to demonstrate on himself while teaching this task. Denckla's suggested instructions: "When I say 'go,' tap your pointer (index finger) and thumb together as fast as you can 'till I stop you." After the child demonstrates the capacity to execute 20 such taps he is asked to repeat the same maneuver again, with the same hand. Accordingly, a total of two sets of 20 taps each are requested. The child is then asked to repeat the same two sets with the nonpreferred hand. Then he is asked to repeat again the two sets with the *nonpreferred hand* (bringing the total with the nonpreferred hand to four sets of 20 taps). He is then asked to return to the preferred hand and again perform two sets of 20 taps (bringing the total to four sets of 20 taps each to the preferred hand). After the child has been given the opportunity to practice the series (two sets of 20 taps each: preferred hand, nonpreferred hand, nonpreferred hand again, preferred hand), he is timed with a stopwatch while performing the task. However, the examiner only starts the stopwatch at the beginning of the *second* 20-tap set performed by each hand. In other words, of the total of eight 20-second sets performed, only four are timed, two with the preferred hand and two with the nonpreferred. The two preferred hand scores are averaged and the two nonpreferred scores are averaged and these are considered to be the child's scores for comparison with the normative data (Table 5.16).

Twenty Successive Finger Movements

Here the child is instructed to oppose the thumb of the preferred hand to each of the four other fingers, starting with the index finger and ending with the fifth. For each repeated trial the child is instructed to start again with the index finger and proceed to the fifth, rather than proceeding backwards from the fifth to the index finger. While demonstrating, the examiner says, "When I say 'go,' make each finger march past the thumb and tap it in turn; don't go backwards, keep marching from pointer (index finger) to pinkie (fifth finger) 'till I stop you." The child is asked to perform six sets of 4 taps each (thumb to

Table 5.16

Time to Perform 20 Repetitive Finger Movements

	Number of Children	Mean	S.D.
Age 5			
Boys:	42		
Right hand		7.30	1.08
Left hand		7.95	1.00
Girls:	41		
Right hand		7.85	1.78
Left hand		8.56	1.86
Age 6			
Boys:	38		
Right hand		6.69	0.82
Left hand		7.44	0.91
Girls:	39		
Right hand		6.51	1.01
Left hand		7.15	0.97
Age 7			
Boys:	39		
Right hand		5.94	0.81
Left hand		6.60	0.83
Girls:	38		
Right hand		5.99	0.70
Left hand		6.83	0.82
Age 8			
Boys:	14		
Right hand		5.99	0.98
Left hand		6.31	0.64
Girls:	14		
Right hand		5.50	0.80
Left hand		6.14	0.88
Age 9			
Boys:	14		
Right hand		5.97	0.72
Left hand		6.35	1.23
Girls:	14		
Right hand		5.84	1.25
Left hand		6.43	0.90
Age 10			
Boys:	14		
Right hand		5.55	1.22
Left hand		6.09	1.11
Girls:	14		
Right hand		5.77	1.38
Left hand		6.27	1.79

Reproduced with permission of the author and Spastics International Medical Publications, the publisher, from M. B. Denckla, "Development of Speed in Repetitive and Successive Finger-Movements in Normal Children," *Developmental Medicine and Child Neurology*, 15:653–645, 1973. M. B. Denckla, "Development of Motor Coordination in Normal Children," *Developmental Medicine and Child Neurology*, 16:729–741, 1974.

Table 5.17

Time to Perform 20 Successive Finger Movements

	Number of Children	Mean	S.D.
Age 5			
Boys:	37		
Right hand		16.70	4.08
Left hand		16.86	5.32
Girls:	40		
Right hand		14.40	2.94
Left hand		14.33	2.20
Age 6			
Boys:	36		
Right hand		14.48	3.23
Left hand		14.26	2.66
Girls:	39		
Right hand		13.13	2.61
Left hand		13.18	3.21
Age 7			
Boys:	39		
Right hand		12.22	2.92
Left hand		12.60	3.05
Girls:	38		
Right hand		11.29	3.18
Left hand		11.68	3.30
Age 8			
Boys:	14		
Right hand		10.41	2.03
Left hand		10.84	2.70
Girls:	14		
Right hand		9.25	2.69
Left hand		9.89	2.76
Age 9			
Boys:	14		
Right hand		10.45	2.95
Left hand		10.94	3.82
Girls:	14		
Right hand		9.59	2.10
Left hand		9.84	2.20
Age 10			
Boys:	14		
Right hand		10.22	2.74
Left hand		10.19	2.65
Girls:	14		
Right hand		8.41	2.37
Left hand		7.99	2.11

Reproduced with permission of the author and Spastics International Medical Publications, the publisher, from M. B. Denckla, "Development of Speed in Repetitive and Successive Finger-Movements in Normal Children," *Developmental Medicine and Child Neurology*, 15:653–645, 1973. M. B. Denckla, "Development of Motor Coordination in Normal Children," *Developmental Medicine and Child Neurology*, 16:729–741, 1974.

index finger, once; thumb to middle finger, once; thumb to ring finger, once; and thumb to fifth finger, once). The total number of taps is therefore 24. However, the examiner only times with the stopwatch the second through the sixth sets (20 taps); the first set of 4 taps are not timed. As with the repetitive taps, the sequence is six sets of 4 taps with the preferred hand, six sets with the nonpreferred, another six sets with the nonpreferred, and six sets again with the preferred. Only sets two through six are timed. The two scores for the preferred hand and the two scores for the nonpreferred hand are averaged and the child's score is compared with the normative data shown in Table 5.17.

GROSS MOTOR COORDINATION

Foot Tally Counter

The aforementioned mounted hand tally counter used by Knights and Moule to measure finger-tapping speed can also be used to measure foot-tapping speed (Knights and Moule, 1967). The child is instructed to place his heel at the edge of the board and to tap the counter with the ball of his foot as rapidly as he can (Figure 5.5). As mentioned, the 6 in. × 10 in. board recommended by Knights and Moule is, in my experience, a little too small because it requires some extra stabilization when used for foot tapping. Again, the dominant and nondominant feet are

Figure 5.5
Foot Tally Counter.

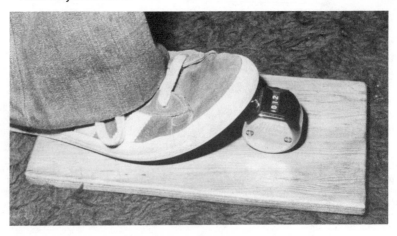

alternated until each foot has been tested four times (10 sec each trial).
The best three scores are averaged to obtain the child's score. Normative
data are presented in Table 5.18.

Table 5.18
Means and Standard Deviations for Foot Tapping for Each Chronological Age

		Chronological Age in Years									
		5.7	6.5	7.5	8.5	9.5	10.5	11.5	12.5	13.5	14.4
Dominant foot	Mean	20.9	27.0	26.3	31.7	32.4	33.6	38.8	40.4	42.1	43.0
	S.D.	4.5	5.7	3.0	4.5	5.7	6.0	5.4	6.8	6.2	5.2
Nondominant foot	Mean	20.2	25.8	24.7	29.9	31.5	31.7	35.0	39.1	40.5	40.4
	S.D.	4.4	6.0	3.6	4.5	4.8	4.3	5.6	6.0	6.3	7.1
		10	12	27	22	19	17	25	11	16	10

Reprinted with permission of author and publisher from Knights, Robert M., and Moule, Allan D. Normative and ability Data on Finger and Foot Tapping in Children. PERCEPTUAL AND MOTOR SKILLS, 1967, 25, 717–720.

Twenty Repetitive Foot Taps

Denckla (1974) has also devised a test for foot-tapping speed. In her
test the child's heel remains fixed on the floor and he is asked to try to
tap his toes (really his forefoot) as rapidly as he can. The stopwatch is
started with tap number 2 and discontinued with tap number 21. Accordingly, the time to execute 20 taps is recorded. Both right and left
feet are given one trial each. Normative data (for which there are 14
children in each age/sex group) is presented in Table 5.19.

Table 5.19
Time to Perform 20 Repetitive Foot Taps

	Right		Left	
Age in Years	Mean	S.D.	Mean	S.D.
Boys				
5	8.57	2.16	8.66	1.86
6	6.83	0.82	7.13	1.31
7	6.31	1.63	6.82	1.40
8	4.71	0.58	5.15	0.71
9	5.75	0.88	6.08	0.90
10	5.84	1.39	6.31	1.10
Girls				
5	8.49	1.35	9.74	3.38
6	6.79	1.45	8.01	2.53
7	6.26	3.01	5.95	1.61
8	6.14	0.96	6.04	1.09
9	5.62	0.84	5.91	1.21
10	6.32	2.03	6.34	1.88

Reproduced with permission of the author and Spastics International Medical Publications, the publisher, from M. B. Denckla, "Development of Motor Coordination in Normal Children," *Developmental Medicine and Child Neurology*, 16:729–741, 1974.

Twenty Heel-Toe Alternating Movements

In this test (Denckla, 1974) neither heel nor toe (actually the forefoot) remains on the floor throughout the test. Rather, the child is asked to try to alternately tap his heel and then his toes on the floor, one after the other. In other words, a rocking movement is requested. Ten pairs of heel-toe taps are recorded, starting with pair number 2 and ending with pair number 11. Both feet are timed, with one trial only being given for each foot. Normative data (for which there are 14 children in each age/sex group) are shown in Table 5.20.

Table 5.20
Time to Perform 20 Heel-Toe Alternating Movements

	Right		Left	
Age in Years	Mean	S.D.	Mean	S.D.
Boys				
5	15.03	3.75	14.50	3.40
6	12.16	1.49	12.93	3.45
7	10.23	2.27	11.70	2.90
8	9.44	2.36	10.14	2.74
9	9.21	1.84	9.84	2.25
10	8.07	1.56	8.61	1.57
Girls				
5	12.71	4.07	13.16	3.94
6	11.75	3.44	12.36	4.11
7	9.22	3.00	9.71	3.14
8	8.71	2.06	8.43	1.72
9	7.44	1.02	8.11	2.33
10	6.90	1.57	7.00	1.49

Reproduced with permission of the author and Spastics International Medical Publications, the publisher, from M. B. Denckla, "Development of Motor Coordination in Normal Children," *Developmental Medicine and Child Neurology*, 16:729–741, 1974.

Hopping on One Foot

In this test of gross motor coordination (Denckla, 1974) the child is simply asked, "Let's see how many times you can hop on one foot in one place, without moving across the floor." The examiner counts the number of times the child hops on the preferred foot until the lifted foot is placed on the floor. The ceiling number of hops is set at 50, and the child's hopping is discontinued when he reaches this limit. The procedure is then repeated for the nonpreferred foot. Table 5.21 data shows the percentage of children succeeding in these tasks at various ages.

Table 5.21

Percentage of Children Succeeding at Hopping on One Foot Up to 50 Times on One or Both Sides

Age [Years]	Number of Children	Percentage Able to Hop Unilaterally 12×	25×	50×	Percentage Able to Perform 50 Hops on Either Foot	Percentage Whose Right and Left Hopping Differs by Less Than 5 Hops
5	28	85			15	50
6	28		85		20	50
7	28			90	90	90
8	28			95	85	90
9	28			90	85	90
10	28			100	95	90

Reproduced with permission of the author and Spastics International Medical Publications, the publisher, from M. B. Denckla, "Development of Motor Coordination in Normal Children," *Developmental Medicine and Child Neurology*, 16:729–741, 1974.

Twenty Repetitive Hand Pats

In this test of gross motor coordination (Denckla, 1974) the child is simply asked to pat his hand on the table as rapidly as he can. After the examiner says "go," the stopwatch is started when the child executes tap number 2 and is stopped when the child executes tap number 21. Accordingly, the total number of times the child taps is 20. Both right and left hands are tested, each only once. Normal scores (for which there are 14 children in each age/sex group) are shown in Table 5.22.

Table 5.22

Time to Perform 20 Repetitive Hand Pats

Age in Years	Right Mean	S.D.	Left Mean	S.D.
Boys				
5	6.25	2.67	5.93	1.19
6	5.57	1.20	5.79	1.41
7	4.82	1.06	5.26	1.42
8	4.17	0.96	4.74	0.82
9	4.57	1.13	4.60	0.62
10	4.31	1.17	4.48	1.26
Girls				
5	5.91	1.26	6.45	1.25
6	5.48	0.72	6.00	1.02
7	5.22	1.44	5.16	1.18
8	4.55	0.48	4.63	0.64
9	4.26	0.72	4.50	0.67
10	5.43	1.81	5.37	1.72

Reproduced with permission of the author and Spastics International Medical Publications, the publisher, from M. B. Denckla, "Development of Motor Coordination in Normal Children," *Developmental Medicine and Child Neurology*, 16:729–741, 1974.

Twenty Hand Flexion-Extension Movements

In this test of gross motor coordination (Denckla, 1974) the child is asked to make a fist and hold his arm extended anteriorly with the dorsum of the fist superior. Without rotating the fist along the long axis of the forearm, the child is asked to flex and then extend his fist at the wrist. In other words, the fist moves up and down while the arm and forearm are rigidly held. Ten pairs of flexion-extension movements are timed, with a total of 20 movements. Stopwatch timing starts at the beginning of the second pair and ends at the time of completion of the eleventh pair, with a total of 10 pairs being timed. One trial each for both the right and left hands are timed. Normative data (for which there are 14 children in each age/sex group) are presented in Table 5.23.

Table 5.23
Time to Perform 20 Hand Flexion-Extension Movements

Age in Years	Right Mean	S.D.	Left Mean	S.D.
Boys				
5	10.34	1.95	10.71	1.90
6	9.79	1.75	11.13	2.63
7	8.93	1.43	9.00	2.23
8	7.39	1.62	7.94	1.53
9	7.84	1.87	8.34	2.01
10	7.66	2.14	8.34	1.52
Girls				
5	10.07	2.47	10.93	2.33
6	9.34	1.17	10.53	2.09
7	7.86	2.05	8.52	1.59
8	8.72	2.20	9.02	2.40
9	8.15	1.35	8.17	1.51
10	7.34	1.43	7.26	1.37

Reproduced with permission of the author and Spastics International Medical Publications, the publisher, from M. B. Denckla, "Development of Motor Coordination in Normal Children," *Developmental Medicine and Child Neurology*, 16:729–741, 1974.

Twenty Arm Pronation-Supination Movements

For this test of gross motor coordination (Denckla, 1974) the child may choose whether or not he wishes to keep his elbow flexed. In either case the forearm is held anteriorly, with the hand flat and the palmer surface of the hand facing the floor. The child is asked to pronate and supinate his forearm as rapidly as possible. The time to execute 10 pairs of pronation-supination movements is recorded. The stopwatch is started at the beginning of the second pair of movements and stopped at the end of the eleventh. One trial each for both the right and left arms are used in determining the child's score. Normative data (for which there are 14 children in each age/sex group) are shown in Table 5.24.

Table 5.24

Time to Perform 20 Arm Pronation-Supination Movements

Age in Years	Right Mean	S.D.	Left Mean	S.D.
Boys				
5	9.32	1.67	9.35	1.64
6	8.37	1.47	8.76	1.17
7	8.59	1.90	8.87	1.93
8	6.83	1.43	7.27	1.08
9	7.59	1.91	7.66	1.76
10	7.09	1.54	7.41	1.73
Girls				
5	9.57	1.56	10.28	1.61
6	9.38	1.51	9.02	1.26
7	7.69	0.88	7.54	1.01
8	7.29	1.33	7.69	1.15
9	6.76	1.30	7.05	1.19
10	7.05	1.36	7.04	1.55

Reproduced with permission of the author and Spastics International Medical Publications, the publisher, from M. B. Denckla, "Development of Motor Coordination in Normal Children," *Developmental Medicine and Child Neurology*, 16:729–741, 1974.

Throwing Balls in A Basket

Ball-throwing accuracy is an excellent test of gross motor coordination (although finger dexterity is also involved to a limited degree). The traditional way in which this function has been tested has been for the examiner to "play catch" with the child and ascertain his competence. Clearly, any conclusions drawn from such a method are subjectively arrived at. Because the examiner's own level of competence affects the child's performance (it is harder for a child to catch an examiner's misplaced throw), conclusions derived from this method are even more suspect. Even if the examiner was faultlessly consistent and accurate with his or her throws, the tester's criteria for healthy and pathological performance on the child's part must still be individual and impressionistic.

The Lincoln-Oseretsky Scale (Sloan, 1955) includes a test of ball-throwing accuracy (test no. 22). The child is asked to throw a regulation tennis ball at a 10-inch square of cardboard placed on a wall exactly 8 ft away. The target is placed at the level of the child's chest and the instructions state that the "ball should be held in the hand close to the shoulder and must be thrown in a straight line" and "must not be tossed or thrown overhand or underhand." The child throws the ball five times with each hand and the examiner records the total number of balls that hit the target.

I believe that this test has a number of drawbacks. Five throws, in my opinion, is far too small a number to measure accurately a child's competence. Each miss changes the child's level by 20%. In this examiner's experience it is sometimes difficult to determine whether or not the ball actually hit the edge of the target or just the adjacent wall. (The contact time is usually a fraction of a second and there is no spot to mark the point where the ball made contact with the wall or target.) The average number of children of each sex used to determine what is normal was 20–23. Although such a number lends itself to statistically useful norms, a larger number in each category would provide the examiner with greater conviction for the reliability of the data. Interpreting the meaning of a child's score is especially cumbersome when utilizing the Lincoln-Oseretsky Scale. For this test a child with 4 or 5 hits is given a score of 3 points; 2 or 3 hits warrants a score of 2 points; 1 hit gets 1 point; and no hits is scored 0. If a 9-year-old girl, for example, gets 3 hits with the right hand she is given a score of 2 points (she would get 2 points for 2 hits as well). One then refers to the chart of normative data and ascertains that the figure that one must use to calculate the meaning of this child's score is 47. This number signifies that the average 9-year-old girl gets a score which is 47% of the maximum score on the test, which is 3 points. In other words, the average 9-year-old girl gets a score of $0.47 \times 3 = 1.41$. We learn then that this girl (with a score of 2 points) is above average with 3 hits, but little more. We know nothing about how far above average. A girl with 2 hits is also above average, but less so.

An even less convincing test relating to ball playing capacity is the Lincoln-Oseretsky test for ball catching (test no. 12). Here, the examiner throws a regulation tennis ball five times to the child, who stands 10 feet away, and records the number of catches. The examiner is instructed to "toss the ball to S with an underhand motion so that when the ball reaches S it is describing a downward curve and S is able to catch the ball in his cupped hand with the palm facing upward. The ball should be 'lobbed' over and not thrown in a straight line. E is to toss the ball toward the hand the subject is to use in making the catch. If E makes a bad toss, the trial is not counted." The decision as to whether the toss was "bad" is up to the examiner. The decision as to whether the ball has traversed the required trajectory is also up to the examiner. There are clearly many misses where even the most astute observer would be hard put to determine whether the child's miss was the result of the examiner's poor throw or the child's poor catch. The only thing that one can conclude when a child does poorly on this test is that *either* the child is poorly coordinated, *or* the examiner is poorly coordinated, *or both are.*

The Denver Developmental Screening Test (Frankenburg and Dodds, 1969) includes a test of ball-throwing capability. The complete instructions: "Child must throw a ball overhand 3 feet to within arm's reach of tester." The scale indicates that normal children begin to develop the capacity to accomplish this task at 15 months; that 50% do it successfully by 20 months; 75% by 23 months; and 90% by 30 months. My experience with this test has been that it is often difficult to determine whether the ball has indeed landed in the target area. No instructions are given regarding the number of trials the child is permitted. Some examiners, I would imagine, allow the child only one trial and others more. Clearly, patients tested by the latter group are more likely to successfully accomplish the task. Furthermore, the target area is determined by the length of the examiner's arm. Accordingly, children with long-armed examiners are going to do better than those whose testers are short-armed.

In the attempt to provide a more objective test for ball throwing accuracy, I decided that a test in which the child is asked to throw balls in a basket would obviate some of the drawbacks of the above-mentioned motor coordination tests (Gardner, 1979). No dependence is placed on the examiner's ball-throwing capacity, ability to judge distance, capacity to observe accurately split-second events, or his or her arm length in determining a child's score. The ball either goes into the basket or it does not. There is no reliance on the examiner's subjective decisions (Did the ball hit the target or not? Did the ball fall within an arm's length of me?).

In the specific test that I designed, 24 regulation size tennis balls are used. The first 3 are used for practice, and the remaining 21 scored. This larger number of balls was selected to prevent the aforementioned defects of a scoring system that uses small numbers of balls. The basket chosen was a common size waste basket manufactured by the Sterilite Corporation (Townsend, Maryland 01469, model no. 1050). The basket is 19¾ in. high, has a base diameter of 11¼ in. (irrelevant to its purposes here), a top inner diameter of 13½ in. (a crucial measurement), and a top outside diameter of 14½ in. (not an important measurement). (The basket comes with a somewhat elaborate sliding cover which is of no value in this test and may have to be purchased only to be discarded.) In all probability, any basket with a top inner diameter of 13½ in. and height 19–21 in. will serve. Other equipment necessary is a yardstick (or other measuring instrument), a bucket for holding the 24 tennis balls, and possibly a second bucket for the examiner to collect missed balls. Lastly, it is preferable to place a brick or some heavy stones in the basket to prevent its being moved during the course of the test. (Obviously the distance between child and basket must remain fixed if the test is to have significance.) All the equipment that is needed to

Figure 5.6
Balls and Basket Test Equipment.

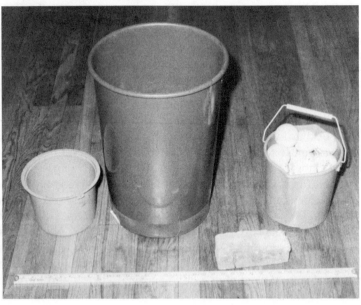

administer the Balls and Basket Test is shown in Figure 5.6.

The basket (with the brick inside) is so positioned that it is not close enough to any walls that might allow balls to rebound into it. If, in spite of these precautions, a ball does rebound into the basket, it is removed and not counted as a point. It is preferable to draw a circle around the base of the basket to ensure that it remains in the same position throughout the testing. A yardstick is placed 6 ft from the basket's center point for all subjects who have not yet reached their ninth birthday, and 9 ft away for all subjects 9 years of age and older. Using a yardstick, rather than any other measuring device, is probably the easiest way to make these distance determinations. To ensure that the distance between the child and the basket remains constant, it is preferable to use the yardstick *and* a chalk line (at the edge closest to the child) as the line beyond which the child must stand. The bucket of 24 balls is placed next to the child.

The child is simply told, "This is a test to see how many balls you can get in the basket. The first 3 balls are for practice. Then I will count the number of balls you get in." The child is permitted to throw overhand, underhand, or sideways; in fact, he may choose any position he wishes. He can lean forward as far as he wants; however, he may not put either foot in front of the ruler and chalk line. If, before throwing a ball, the child's foot goes in front of the line, the ball is not counted

Figure 5.7
Testing Arrangement of the Balls and Basket Test.

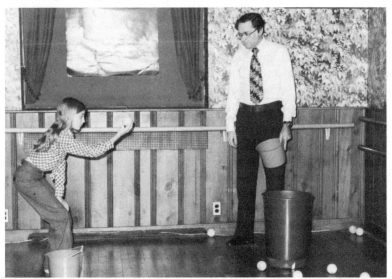

(whether or not it gets into the basket) and the throw is repeated. After all balls are thrown, the examiner merely counts the number that successfully landed in the basket. A typical testing arrangement is shown in Figure 5.7.

My associates and I administered the test to 1,350 school children ages 5 to 16 (670 boys and 680 girls). The children all attended public schools in Bergen County, New Jersey (the same schools from which Purdue Pegboard data were collected). Only children in regular classes were included. Children in special educational classes or those known to have any special handicaps were excluded from the study. The children were from blue-collar and white-collar families in schools where the students tended to score in the average to slightly-above-average range on national standardized tests.

The subjects of each sex were divided into 22 groups, each group consisting of children at the same half-year level: the youngest group, ages 5-0 to 5-6; the oldest, ages 15-6 to 15-11. Ranges, means, standard deviations, and percentile ranks for boys are presented in Tables 5.25 and 5.26. Similar information for girls is presented in Tables 5.27 and 5.28. The distances chosen for the two age brackets (below and above 9 years of age) appear to have been judicious. Few got no balls in and none got in all 21 (there were some 19s). The spread of scores also appears to be balanced. The results indicate also a leveling off of the scores after age 11, with insignificant differences between the performance of children at subsequent ages. The data for 14 and 15 year olds, then, are probably applicable to older children and adults. My experiences with the test for older youngsters and adults tend to confirm this.

A boy, for example, age 8 years 8 months successfully gets 5 balls in the basket. Referring to Table 5.25, we see that the normal range for boys that age is from 7 to 16, with a mean score of 11.37 and a standard deviation of 2.57. The boy's score is 6.37 points below the mean (11.37 − 5.00 = 6.37), or 2.48 standard deviations (6.37/2.57 = 2.48) below the mean. Referring to Table 5.26, we see that a score of 8 is at the tenth percentile level of normals and the boy's score of 5 is far below that. The results strongly suggest that this child has a gross-motor-coordination deficit.

Table 5.25
Balls and Basket Test—Boys

Age	N	Low	High	Mean	S.D.
Balls Thrown from 6 Feet					
5-0 to 5-5	30	0	11	6.37	3.00
5-6 to 5-11	30	2	14	6.27	2.61
6-0 to 6-5	30	1	14	6.17	3.38
6-6 to 6-11	30	3	15	8.67	3.13
7-0 to 7-5	30	3	17	10.33	3.47
7-6 to 7-11	30	0	16	9.83	4.76
8-0 to 8-5	30	3	16	11.40	3.21
8-6 to 8-11	30	7	16	11.37	2.57
Balls Thrown from 9 Feet					
9-0 to 9-5	30	2	14	7.40	3.02
9-6 to 9-11	30	3	15	9.03	3.25
10-0 to 10-5	30	3	13	8.70	2.53
10-6 to 10-11	30	4	17	9.73	3.08
11-0 to 11-5	30	3	17	9.57	3.46
11-6 to 11-11	30	5	17	11.03	2.80
12-0 to 12-5	30	5	16	11.33	2.92
12-6 to 12-11	30	4	16	11.17	2.96
13-0 to 13-5	40	5	16	11.35	2.86
13-6 to 13-11	30	4	19	11.13	3.70
14-0 to 14-5	30	4	19	12.70	3.22
14-6 to 14-11	30	2	19	11.27	3.42
15-0 to 15-5	30	8	17	12.53	2.54
15-6 to 15-11	30	9	19	12.47	2.37
	670				

Table 5.26

Balls and Basket Test: Percentiles for Boys

Age	N	10	20	30	40	50	60	70	80	90
				Balls Thrown from 6 Feet						
5-0 to 5-5	30	2.1	3.0	5.0	6.0	6.5	7.6	8.0	9.0	10.9
5-6 to 5-11	30	3.1	4.0	4.3	6.0	6.0	7.0	7.0	8.8	9.9
6-0 to 6-5	30	3.0	3.0	4.0	5.0	5.0	6.6	7.7	9.0	11.8
6-6 to 6-11	30	4.0	5.0	7.0	8.4	9.0	10.0	10.7	11.0	12.9
7-0 to 7-5	30	5.1	7.0	9.0	10.0	10.5	11.0	12.7	13.8	14.9
7-6 to 7-11	30	1.3	6.0	8.0	8.0	10.0	11.0	14.0	15.0	16.0
8-0 to 8-5	30	7.1	8.2	10.0	11.4	12.0	12.6	13.7	14.8	15.0
8-6 to 8-11	30	8.0	9.0	10.0	11.0	11.0	12.0	12.7	14.0	15.0
				Balls Thrown from 9 Feet						
9-0 to 9-5	30	3.1	5.0	6.0	6.0	7.5	8.0	9.0	10.8	11.0
9-6 to 9-11	30	4.1	6.2	7.0	7.4	9.0	10.0	11.0	12.0	13.9
10-0 to 10-5	30	5.0	6.2	7.0	8.4	9.0	10.0	10.0	11.0	11.9
10-6 to 10-11	30	7.0	7.0	7.3	8.0	9.0	10.6	11.7	12.0	13.0
11-0 to 11-5	30	6.0	6.0	7.3	8.0	9.5	11.0	11.0	12.0	14.9
11-6 to 11-11	30	8.0	8.0	9.0	10.0	11.0	12.0	13.0	13.8	14.9
12-0 to 12-5	30	7.0	9.2	10.0	11.0	11.0	12.0	14.0	14.0	14.0
12-6 to 12-11	30	7.0	9.0	9.3	11.0	11.0	12.6	13.0	14.0	15.0
13-0 to 13-5	40	6.1	9.2	10.0	11.0	12.0	12.0	13.0	14.0	15.0
13-6 to 13-11	30	5.1	8.0	9.3	10.0	11.5	12.0	13.0	14.8	16.0
14-0 to 14-5	30	10.0	10.0	10.0	11.0	13.0	13.6	14.0	15.0	17.9
14-6 to 14-11	30	7.0	8.2	9.3	11.0	11.0	12.0	13.0	14.0	15.8
15-0 to 15-5	30	9.1	10.0	11.0	12.0	12.5	13.0	14.0	15.0	16.0
15-6 to 15-11	30	9.0	10.2	11.0	12.0	12.0	13.0	14.0	14.0	15.9
	670									

Referring to Table 5.27, we see the range for girls her age is from 1 to 10, mean 6.13, standard deviation 2.45. Her score then is over 1 standard deviation above the mean. Referring to Table 5.28, we see that a score of 9 is above the eightieth percentile level. Accordingly, we can conclude that a gross-motor-coordination problem (at least one that would impair ball throwing) is unlikely.

In my experience, coordination problems are among the more common difficulties suffered by children with MBD. Yet hearsay information and subjective impressions have often been relied upon to conclude that a child is exhibiting such deficits. The examiner does well to utilize tests of the kinds described in this chapter to provide more solid and convincing evidence regarding whether or not a child has a coordination deficit.

Table 5.27

Balls and Basket Test—Girls

Age	N	Low	High	Mean	S.D.
		Balls Thrown from 6 Feet			
5-0 to 5-5	30	1	12	4.53	2.50
5-6 to 5-11	30	1	11	5.07	2.52
6-0 to 6-5	30	2	13	7.37	2.94
6-6 to 6-11	30	2	14	8.33	3.58
7-0 to 7-5	30	2	12	7.67	2.89
7-6 to 7-11	30	1	17	9.90	3.70
8-0 to 8-5	30	1	19	8.70	3.99
8-6 to 8-11	30	5	14	10.70	2.82
		Balls Thrown from 9 Feet			
9-0 to 9-5	30	1	10	6.13	2.45
9-6 to 9-11	30	2	12	7.10	2.34
10-0 to 10-5	30	3	16	7.50	2.85
10-6 to 10-11	30	3	15	8.47	3.47
11-0 to 11-5	30	3	14	8.07	2.82
11-6 to 11-11	30	4	14	8.37	2.33
12-0 to 12-5	30	4	15	9.87	2.70
12-6 to 12-11	30	4	16	9.90	3.02
13-0 to 13-5	50	5	15	10.36	2.60
13-6 to 13-11	30	5	17	12.07	3.20
14-0 to 14-5	30	4	16	10.07	2.90
14-6 to 14-11	30	5	19	9.67	3.07
15-0 to 15-5	30	6	18	10.90	2.48
15-6 to 15-11	30	4	14	9.73	2.50
	680				

CONCLUDING COMMENTS

Of all the signs and symptoms of MBD, it is probable that hyperactivity and coordination problems are the ones that are most frequently diagnosed on the basis of subjective criteria. The examiner is more likely to use heresay evidence when making the diagnosis of hyperactivity. He or she may rely on parents' and teachers' observations because such children do not often exhibit hyperactivity in the one-to-one office situation. When diagnosing coordination deficits, the examiner may use heresay as clues ("He's always been clumsy." "He's the last one chosen in baseball and basketball games."), but is likely to perform some kind of examination as well. Often the conclusions derived from such an assessment are subjective and impressionistic.

Fine motor coordination is usually tested by asking the child to oppose successively, as rapidly as he can, the tip of his thumb to the tips of each of his other four fingers. On the basis of his accumulated experience, the examiner attempts to ascertain whether the child's error frequency and speed is in the normal or abnormal range. A preferable

Table 5.28

Balls and Basket Test: Percentiles for Girls

Age	N	10	20	30	40	50	60	70	80	90
				Balls Thrown from 6 Feet						
5-0 to 5-5	30	2.0	2.2	3.0	3.0	4.0	5.0	6.0	6.0	8.0
5-6 to 5-11	30	2.0	2.2	3.0	4.0	5.5	6.0	6.7	7.0	8.9
6-0 to 6-5	30	4.0	4.2	5.3	6.4	7.5	8.0	9.0	10.0	11.9
6-6 to 6-11	30	4.0	5.0	6.0	7.0	7.5	10.0	11.0	12.0	13.0
7-0 to 7-5	30	2.1	5.2	6.3	7.4	8.0	8.6	9.0	10.8	11.0
7-6 to 7-11	30	5.0	7.0	8.3	9.0	10.0	11.6	12.0	13.0	14.9
8-0 to 8-5	30	4.0	4.2	7.0	8.0	8.0	9.6	10.7	11.8	14.0
8-6 to 8-11	30	6.1	8.0	9.0	10.0	11.5	12.0	12.7	14.0	14.0
				Balls Thrown from 9 Feet						
9-0 to 9-5	30	3.1	4.0	4.3	5.4	6.0	6.6	7.7	8.8	10.0
9-6 to 9-11	30	4.0	5.0	6.0	7.0	8.0	8.0	8.0	9.0	10.0
10-0 to 10-5	30	4.1	5.0	6.0	6.4	7.0	7.0	9.0	9.8	11.9
10-6 to 10-11	30	4.1	5.2	6.0	7.0	7.5	9.6	11.0	12.0	13.9
11-0 to 11-5	30	4.1	6.0	7.0	7.4	8.0	8.0	9.0	10.8	12.9
11-6 to 11-11	30	5.1	6.0	7.0	8.0	8.0	9.0	9.0	10.0	11.9
12-0 to 12-5	30	5.1	7.2	9.0	10.0	10.0	11.0	11.0	12.0	13.9
12-6 to 12-11	30	5.1	7.0	9.0	10.0	10.0	11.0	11.0	12.0	14.0
13-0 to 13-5	50	7.0	8.2	9.0	10.0	10.0	11.0	12.0	13.0	13.9
13-6 to 13-11	30	8.0	8.2	10.0	12.0	13.0	13.0	14.0	15.8	16.0
14-0 to 14-5	30	6.0	7.2	8.0	9.0	10.0	11.6	12.0	13.0	13.0
14-6 to 14-11	30	6.0	7.2	8.0	9.0	9.0	10.0	11.0	11.8	13.0
15-0 to 15-5	30	8.0	9.0	9.0	10.0	11.0	12.0	12.0	12.0	14.0
15-6 to 15-11	30	6.1	7.2	8.3	9.4	10.0	11.0	11.0	11.8	13.0
	680									

way of assessing this function is to utilize the hand tally counter, the Eye-Motor Coordination subtest of the Frostig Test of Visual Perception, Denckla's repetitive and successive finger movement tests, or the Purdue Pegboard. The latter is especially sensitive to such deficits, especially with the normative data on over 1,300 children that is now available. The examiner should administer a few of these tests, rather than only one, in order to have more confidence in his or her conclusions.

Gross motor coordination is frequently evaluated by observing the child's gait while walking and "playing catch" with him. Both rely on subjective impressions by the examiner regarding what is normal and what is abnormal. And the ball-playing method is based on the assumption that it is the child's, not the examiner's, impairment that is responsible for the child's failure to catch the ball. The foot tally counter, Denckla's series of gross-motor-coordination tests, and the Balls and Basket Test are much more likely to provide an objective assessment of gross-motor-coordination function. The Balls and Basket Test is especially valuable for such assessment because of the availability of data on over 1,300 children on which it is standardized.

6

⬚○ Soft Neurological
Signs

In a sense, every sign described in this book could justifiably be called a soft neurological sign. Minimal brain dysfunction, by definition, is a collection of mild neurological syndromes (still to be clearly delineated from one another) that share in common varying degrees of minimal, but definite, neurological impairment. At this time, however, a certain subgroup of MBD is referred to by the term soft neurological signs. Because of the widespread use of the term, I will also subscribe to the convention, but recognize that the term is a poor one and that we do better to describe more specifically each of the entities subsumed under the rubric than to artificially pull together certain clusters as if the members had a certain special relationship.

The term soft neurological signs was, to the best of my knowledge, first introduced by Bender (1947) in a discussion of minor neurological impairments seen in children with schizophrenia. Although many authors do not make the differentiation, most presently use the term to refer to two classes of mild neurological impairments. The first type are manifestations of developmental lags such as lateness in suppressing such primitive signs as the Babinski and tonic neck reflexes; significant lateness in such developmental milestones as standing, walking, talking, and bowel and bladder training; and persistence of immature speech patterns on a neurological (as opposed to a psychogenic) basis. Such signs have to be elicited during the period in which they should have disappeared, but *before* they belatedly do so. For example, the average child begins to walk during the 10–14 month period. A child who is still not walking at 19 months would be considered by most examiners to have a neurological developmental lag that many would label a soft neurological sign. If at 20 months the child began to walk, the sign would no longer be present. If the child was first seen at 20 months then one would have to make some judgment about the parents' reliability in order to decide whether or not such a sign *was* present. (Signs, by definition, are manifestations observed by the examiner.) This introduces a subjective element at times which may compromise the credibility of those who report such signs. Denckla and Rudel (unpublished manuscript) refer to these as the *soft developmental type* of soft neurological sign and this is the term I will use here.

The second type of soft neurological sign includes mild abnormalities that one may find when conducting a traditional neurological examination. They include such findings as reflex asymmetries, hypo- and hyperreflexia, mild tremors and choreiform movements, motor overflow, and mild coordination deficits. Again, subjective elements may enter when making such decisions. For example, one examiner may consider a child to have 2 + deep tendon reflexes (normal) and another may decide that they are 3 + (hyperreflexic). It is in this second group, even more than in the first, that subjective factors may play a significant role in the examiner's decision as to whether such a sign is present. Denckla and Rudel refer to these as the *soft neurological type* of soft neurological sign and I will employ this term here.

Many, such as Ingram (1973), do not believe in the existence of such signs and consider use of the term a manifestation of "soft thinking" on the part of those examiners who believe in the concept. Schain (1975) is also dubious about the existence of soft neurological signs because of the vague criteria upon which they are often based and low interexaminer agreement found when multiple examinations of the same patient are conducted. These drawbacks to identification notwithstanding, I personally am an adherent to the concept. It seems reasonable to me that for many signs and symptoms there should be borderline and intermediate states, rather than just a present or absent situation. The best way to settle this conflict is to conduct objective studies of both normals and those with MBD, in which one *quantifies* the findings. In many areas such data are already available (and will be presented in various parts of this chapter) and readily confirm, in my opinion, the existence of such intermediate states. For many other soft neurological signs, studies still need to be done to determine whether or not they, in fact, do exist. The central problem facing those who would try to define such signs is where to draw the line that demarcates the normal from the abnormal. Let us say that in a given population the average male's height is 5 ft. 6 in. At what point does one say that a male is "short"? Does one use 5 ft. 0 in., 4 ft. 10 in., 3 ft. 8 in., or any other particular height? Similarly, what cut-off point does one use to define a person as "tall"? Clearly, such points of differentiation are arbitrary. The best solution to this problem is to present a value in terms of *standard deviation from the mean* or *percentile rank.* With such data the examiner can decide for himself what significance he wishes to ascribe to the data; he can decide himself how many standard deviations from the mean or what percentile warrants a particular label. Accordingly, the examiner can state, for example, "90% of children Robert's age can stand longer on one foot than he can" or "the age at which Jane began to walk is 2 standard deviations later than the average for girls."

The factors that can cause soft neurological signs are essentially all those etiological agents described in chapter 1, which can interfere with central-nervous-system functioning. Any entity that deleteriously affects nerve cells, central nervous system connective tissue, cerebral blood and spinal fluids, and brain and skull size may impair neurological functioning. Nerve cell myelinization provides one example of the way in which the developmental type of soft neurological sign may be brought about. Yakovlev and Lecours (1967), in an excellent study, have demonstrated that there is great variation among the parts of the brain with regard to the age when myelinization is completed. Myelinization begins during fetal life and terminates at different times in different parts of the brain. Although most nerve fibers in the brain are completely myelinated by the third to fourth year of life, certain sections of the brain do not complete the process until many years later. The reticular formation, for example, is not fully myelinated until the teens and many intracortical association fibers only complete the process *during the fourth decade of life.* It is reasonable to assume that nerve fibers do not function optimally until completely myelinated and that children whose myelinization is particularly slow will manifest various types of neurological immaturity. Some children with such lags may only represent the lower end of the bell-shaped curve for myelinization rate. In others, disease processes may have caused the retarded myelin development. And in others there may be a combination of factors: myelinization lag *and* exposure to detrimental extrinsic influences may bring about developmental lag. The soft neurological type of neurological sign is in all likelihood the result of disease processes affecting isolated areas rather than myelinization lags.

THE SOFT DEVELOPMENTAL TYPE OF SOFT
NEUROLOGICAL SIGN

Primitive Reflexes

The appearance and disappearance of certain primitive reflexes provide an excellent example of the developmental type of soft neurological sign. These primitive reflexes can be divided into two categories: (1) those that disappear with age and (2) those that appear with age. A soft neurological sign is considered to be present when the reflex is still present a significant time after the overwhelming majority of children have lost it or when it fails to appear when most, if not all, normal children exhibit it.

An example of the first category of primitive reflex is the *Moro reflex*. If a newborn infant is placed on its back and one slams down sharply on its bed or table, the infant's arms extend and then abduct as if it were embracing someone, its fingers spread, and its femora become flexed on the pelvis. It is as if the infant were trying to climb up a pole. The same reaction can be elicited by maneuvers that cause a sudden extension of the infant's head on its spine. Accordingly, if the baby is pulled up by the arms from the supine position, while allowing the head to remain on the table, the reflex will be exhibited when the arms are dropped. Or if the child is held with the examiner's right hand supporting its head and the left hand supporting its trunk, the reflex will exhibit itself if the right hand is quickly dropped so that the infant's head can fall back 20–30°. Paine and Oppé (1966) provide data regarding the ages at which this reflex becomes suppressed by the infant's developing brain. According to their findings, about 93% of infants will still exhibit the reflex by 1 month, only 22% by 5 months, and by 6 months all normal children should no longer manifest the sign. Its presence beyond that time is strongly suggestive of neurological impairment.

The *tonic neck reflex* is a more complex mechanism that is of greater predictive value than the Moro with regard to neurological dysfunction. When the infant is placed in the supine position, and its neck sharply rotated along the long axis of its body, the extremities on the same side as the child's chin become extended whereas those on the side of its occiput become flexed. According to Paine and Oppé's data this reflex may or may not be present at birth. If not, it should develop quickly so that by 1 month it is present in 67% of children. It reaches its peak frequency at 2 months, with 90% of children manifesting it. Its frequency then declines so that by 6 months only

11% exhibit it and by 7 months it was not present in any of the children they studied. Its presence beyond that time is strongly suggestive of neurological impairment. The reflex is probably a residuum of the withdrawal reaction that lower animals exhibit when suddenly surprised by an enemy. Imagine, for example, an animal sleeping in the prone position, suddenly being awakened by a foe. It does well to face the source of alarm while recoiling from the danger. This is best done by extending the limbs close to the enemy which the animal is facing and flexing those that are most distant from the foe. In this way the animal falls back and removes itself somewhat from the danger, while still maintaining itself in the best position to observe it.

Although Paine and Oppé consider the tonic neck reflex to be normally obliterated by 7 months, and Critchley (1970) states that he has never seen it beyond 8 months of age in normal children, Bender (1947) holds that it can persist in modified form until the age of 6 years. She believes that when a normal child of 4 or 5 years of age is asked to stand erect with his arms extended, and the examiner twists the child's head, the arm that the child then faces will extend and the other arm will flex slightly. She considers the presence of arm movements beyond age 6 to be a sign of neurological impairment. This is especially true of schizophrenic children whom Bender believes to be suffering primarily with a neurophysiological disorder. She goes further and holds that the whirling that these children sometimes exhibit is an exaggeration of the tonic neck reflex, with the whole body moving on its longitudinal axis, rather than merely the extremities.

The pattern of loss of the Babinski reflex provides another example of this type of soft neurological sign. Paine and Oppé state that the Babinski sign is generally present at birth and is usually suppressed by the age of 1 year. However, Brain and Wilkinson's excellent study (1959) reveals that things are not so simple. They found that a child may lose the Babinski sign as early as 9 months and as late as 24 months. However, the period of diminution of the reflex is broad. Whereas in the newborn the reflex can be elicited from a wide variety of stimuli as high as the abdomen and the thighs, as the child grows older the area from which the Babinski can be evoked gradually contracts until it confines itself to the sole of the foot. In addition, during the period when the reflex is becoming obliterated there are times when it may be elicited and times when it may not be. The only thing that one can say with certainty is that by 24 months it should no longer be present and that children who exhibit it beyond that time are strongly suspect for neurological dysfunction.

The development of the ability to oppose the thumb to the forefinger (pincer grasp) is an example of a sign that appears with age. At birth the normal child will exhibit a grasp reflex, i.e., there is reflex grasping to palmer stimulation. By 4–6 months the child should develop the capacity to voluntarily (rather than reflexly) grasp an object by grossly clenching it, but not with forefinger-thumb opposition (Escalona and Stone, 1968). Around the sixth month some children will start to be able to grasp voluntarily utilizing forefinger-thumb grasp. According to Paine and Oppé 16% of children do this by 7 months, 63% by 9 months, 95% by 11 months, and 100% by the age of 12 months. Accordingly, a child who cannot utilize a pincer grasp after 1 year of age is probably suffering with a neurological impairment.

The Developmental Milestones

Although the preceding discussion dealt with phenomena that might justifiably be referred to as developmental milestones (and my subsequent discussion will include such material as well), the term is generally reserved for those landmarks that one usually inquires about in routine history-taking in pediatrics and child psychiatry. The milestones that I generally inquire about and the age ranges at which they take place have been discussed in chapter 1. It is important that the examiner appreciate that these milestones are rough averages and that children vary greatly with regard to the ages at which they accomplish these tasks. Most examiners recognize that parents may be extremely unreliable regarding the dates at which the child reached each of the landmarks. In fact, it is probably only a rare parent who will be accurate regarding most of them. It is common for a parent to guess an answer rather than say that he or she doesn't recall the specific time when the child first exhibited the behavior inquired about. The questionnaire that I utilize gives the parent who does not recall the data a chance to state that it was early, normal, or late to the best of his or her recollection. My experience has been that the age of the first words and the age when the child first walked unaided are best remembered. In addition, parents usually have better recall for their first-born children than for those who came subsequently. By the time the third or fourth child appears, each step is no longer a unique event for the parents and so is less likely to be recalled years later. Bernstein, Page, and Janicki (1974) found that 62% of 413 hyperactive children they studied had lags in their developmental milestones.

Speech

It is important to differentiate between speech and language if one is to properly understand the difficulties of children with MBD. Language refers to the process by which one forms and processes the symbols for various entities. Speech refers to the articulation and verbalization of such symbols. For example, when a child is shown a pen and asked what it is, he must first have learned which linguistic symbols his particular society utilizes to refer to that particular object. If he speaks English, and has no cerebral impairment, he will think of the word pen. If he is French he will think of plume. If he is German the word Feder will come to mind. Each culture and society may devise its own linguistic symbol for an object. When the child then utters the word for the object he uses speech, and it is this aspect of the sequence, the phase of articulation, that I will be focusing upon here. (I will subsequently discuss certain aspects of language development as well.)

Because of the great variability of speech development among normal children, a child's level of speech maturation may be a poor criterion upon which to base a diagnosis of MBD (Charlton, 1973). In addition, psychological factors play an immensely important role in the rate at which a child will learn to speak and the level of maturity he will attain. Wyatt (1969) and de Hirsch (1974) have emphasized how the mother's feedback, her availability as a speech model, and her involvement with the child play a vital role in speech development. Furthermore, regression of speech and fixation at immature speech levels are common manifestations of psychogenic disorders of childhood. Accordingly, delineating the purely neurological factors in abnormal speech development may be especially difficult. Yet, there are normal sequences of speech development that are neurologically based, and it behooves the examiner to be familiar with them if he or she is to properly evaluate the child with MBD.

De Hirsch (1974) describes the following stages in the normal development of speech: cooing, birth–3 months; babbling, 5–10 months; echolalia, 10–12 months; single words; two word sentences; and more complex grammatical forms. Children with neurodevelopmental speech disorders may reveal speech patterns immature for their age. In addition, they may present with a history of sucking difficulties, chewing problems, excessive and prolonged drooling, a long history of nasality, and delayed onset of speech. With regard to the latter, most clinicians hold that a child should start utilizing meaningful speech by the age of 3. If a child is not speaking by 4 one must consider serious pathology, but it is possible that only minor psychogenic disturbance is present. However, most agree that if a child is not using meaningful speech by 5 then he or she is suffering with a serious psychiatric disturbance and one must think of such disorders as schizophrenia, mental retardation, and autism.

The clinician who is not trained in speech pathology may find useful the articulatory criteria proposed by Shank (1964) who holds that children should have mastered the sounds delineated in Table 6.1 at each of the indicated ages. In this table s and z appear twice because the loss of the central incisors between 6 and 7 causes the child to mispronounce these letters during this period. A 4-year-old child, for example, is likely to have mastered the b sound but not the v. Accordingly, he may say *glub* instead of *glove*. Proper pronunciation of the r comes late and a w is often easier for the child to substitute. Accordingly, *rabbit* becomes *wabbit,* and *tree* becomes *twee.* Another useful test of speech development is that utilized by Peters et al. (1973). The child is shown a series of 24 pictures (Figures 6.1 and 6.2) of objects easily recognized by most children (e.g., dress, flag, clown, star, tree, dog, and thumb). He is merely asked to name the pictures as the examiner points to them. Points are given for each correctly pronounced word and points deducted for each word that is not accurately articulated (Figure 6.3). Although the normative data are rough for each age bracket (2½–3½, 4–6, and 7 +), the test does provide the examiner with a general level of the child's articulatory maturity.

Table 6.1
Developmental Norms of Speech Articulation[a]

By 3½	By 4½	By 5½	By 6½	By 8
p: papa	t: toy	f: foot	sh: shop	ch: chop
b: bird	d: daddy	v: voice	zh: rouge	r: rabbit
m: mommy	n: no	s: sister	l: last	wh: where
w: water	g: grandma	z: zoo	th: the	
h: house	k: car			
	ng: sing			
	y: you			

[a] Based on information from K. H. Shank, "Recognition of Articulatory Disorders in Children," *Clinical Pediatrics,* 3:333–334, 1964.

Speech problems are common among children with MBD. They are related to the language difficulties so commonly seen in these children as well as other neurological impairments. Owen et al. (1971) found that 42% of the educationally handicapped children in their study needed speech therapy, whereas only 20% of the normal control group required such treatment.

Figure 6.1
Articulation Test Card.

Articulation test card

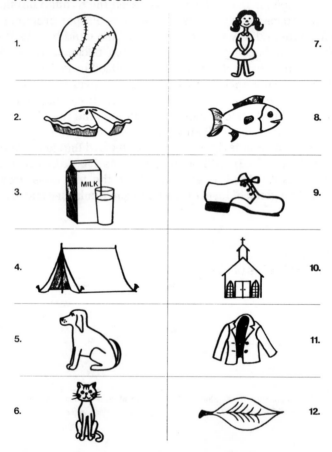

1.
2.
3.
4.
5.
6.
7.
8.
9.
10.
11.
12.

Reproduced with the permission of Peters et al., *Physician's Handbook: Screening for MBD.* Summitt, New Jersey: CIBA Pharmaceuticals, Inc.

Figure 6.2
Articulation Test Card (continued).

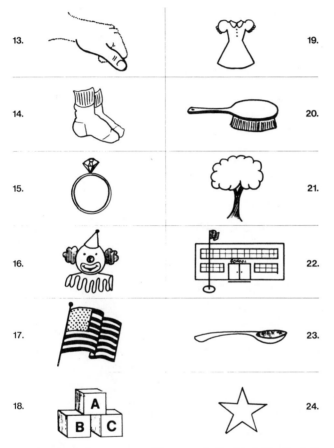

13.

14.

15.

16.

17.

18.

19.

20.

21.

22.

23.

24.

Reproduced with the permission of Peters et al., *Physician's Handbook: Screening for MBD.* Summitt, New Jersey: CIBA Pharmaceuticals, Inc.

Figure 6.3
Articulation Screening Test.

Articulation screening test

Examiner's Record Form

Child's name_____Date_____ Examiner_____

I. *Table for determining test scores*

Child's chronologic age   Points needed:

2½ through 3½ years_____Should score at least [5] points on *pictures 1-8.*

4 years through 6 years _____Should score at least [12] points on *pictures 1-15* only.

7 years and older_____Should score at least [21] points on *pictures 1-24* only.

II. *To determine sound mastery level*

Child's chronologic age_____

Points earned for age_____

Points needed for age_____

III. *Sound mastery level*

Above age_____

At age_____

Below age_____

Record child's responses below

_____ 1. **ball**	_____ 13. **thumb**	
_____ 2. **pie**	_____ 14. **socks**	
_____ 3. **milk**	_____ 15. ring	
_____ 4. tent	_____ 16. **clown**	
_____ 5. **dog**	_____ 17. **flag**	
_____ 6. cat	_____ 18. **block**	
_____ 7. **girl**	_____ 19. **dress**	
_____ 8. **fish**	_____ 20. **brush**	
9. **shoe**	_____ 21. tree	
_____ 10. **church**	_____ 22. **school**	
_____ 11. **jacket**	_____ 23. **spoon**	
_____ 12. **leaf**	_____ 24. **star**	

Reproduced with the permission of Peters et al., *Physican's Handbook: Screening for MBD.* Summitt, New Jersey: CIBA Pharmaceuticals, Inc.

Pencil Grasp

Earlier in this chapter I discussed the grasp reflex of the newborn and the development during the first year of life of the ability to oppose the thumb to the index finger. This capacity enables the individual to perform a variety of fine motor manipulations that are impossible for lower animals. The utilization of this capability to grasp a writing implement is vital for children growing up in a world where writing is such an important function. According to Frankenberg and Dodds (1969) some children will start to scribble with a crayon as early as twelve months of age. Fifty percent can do this at 16 months and 90% by 24 months. They make no mention, however, in their developmental battery of the *way* in which the child holds the crayon at these various ages. Gesell (1940), Gesell and Ilg (1946), and Gesell and Amatruda (1947) describe in great detail the ages at which the normal child develops the capacity for various forms of prehension such as grasping a cube (28 weeks) and dropping a pellet in a bottle (15 months). Unfortunately, they do not describe in any significant detail the stages in the development of the various types of pencil grasp. In addition, the Gesell data is presented in a way that would not be satisfactory to most examiners today. Typically, they present their observations in the following form: The normal child at 28 weeks does such and such ... , and The normal child of two years does so and so.... We appreciate today that such thresholds are not too useful. We are more appreciative of the fact that there is great variability among normal children as to when they attain various developmental capacities. We find data that provide ranges and percentages much more useful clinically.

Touwen and Prechtl (1970) state that the child (age not given) will often pick up a pencil "with the thumb in opposition to three or four fingers." They go on to state: "Children of five years and more should be able to hold a pencil between the thumb and index finger, whereas younger children often hold it between the second and third finger, and very young or severely retarded children may use the whole hand for drawing." Gold (1976) states that by 5 years of age the normal child should be able to hold a pencil in a rigid tripod position with the first three fingers. By 8 the pencil should be held in a more dynamic position with the flexibility of the adult. Denckla (1976) considers the normal child to utilize the fist-type (simian) grasp until about the age of 3. Between 3 and 5, the normal child will use a rigid tripod grasp in which the distal interphalangeal joints of the second and third fingers are hyperextended. After 5 the normal child will exhibit the adult-type tripod grasp with flexion of the interphalangeal joints of all the fingers. Both Gold and Denckla (like most pediatric neurologists) use guidelines based on clinical experience and recognize that normative data on pencil grasp development would be of use.

In an attempt to collect such data, I studied three types of pencil grasp (those I found to be most common) and focused specifically on the presence or absence of the most salient features of each type. I recognized that the study did not include all possible forms of pencil grasp utilized by normal children. Each of the three grasps will first be described in detail and the salient features focused upon for the purposes of the study will be delineated.

In this type of grasp the child holds the writing instrument with a closed fist. This type of grip is often referred to as the simian grasp because it is similar to the way apes hold a rod or similarly shaped implement. It is also called the *ulnar grasp* because the ulnar fingers (fourth and fifth) are utilized. As will be described, in the more mature grasps, only the radial fingers (first through third) are used. In the simian grasp, the child holds the pencil or crayon in the clenched fist with the thumb often covering the index finger (Figure 6.4). An important manifestation of this type of grasp is that all five fingers are flexed at the distal interphalangeal joints. Commonly, the pencil protrudes from the clenched fist between the second and third fingers (Figure 6.4).

Figure 6.4
Simian Grasp.

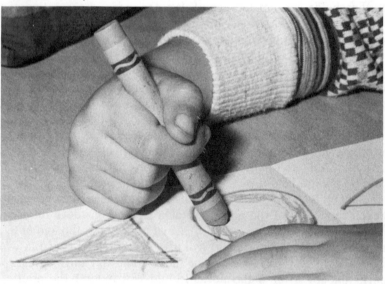

However, frequently the third, fourth, and even the fifth fingers may surround the writing implement (Figures 6.5 and 6.6). When writing (or scribbling, which is far more common prior to three) there is little movement of the muscles of the fingers, hand, or forearm. Rather, most of the pencil movement results from motions of the arm above the elbow. All muscles distal to the elbow are held quite rigidly. It is primarily a gross motor movement with little peripheral fine motor movement.

Figure 6.5
Simian Grasp.

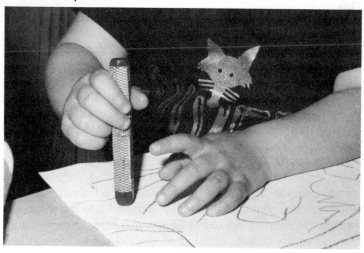

Figure 6.6
Simian Grasp.

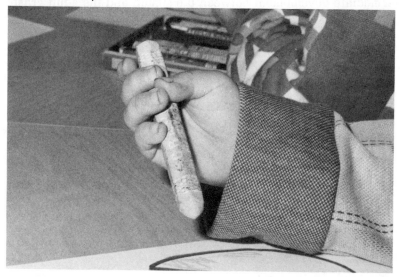

Grasp With Extended Distal Interphalangeal Joints (Intermediate Grasp)

This type of grasp, which most consider a progression from the simian, is essentially a three-fingered grasp. The pencil is held between the thumb, index, and third fingers. The term radial grasp is sometimes used to refer to this and the third type (adult) because radial (as opposed to ulnar) fingers are utilized. Of significance in this type of grasp is the fact that the distal interphalangeal joints of the second and third fingers are *hyperextended* (Figure 6.7) rather than flexed as is the case with the simian and the adult grasps. Occasionally the fourth finger as well is extended (Figure 6.8). Accordingly, the palmer surfaces of the distal phalanges of the second and third (and possibly the fourth) fingers are in extensive contact with the writing instrument. In the adult grasp only the tips of the second and third fingers are generally in contact with the pencil. The pencil is jammed into the webbed space between the thumb and the index finger or it may be pressed against the extended index finger. Because of the extensive contact between the surfaces of the pencil and the fingers, the pencil cannot be easily wiggled by the examiner; rather, it is rigidly held. When writing, the primary movement is from the forearm, rather than from the utilization of the intrinsic muscles of the hand and fingers. In this grasp one can see a progression from the gross arm movements of the simian grasp to the more peripheral fine motor movements of the adult grasp. It is an intermediate development between the simian and the adult grasps.

Figure 6.7
Intermediate Grasp.

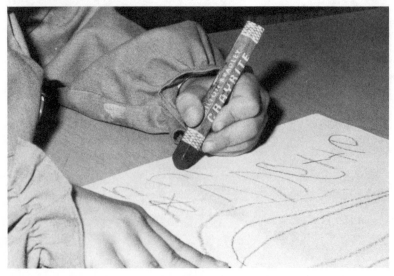

Figure 6.8
Intermediate Grasp.

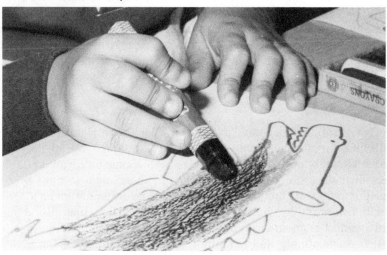

The Pincer (Tripod) Grasp

This is the grasp used by most adults. The distal joints of the thumb, index, and third fingers are flexed (Figure 6.9). Accordingly, the points of contact between the hand and the pencil are primarily at the tips of the first three fingers and at the point where the pencil rests on the web between the first and the index fingers. It is because of this

Figure 6.9
The Pincer (Tripod) Grasp.

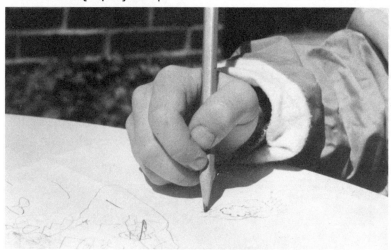

three-point contact that the grasp is referred to as the *pincer* or *tripod* grasp. The pencil is loosely held and can easily be wiggled by the examiner. The primary movements of the pencil originate from the first three fingers, not the hand, and not the forearm. This grasp represents the final step in the progression from the gross arm movements of the simian grasp to the highly sophisticated fine motor movements of the adult pencil grasp.

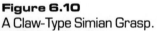

Further Considerations about Grasp

Not all children's pencil grasps will fit neatly into one of the above-mentioned categories. Some children at the simian grasp level will use the whole hand like a claw (Figure 6.10). Some children do not progress through a stage of hyperextension. They seem to pass directly from the simian to the adult-type grasp. And other children's grasps seem to be unique products of their own imagination. In addition, many children shift from one grasp to another, even while drawing the same picture. Accordingly, the examiner does well to observe the child on a few occasions before coming to any conclusions regarding grasp maturity.

A child whose muscles are hypotonic may go through the above progressions; however, in no phase is the pencil held tightly. Rather, it is loosely held and often dangles. It can easily be removed from the hand and may often be dropped.

On occasion one will see an adult who is completely normal neuro-developmentally and yet he or she will hold a pencil with collapsed (ex-

Figure 6.10
A Claw-Type Simian Grasp.

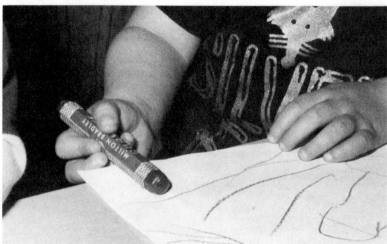

tended) interphalangeal joints of the second and third fingers. There are some adults who even use a simian grasp or some modification of it. Such "immaturity" may be a manifestation of the retention of an earlier habit on a psychogenic basis, rather than the result of a neuro-developmental lag. Many forms of behavior manifest such habit retention. For example, we generally retain throughout life the accents of our childhood even though most of our adult years may be spent in another environment. We may retain the childhood names of our siblings when they themselves have long given up such names and others never use them.

The ability to oppose the thumb to the forefinger (and the other three fingers) is a uniquely human quality. The higher apes can only use a simian grasp. This ability was not only useful for primitive man in the development and utilization of tools but, more recently, it has been crucial to the progress of modern industrial society. Without this capacity most of the intricate maneuvers necessary to the performance of complex manual tasks would be impossible. This capacity, along with more complex and sophisticated cerebral functioning, are the primary differentiating factors between man and lower animals and has enabled mankind to surpass all lower forms of life in adaptation and creativity.

Normative Data on Grasp Type

In order to ascertain the frequencies of each of these types of grasp, my assistants and I conducted a study of grasp type on 307 normal children ages 5 through 15. Each child was observed as to whether he or she utilized the simian (referred to as type 1), the intermediate (type 2), or the pincer (type 3) grasp. Children whose grasps did not fit into one of these three categories (about 5%) were not included in the study. The results are tabulated in Table 6.2. As can be seen, the general rule of thumb that most normal children exhibit the pincer grasp by 5 or 5½ years of age does not seem to be borne out by these findings. At age 8, 14.3% of the normal children studied here still exhibited the type 1 grasp, and 10.5% of children exhibited the type 2 grasp at age 11. However, the number of subjects in each of the categories was quite small (only two children are in the type 2 grasp category for 11 year olds) so that one must be quite cautious before coming to any conclusions regarding the ages at which grasp types 1 and 2 reach insignificant levels. One can say, however, that the distributions of frequencies of the three types of pencil grasp change significantly with age and that as children get older more assume the type 3 grasp $(p < .001)$.

Breakdown of the pencil grasp type between boys and girls did not reveal any significant difference between the sexes. Table 6.3 presents this breakdown into the 171 boys and 136 girls studied $(p < .180)$.

Table 6.2

Pencil Grasp Type of Normal Children [Boys and Girls Combined][a]

Age		Simian [1]	Intermediate [2]	Pincer [3]	Totals
5-0 to 5-11	N	6	14	27	47
	%	12.8	29.8	57.4	
6-0 to 6-11	N	5	17	26	48
	%	10.4	35.4	54.2	
7-0 to 7-11	N	3	5	19	27
	%	11.1	18.5	70.4	
8-0 to 8-11	N	5	3	27	35
	%	14.3	8.6	77.1	
9-0 to 9-11	N	1	4	28	33
	%	3.0	12.1	84.8	
10-0 to 10-11	N	0	2	20	22
	%	0.0	9.1	90.9	
11-0 to 11-11	N	2	2	15	19
	%	10.5	10.5	78.9	
12-0 to 12-11	N	0	1	20	21
	%	0.0	4.8	95.2	
13-0 to 13-11	N	2	0	31	33
	%	6.1	0.0	93.9	
14-0 to 14-11	N	0	0	22	22
	%	0.0	0.0	100.0	
Totals	N	24	48	235	307
	%	7.8	15.6	76.5	100.0

[a] Chi square = 51.418 with 18 degrees of freedom, $p < .001$.

Table 6.3

Pencil Grasp Type of Normal Children [Boys and Girls Compared][a]

Sex		Simian [1]	Intermediate [2]	Pincer [3]	Totals
Boys	N	13	21	137	171
	%	7.6	12.3	80.1	
Girls	N	11	27	98	136
	%	8.1	19.9	72.1	
Totals	N	24	48	235	307
	%	7.8	15.6	76.5	100.0

[a] Chi square = 3.443 with 2 degrees of freedom, $p < .180$.

The pencil grasp type of 308 MBD children was also studied. These children were all in special classes or schools designed for the education of children with learning disabilities considered to be a manifestation of neurophysiological impairment. Their IQs were generally in the 85 to 95 range. Most were one to three years behind their expected reading level for age. They exhibited such signs and symptoms as impulsivity, impaired ability to sustain concentration, gross and fine motor coordination deficits, and an assortment of auditory and visual processing deficits. Children with a history of an MBD diagnosis who were in regular classes ("mainstreamed") were not included in the study. The frequencies for the three types of pencil grasp are shown in Table 6.4. Scanning the data one sees a general shift from type 1 to type

Table 6.4
Pencil Grasp Type of MBD Children [Boys and Girls Combined][a]

Age		Simian [1]	Intermediate [2]	Pincer [3]	Totals
5-0 to 5-11	N	0	2	4	6
	%	0.0	33.3	66.7	
6-0 to 6-11	N	6	2	14	22
	%	27.3	9.1	63.6	
7-0 to 7-11	N	7	2	28	37
	%	18.9	5.4	75.7	
8-0 to 8-11	N	2	4	30	36
	%	5.6	11.1	83.3	
9-0 to 9-11	N	7	3	26	36
	%	19.4	8.3	72.2	
10-0 to 10-11	N	2	0	33	35
	%	5.7	0.0	94.3	
11-0 to 11-11	N	3	3	31	37
	%	8.1	8.1	83.8	
12-0 to 12-11	N	3	3	27	33
	%	9.1	9.1	81.8	
13-0 to 13-11	N	6	5	24	35
	%	17.1	14.3	68.6	
14-0 to 15-9	N	3	12	16	31
	%	9.7	38.7	51.6	
Totals	N	39	36	233	308
	%	12.7	11.7	75.6	100.0

[a] Chi square = 45.311 with 18 degrees of freedom, $p < .001$.

3 grasp with increasing age. This trend proved significant (p < .001). Whereas there was no significant difference between normal boys and girls with regard to the distribution of the three types of pencil grasp (Table 6.3), there was a significant difference between the boys and girls in the MBD group. As can be seen from Table 6.5, MBD girls were more likely than MBD boys to exhibit the type 1 grasp and less likely to exhibit the type 2 grasp (p < .001). In Chapter 2 I have discussed how girls in MBD classes did significantly worse than the boys on the steadiness tester. One can only speculate why girls should do worse than boys on certain tests of neurological functioning. One possible reason for these findings might relate to the process by which youngsters are selected for placement in these special classes and schools. We tend to be more protective of girls than boys. A girl, therefore, has to exhibit more pathology than a boy before being recommended to a special class or school for the learning disabled. Or, it might be that a girl has to have more underlying neurological impairment before developing signs of MBD.

Table 6.5
Pencil Grasp Type of MBD Children [Boys and Girls Compared][a]

Sex		Simian [1]	Intermediate [2]	Pincer [3]	Totals
Boys	N	19	31	168	218
	%	8.7	14.2	77.1	
Girls	N	20	5	65	90
	%	22.2	5.6	72.2	
Totals	N	39	36	233	308
	%	12.7	11.7	75.6	100.0

[a] Chi square = 13.467 with 2 degrees of freedom, p < .001.

Grasps of Normal and MBD
Children Compared

When the total MBD group was compared with the total normal group (Table 6.6), the two groups showed a tendency approaching significance to differ in the frequencies of the three types of grasps (p < .07). Within the age levels studied, further comparisons were carried out on MBD and normal subjects broken down by types 1 and 2 versus type 3 grasp, and by type 1 versus types 2 and 3 grasp. These comparisons reveal that there is a significant difference between 6-year-old MBD and normal children in the frequency with which type 1 grasp is observed (type 1 being more predominant in the MBD group, p < .05). At age levels 13 and 14–15½ the two groups differ in the proportion of subjects exhibiting type 3 grasp, the MBD group lagging significantly behind the normal group for this grasp type (p < .025 and p < .001, respectively).

Table 6.6

Pencil Grasp Types of Normal and MBD Groups Compared

Group	Simian [1]	Intermediate [2]	Pincer [3]	Totals
Normal	24	48	235	307
MBD	39	36	233	308
Totals	63	84	468	615

Chi square = 5.293 with 2 degrees of freedom, $p < .07$.

The two groups differ in the frequency with which the most advanced, type 3 grasp, is exhibited only after age 12 but not before. There are two possible explanations for this finding. One relates to the possibility that MBD children seen in special schools after the 12-year level are in some way different from the younger children in the same school, i.e., more severely impaired than the younger MBD children. Alternatively, it is possible that the development of type 3 grasp may only show a lag in the MBD population at the older age levels, 13 and up. The clinical significance of this finding is clear. *A child past the age of 12 who still uses the simian or intermediate grasp is highly suspect for the kind of neurodevelopmental lag described in MBD.* The traditional rule of thumb that after 5 or 5½ the use of types 1 or 2 grasp is pathological is not useful as a guideline. Only after the pubertal period can one consider the use of type 1 and 2 grasps to be a pathological sign.

Hand Preference and Grasp Type

While conducting the above studies, the examiner noted which hand the child used while writing. Among normal children, 91.5% wrote with the right hand and 8.5% with the left hand. Among MBD children, these proportions were 79.9% and 20.1%, respectively. For all 615 subjects combined, left-handed and right-handed children did not differ in the frequencies of the three types of pencil grasp ($p < 0.152$). However, for the normal children, but not for the MBD group, differences between left- and right-handed children were significant, with a greater proportion of left-handed children assuming the type 1 grasp and more right-handed children assuming the type 2 grasp ($p < .05$). One can only speculate on the significance of these findings. Left-handedness in some individuals appears to reflect atypical cerebral organization, with some abilities less lateralized to the left or right hemisphere than is the case in right-handed individuals (Hardyck and Petrinovich, 1977). The mechanism underlying the relationship between such presumed atypical cerebral organization with atypical pencil grasp is unclear. The difference between the normal and MBD samples regarding the association of handedness and pencil grasp is also not clear.

THE SOFT NEUROLOGICAL TYPE
OF SOFT NEUROLOGICAL SIGN

As mentioned earlier in this chapter, the soft neurological type of soft neurological sign includes mild abnormalities that one may find when conducting a traditional neurological examination. They include such abnormalities as reflex asymmetries, hypo- and hyperreflexia, hypo- and hypertonia, minor cerebellar coordination deficits, mild spasticity or rigidity of muscles, minimal eso- or exotropia, and mild nystagmus. As mentioned, quantification of such findings is difficult and agreement among examiners about such findings is not common. Four of the abnormalities generally considered to be in this category are described here: tremors and choreiform movements, motor impersistence, motor overflow, and eye-head dissociation. They have been selected because they lend themselves more easily to objectification and normative data have been collected on them.

Tremors and Choreiform Movements

Brock (1945) defines a *tremor* as a "regular rhythmic, alternating contraction of muscle group or groups and their antagonists." Tremors are generally considered to be a manifestation of disease of the basal ganglia. Paine and Oppé (1966) describe two categories of tremors: fine and course. Fine tremors are generally of 9–10/sec frequency. They may be familial in origin and may be seen in hperthyroidism. Course tremors are slower, 3–5/sec, and may be seen with other manifestations of basal ganglia disease such as chorea, athetosis, dystonia, and hemiballismus. According to Paine and Oppé, if a tremor is not of one of the aforementioned frequencies, it cannot justifiably be referred to as a tremor, and psychogenic etiology or other disorder must be considered. Tremors are generally detected by observing the child's outstretched hands. Course tremors may be observed this way, but fine tremors may not be so readily seen. This is especially the case when the tremors are mild. In such cases electromyographic (EMG) studies may be useful in determining whether the child has tremors. Some of the children with high scores on the steadiness tester described in chapter 2 have tremors. Although I have not yet conducted any studies to determine what percentage of the high scorers have tremors, my guess would be that it is small. However, as mentioned in chapter 2, tremor is one of the causes of such high scores and should be considered before coming to any definite conclusions regarding the meaning of an elevated steadiness-tester score.

Chorea is defined by Brock (1945) as "brief, explosive, unsustained, abrupt movements, possessing a coordination comparable to that seen in voluntary movement." Unlike tremors, they do not have a fixed frequency; rather they are aperiodic. Brock describes them as "subjectively purposeful, but objectively aimless," i.e., the patient may attempt to rationalize them as having a function in order to deny their involuntary nature. Chorea is also the result of basal ganglia disease. Children with MBD sometimes exhibit mild chorea movements that are often referred to as choreiform movements. Prechtl and Stemmer (1962) consider such movements to be an important factor in hyperactive behavior. However, they do not present any evidence regarding the exact percentage of hyperactive children they consider to be excessively active because of choreiform movements.

Such movements were originally brought to their attention as artifacts during electroencephalographic studies of children with poor school performance. "Many" (percentage not given) of these children exhibited "chorea-like twitchings of the extremities and head, which showed up on the EEG as muscle artifacts from the cervical and temporal muscles." Electromyographic studies of these particular children revealed aperiodic phasic discharges, of sudden occurrence and short duration (½–2 sec). They were of the type normally produced only by the tendon reflexes, e.g., from the quadriceps in the knee-jerk. They were not only seen in contracted muscles, where the movement they produced could be observed, but in fully relaxed muscles in which there was no visible movement. The authors consider this group of children common enough to warrant their being categorized as a subgroup of hyperactive children and suggested the name "choreiform syndrome." Although many in the field recognize that choreiform movements may be a manifestation of MBD, and may even be playing a role in such children's hyperactivity, the view that this symptom is common among such children has never been widespread. Accordingly, the term "choreiform syndrome" is not commonly heard.

I believe that EMG studies of large numbers of normal and MBD children would shed some light on this question. I suspect that the percentage of children who would be found to exhibit choreiform movements would be small. At this point I believe that is reasonable for the examiner to attempt to detect choreiform movements by observing the child's hands while they are resting in his lap. If a child appears to be exhibiting such movements and if, in addition, the child exhibits a high score on the steadiness tester, then one might want to conduct EMG studies. One might be convinced of the presence of the sign purely on the basis of direct observation. However, for both confirmation and quantification, one may wish to have the EMG studies done as well.

Motor Impersistence

Younger children cannot maintain a state of muscle contraction as long as older children. For example, they cannot stand on one foot, clench their fists, or keep their eyes shut as long as older ones. There is a developmental progression of the capacity to maintain muscle tension on a voluntary basis and children with MBD may exhibit lags in such progression. The term *motor impersistence* was first used by Fisher (1956) to refer to the impairment in this function. The phenomenon was defined by Garfield et al. (1966) as the "inability to sustain certain voluntary motor acts initiated on verbal command." They considered the impairment to be the result of a primary defect in sustaining attention. Benton (1970) subsequently used the following definition: "the inability to sustain an act that has been initiated on command."

Denckla's Test of Balancing on One Foot

One good test of motor persistence (or for the presence of motor impersistence) is the child's ability to stand on one foot. Of course, other functions (such as vestibular and proprioceptive) are being tested here as well, but the persistence capacity is prominent. Denckla (1974) has provided normative data on the length of time children from 5 to 10 can be expected to stand on one leg. Her data is based on testing 168 children, 28 at each of the 6 age levels from 5 to 10. The child is asked to balance himself on one leg for as long as he can. The number of seconds the child can successfully maintain balance is recorded. After 30 seconds he is told to replace the upheld foot on the floor (if he hasn't already lost balance). He is then instructed to repeat the same task with the other foot. Table 6.7 presents Denckla's findings. As can

Table 6.7

Balancing on One Foot for 30 Sec: Percentage of Children Succeeding on One or Both Sides

Age [Years]	Number of Children	Percentage Able to Balance Unilaterally			Percentage Able to Balance on Either Foot	Percentage with Right-Left Difference for Balance Less than 5 Sec
		10 sec	20 sec	30 sec	30 sec	
5	28	85			25	65
6	28		85		30	65
7	28			90	70	70
8	28			95	80	90
9	28			90	85	90
10	28			100	95	100

Reproduced with permission of the author and Spastics International Medical Publications, the publisher, from M. B. Denckla, "Development of Motor Coordination in Normal Children," *Developmental Medicine and Child Neurology*. 16:729–741, 1974.

be seen, her data indicate that 85% of 5-year-olds can balance themselves on the dominant foot for 10 sec; 85% of 6-year-olds can do so for 20 sec; and 90% of 7-year-olds can do so for 30 sec. Touwen and Prechtl (1970) have also provided such data, which is expressed in terms of the number of seconds that the average child at ages 3–7 should be able to stand on one leg. For example, the average 3-year-old cannot perform this task well, if at all. The average 4-year-old should be able to stand on one leg for 5–10 sec; the 5-year-old 10–12 sec; and the 6-year-old 13–16 sec. The authors do not, however, indicate the number of children studied in order to come to their conclusions.

Lincoln-Oseretsky Scale
[Test 32]

Test 32 of the Lincoln-Oseretsky Scale (Sloan, 1955) also provides normative data for standing on one foot. This test involves more specific instructions than Deckla or Touwen and Prechtl on the child's positioning. They require the child's eyes to be closed. This is an important determinant of the child's success at this task because balance time is shortened significantly when the eyes are closed. Accordingly, data collected under these two different conditions are not comparable. Whereas the aforementioned examiners have no requirements regarding how the child positions the leg that is lifted off the floor, the Lincoln-Oseretsky test requires the child to place the sole of the uplifted leg against the inner aspect of the weight-supporting leg at the level of the knee. Only one trial is allowed for each leg and the examiner determines whether or not the child has been successful in maintaining balance for 10 sec.

The cumbersome scoring system and the rather flimsy conclusions one finally derives from this test have ben described in chapter 5. For example, a 9-year-old boy who was successful in standing 10 sec on his right leg would get 3 points. (Failure gets 0 points; there is no 1 or 2 point score here.) The subtest tables indicate that a numerical value of 39 is warranted here. When translated, this means that the average 9-year-old boy gets a score of 39% of 3, or 1.17. So all we know, then, is that the score of 3 is above average, as are a host of other scores. No information like the kind that is provided by percentile ranks or standard deviations is given. Accordingly, I consider this to be a poor test.

Denver Development Screening Test
[Foot Balancing]

The Denver Developmental Screening Test (Frankenburg and Dodds, 1969) also includes a test of the child's ability to balance on one foot. According to these authors the child begins to develop the capacity to perform this function at 3 years of age. By 4½, 50% of children should be able to sustain such balance for two or three 10-sec trials. By 5, 75% should be able to do this and by 6, 90%.

McCarron Assessment of Neuromuscular Development [Foot Balancing]

The test for one-foot balancing that I find particularly useful is McCarron's (1976). His data is based on over 2000 children ages 3½ to young adult. The child is placed in the center of the room (away from walls and furniture) and is simply told "Stand on one foot as long as you can." The arms are free to move for balance. Timing begins as soon as the child lifts his leg. Timing stops when the lifted leg returns to the floor. If this has not occurred by 30 sec the test is then stopped. One trial for each leg is given, first with eyes open, then with eyes closed. The total score is the total number of seconds of successful leg-raising performance. Accordingly, a maximum score of 120 (30 × 4) is possible. If during any trial a child fails to keep a leg aloft for 10 sec, a second trial is allowed and the better of the two scores is the one used.

Normative data are provided at half-year levels from 3 years 6 months through 18 years 0 months. In addition, scores for young adults and mentally disabled adults are also provided. Data for males and females are combined. The raw score is converted to a scaled score by referring to the table for the child's age bracket. A scaled score of 10 corresponds to the mean of the raw scores, i.e., the average range for that age group. A scaled score deviation of 3 is the equivalent of 1 standard deviation. For example, an 8-year-3-month-old boy achieves the following: Eyes open, right leg—13 sec; left leg—12 sec. Eyes closed, right leg—10 sec; left leg—9 sec. The child's raw score, therefore, is 44 sec. Referring to the 8- to 8½-year norms one sees that this corresponds to a scaled score of 4, which is 6 points below 10, or 2 standard deviations below the mean. Such a score would be strongly suggestive of some kind of neuromuscular deficit, one possibility being motor impersistence. One drawback of the McCarron test is that one must combine the eyes-open and eyes-closed scores. This deprives the examiner of the extra information that might be obtained (regarding vestibular system impairment, for example) from separate scores.

Southern California Perceptual-Motor Tests [Standing Balance]

The Southern California Perceptual-Motor Tests (Ayres, 1968) includes a test of the child's capacity to stand on one foot and treats the capacity to do so with eyes open and eyes closed as two separate tests. The test was standardized on 1004 children age ranges 4-0 through

8-11. One of the disadvantages of the McCarron and Denckla tests is that they do not require the child to stand longer than 30 sec. Accordingly, their instruments do not differentiate among those who do well. The Standing Balance Subtest of the Southern California Perceptual-Motor Tests (SCPMT) requires the child to stand on one leg for 180 sec. This duration ensures that differentiation will be made among those who do well on this test.

The test is divided into two parts: Standing Balance, Eyes Open (SBO) and Standing Balance, Eyes Closed (SBC). The patient is placed in the center of the room, away from walls and furniture. He is asked to stand with arms folded, elbows flexed, and hands tucked in and held against the chest. Nothing is said about the child keeping his eyes open, as he generally does so in this section of the test. (Of course, if he does close his eyes, he is intructed to open them.) The examiner then touches the child's left leg, near the foot, and says, "Lift this foot. Don't hop or move around." If the child has not adequately attended to maintaining his balance or falls after a few seconds he is given a second chance (but not a third). The examiner records the time the child has been able to maintain balance, up to 180 sec. The child is then instructed to repeat the same task with the right leg. A maximum raw score of 360 can be obtained. By reference to the appropriate chart, the examiner can ascertain the child's standard score (standard deviation to the first decimal place). For example, an 8-years-3-months-old boy successfully stands for 37 sec on his left foot and 44 sec on his right foot. His total score is 81 sec. His standard score is found to be -0.2 standard deviations, a little below the mean but certainly not suggestive of a motor impersistence problem. A 5-year-3-month-old child with this score would be 2.5 standard deviations above the mean and would hardly be a candidate for the label of motor impersistence. A 4-year-old whose total raw score was 2 sec would be 1.4 standard deviations below the mean. The question of motor impersistence would certainly have to be raised for such a child.

The test is then repeated with the child instructed to keep his *eyes closed* while balancing on one foot. It is generally helpful to advise the child that this task is much harder to perform with the eyes closed than with his eyes open. Again, 360 is the maximum obtainable score. However, it would be a very rare child who would even come close to this score. The 8-year-11 month old whose raw score was 30 sec would only be 1.6 standard deviations above the mean for his age bracket.

Garfield's Tests

The ability to stand on one leg, of course, is only one way of measuring motor impersistence. Other muscle systems have been utilized. Garfield (1964) collected data on a variety of muscle-contraction tasks on 140 normal children (10 boys and 10 girls at each of the seven age levels from 5–11). Of the tests he utilized, I find the following to be the most useful (the drawbacks to be mentioned below notwithstanding).

1. **Keeping the eyes closed.** The child is instructed to close both eyes and keep them closed as long as he can. After 20 sec the child is told to open his eyes (if he hasn't already). Then a second 20-sec trial is given.
2. **Protruding tongue (subject blindfolded).** While blindfolded the child is asked to protrude his tongue as long as he can. Two 20-sec trials are administered.
3. **Protruding tongue (eyes open).** Same as above, except this time the child is not blindfolded and the eyes are kept open.
4. **Keeping mouth open.** The child is instructed to keep his mouth open as long as he can. Two 20-sec trials are administered.

Although specific norms are not given (the study compared normal and brain-damaged children on these and other motor persistence tasks), the authors describe a gradual improvement in performing these functions between ages 5 and 7, after which they should be performed without difficulty by normal children.

The Gardner Steadiness Tester

As described in chapter 2, the Gardner steadiness tester measures (among other things) motor impersistence. Its primary purpose, however, is to measure hyperactivity and the impaired ability to sustain concentration. If a very high scoring subject (scoring beyond the level seen in anxious and tense children) proved to have a normal activity level, no impaired ability to sustain attention, and no evidence for resting tremors or choreiform movements, then one could reasonably presume that the high score was related to motor impersistence. In order to demonstrate normal activity level one would have to use some of the sophisticated laboratory devices described in chapters 2 and 3 (devices such as radio telemetry and the continuous-performance task). One would also have to rule out resting tremors and choreiform movements. One might attempt this clinically, but electromyographic studies would be more objective (again expensive laboratory equipment has to be utilized). All this is theoretical, however, and I have had no occasion to track down impersistence so exhaustively. Perhaps children with motor impersistence would show a deterioration of performance on the steadiness tester as they progressed along each of the three 60-sec trials. The device lends itself well to such studies, and perhaps they will be conducted in the future. However, because the symptom is not a cause for significant concern, and because it is probably one of the less common manifestations of MBD, there is little motivation for investigators (including me) to pursue such studies.

In practice, then, I use the McCarron and Ayres tests as my primary sources of information about motor impersistence, and occasionally I use the Denckla and Garfield tests as well. The examiner does well to appreciate that in all of these tests of motor persistence an attentional deficit may produce false positive results. And, as we must ever remind ourselves, the attentional deficit can produce false positives for the great majority of tests described in this book.

Motor Overflow

The term *motor overflow* refers to the involuntary movements that occur in association with and in addition to a specific act that the child has been requested to perform. They are unnecessary to the performance of the task at hand and generally serve no ostensibly useful purpose. For example, when the child is asked to oppose repetitiously his thumb to the index finger, the other fingers of the hand move repetitiously as well. At the same time the child may stick his or her tongue out of the mouth, there may be movements of the arms and shoulder, twitches and grimacing may be observed, and the fingers on the other hand may go through the identical motions. These other motions are generally referred to as *associated movements* or *adventitious movements*. The phenomenon is usually referred to as *motor overflow* or *motor spread*. The term *synkinesia* refers to the ipsilateral overflow of such movements and the term *mirror movements* is generally used when the overflow is contralateral in the homologous extremity or symmetrical part of the body. Most examiners agree that the younger the child the greater the number of adventitious movements one will observe, and that by adolescence they are usually not present. Most examiners agree, as well, that such movements are likely to be more common in children with MBD than their peers of the same age, and that this relates to the failure of the brains of such children to have suppressed this primitive response.

Touwen and Prechtl Mouth-Opening Finger-Spreading Phenomenon

Touwen and Prechtl (1970) describe what they refer to as the *mouth-opening finger-spreading phenomenon*. The examiner supports the child's relaxed arms on his or her forearm. The child is asked to close his eyes, open his mouth, and stick out his tongue. Up to the age of 3 or 4 there will be associated spreading and extension of the fingers. This phenomenon will be present with less frequency at ages 5 to 6, and should no longer be present by 7 to 8. Its presence beyond that age is suggestive of neurological impairment. In another test for the presence of adventitious movements, the child is asked to walk on tiptoe 20 continuous paces back and forth. Children up to 7 will generally exhibit associated movements. Commonly the arms extend and clenched fists may be made. Lip and tongue movements may also be seen. Touwen and Prechtl consider the presence of such movements beyond 7 to 8 years of age to be a sign of neurological impairment.

Kinsbourne's Finger Stick Test

Kinsbourne (1973) describes a *finger stick test* for the presence of associated movements. The child is positioned wih arms extended. Four light sticks or ball point pens are placed between the fingers of each hand (a total of eight sticks). When all the sticks are securely held the child is asked to drop *one stick only* from the dominant hand, while trying to hold onto the other seven. In each of the six trials, the examiner counts the number of sticks dropped by the *nondominant hand* (although sticks may be dropped by the dominant hand these are not counted). In six trials the maximum number of sticks that might be dropped by the nondominant hand is 24. According to Kinsbourne the normal 6-year-old should not drop more than a total of five sticks in the six trials. To do so is suggestive of neurological impairment.

Abercrombie, Lindon, and Tyson's Finger Movement Test

Abercrombie, Lindon, and Tyson (1964) describe what appears to have potential as a good test of motor overflow. The child places both hands on the table with the palmer surfaces down. The examiner points to each finger in succession and asks the child to raise that finger and *only* that finger. Observation is made of both homolateral and contralateral raising of other fingers. This test appears to have merit in that one can readily objectify the observations. Unfortunately, the authors are not clear regarding the scoring system and they provide data on only 6- and 9-year-olds (25 in each group).

Cohen et al. Tests of Motor Overflow

Cohen, Taft, Mahadeviah, and Birch (1967) have done the most extensive and objective work that I know of in providing objective normative data for motor overflow as well as comparing normal children with those with MBD. In their examination, the child (with eyes closed) is asked to perform five tasks:

1. Repetitive opposition of the thumb and forefinger for 15 sec.
2. Repetitive opposition of the thumb and fifth finger for 15 sec.
3. Successive opposition of the thumb to each of the other four fingers for 15 sec.
4. Alternate squeezing and relaxing of a rubber toy which is held in the hand for 15 sec.
5. Rapid alternation and supination of the hand for 15 sec.

The presence of adventitious movements (on either side) is recorded for each of the sections on a scale of 0 to 3 (with 0 signifying no adventitious movements, and 3 representing maximum associated movements). The child, therefore, can obtain a maximum score of 15. The test is repeated for the other hand for which there is also a maximum score of 15 (total possible score is therefore 30). In performing this test, the examiner does well to look carefully for the presence of adventitious movements. Many are subtle and mild. For example, a short jerking movement of the contralateral extremity may easily be missed or the examiner may not have noticed that the child's tongue is out while performing a hand maneuver. To ignore these will result in inaccurate scoring. Normative data is provided for children from 6 through 12 (the number varies from 31 to 72) as well as for children with signs of CNS impairment (the number varies from 12 to 28) (Table 6.8). The authors found that there was no significant difference between the normal and neurologically impaired groups below the age of 9. After that the organically impaired group exhibited significantly more adventitious movements. Twitchell et al. (1966) similarly conclude that such movements are no longer present in normal children after the age of 9.

Table 6.8
Motor Overflow at Different Ages for Normal and CNS Impaired Children

Age[a] [Years]	Normal Group Number of Subjects	Normal Group Mean Overflow Score	Age [Years]	CNS Impaired Group Number of Subjects	CNS Impaired Group Mean Overflow Score
6- 7	31	17.0 ± 1.08	6- 7	13	16.7 ± 1.02
7- 8	39	16.6 ± 0.88	7- 8	16	14.9 ± 1.34
8- 9	31	12.1 ± 1.01	8- 9	18	13.3 ± 1.48
9-10	32	5.5 ± 0.90	9-10	21	12.8 ± 1.53
10-12	72	3.3 ± 0.33	10-12	28	11.8 ± 1.12
12-14	—	—	12-14	16	10.6 ± 1.59
14-16	—	—	14-16	12	7.6 ± 1.65
Total	205			124	

[a] Beyond 9 years of age all differences significant at a $p < 0.01$ level.

Reprinted with permission of publisher and authors from H. J. Cohen, L. T. Taft, M. S. Mahadeviah, and H. G. Birch, "Developmental Changes in Overflow in Normal and Aberrantly Functioning Children," *Journal of Pediatrics*, 71:39–47, 1967.

Eye-Head Dissociation

In the routine examination of the extraocular muscles of a 5-year-old child the examiner traditionally asks the child to keep his head still while the eyes follow an object that traverses the various visual fields. Typically such a child will move his head in order to view the object, rather than just move the eyes while the head is still. If the examiner urges the child to keep the head still he will usually still not "cooperate." Even if the child's head is held by a nurse or the mother, the child will attempt to move the head in order to view the moving object. Such a child is not being negative; he is generally not capable of dissociating head from eye movements at that age. It is only by age 7 that most children can do this. The child above 7 who cannot probably has some neurological impairment (Peters et al., 1973).

The normal 5- and 6-year-old may read a book with the whole head going back and forth in order for the eyes to properly scan the printed page. (This phenomenon is sometimes compared to the carriage on the typewriter which must shift back totally to the left with each new line.) Some MBD children still exhibit this phenomenon after the age of 7 and may receive optometric treatment to correct this "deficiency." I believe that such treatment *for this condition* is unwarranted. It is generally a manifestation of a developmental lag and usually corrects itself by 8 or 9, in my experience. If after a year of such treatment the child is "cured," the parents will usually consider the improvement to be the result of the therapy. Actually, the therapy probably had absolutely no influence on the acquisition of this ability and the improvement would have occurred anyway. In addition, even if the impairment were to remain, it is not a particularly debilitating handicap and is certainly not worth the time and expense that its "treatment" often entails.

7

□○ Auditory Processing

By auditory processing, I refer to the series of events that occur between the time an auditory stimulus reaches the external ear and the time the stimulus is recognized and stored. There are various points along this path (or more properly paths) where pathological processes can interfere with normal functioning. The examiner should try to identify the level of such dysfunction. The instruments described in this chapter will be presented in the sequence that begins at the ear with tests of auditory acuity and ends with a discussion of the complex functions of language appreciation and integration with other sensory modalities. Although the tests attempt to focus on particular steps along this pathway they are by no means so discrete; rather they usually involve other functions as well, which may not even be auditory.

Auditory processing deficits can seriously compromise a child's capacity to communicate. Children's first knowledge of language comes via the auditory channel. The child does not generally begin to speak until there has been a significant degree of familiarity with and incorporation of the language spoken by others. And the child generally does not write until there has been longstanding familiarity with the spoken language, both receptive and expressive. One can easily see then how an impairment in auditory functioning can interfere significantly with the child's subsequent linguistic development and the capacity to communicate. I recall at this point an experience that occurred when I was in medical school. Following a lecture in otolaryngology, a classmate of mine asked the instructor what was the earliest age at which he would prescribe a hearing aid. The answer was, "If the child's delivery is breech, I'd wait until the head came out."

AUDITORY ACUITY

If an auditory stimulus is not heard, that is, if it is not received, it is not going to proceed along the other phases of auditory processing. Problems in auditory acuity can occur when there is pathology in the external, middle, and inner ears, as well as the cochlear (VIII) nerve that conducts auditory stimuli into the brain. It has been this examiner's experience that only an insignificant fraction of MBD children have auditory acuity problems. Nevertheless, examining for such loss is part of the thorough evaluation of such children. Merely surmising that there is no such loss because the child seems to hear well in the clinical interview is not adequate. A patient may have significant hearing loss in one ear and still appear to hear adequately because the intact ear functions well enough to compensate for the loss.

A Screening Test for Auditory Acuity

The person with intact hearing should be able to identify correctly words spoken from a distance of 20 ft and words whispered from a distance of 15 ft (Boies, 1954). A child's auditory acuity, then, may be roughly tested by occluding one ear with cotton (older children can usually be trusted to do this with their own fingers) and so seating the child that the free ear is facing the examiner, who stands 20 ft away for voice testing and 15 ft away for whisper testing. The test is then repeated with the other ear. Of course, this is a rough test. There is no standardization of the intensity and frequency of the sounds being transmitted to the child. Male and female examiners provide the child with different tests. However, it does have value as a screening test, its deficiencies notwithstanding. If there is any suspicion that the child has an impairment in auditory acuity, then a formal audiometric examination should be obtained.

The Audiometric Examination

The audiometer is an instrument that can provide tones over a variety of frequencies and intensities. Earphones are worn by the examinee to prevent distracting sounds from compromising the test. The instruments most commonly in use today provide frequencies from 125 to 8000 Hz (cycles/sec). In the usual testing situation up to 10 frequencies are tested: 250, 500, 750, 1000, 1500, 2000, 3000, 4000, 6000, and 8,000 Hz. Each frequency can be presented over a range of intensities up to 100 db. (A decibel is a measure of the pressure intensity of the sound wave. One decibel is the smallest difference in sound intensity that can be appreciated by the normal human ear.) At each frequency tested, the examiner increases the intensity of the tone until the patient indicates by word or gesture that he hears it; or the examiner decreases the intensity until the patient no longer provides any indication that a tone is being heard. In this way a threshold is obtained that is the lowest intensity (decibel level) that is audible at the given frequency. The audiogram presents a curve of such decibel levels at the various frequencies. Generally, a normal person should not require more than 30 db to perceive one of the frequencies presented. If a greater sound intensity is required, especially over a range of frequencies, then further investigation is warranted to determine the etiology of the hearing loss.

The complete audiogram will often provide other information such as bone conduction vs. air conduction, Weber test, Rinne test, and speech audiometry (in addition to the tone audiometry described above). Such information provides insight into the nature of hearing deficits that might be revealed by an abnormal audiogram. Evaluation of these factors goes beyond what I would consider reasonable for most examiners involved in MBD diagnosis and therefore beyond the purpose of this book.

AUDITORY ATTENTION

Once the examiner is convinced that the ear, the external hearing transducer, is normal, the next area to be investigated is that of auditory attention. Without adequate attention, the auditory stimuli will not be properly transmitted.

The Goldman-Fristoe-Woodcock Auditory Selective Attention Test

Basically this instrument evaluates the child's ability to identify an auditory stimulus in competition with increasingly intensifying distracting sounds. A voice recorded on a cassette tape instructs the child to point to one of four pictures displayed on a stand in front of the child. A sample picture display is shown in Figure 7.1. The child is simply told, "Put your finger on ... rake." The examiner then records whether or not the child has correctly identified the object named on the tape.

Figure 7.1

The Goldman-Fristoe-Woodcock Selective Attention Test.

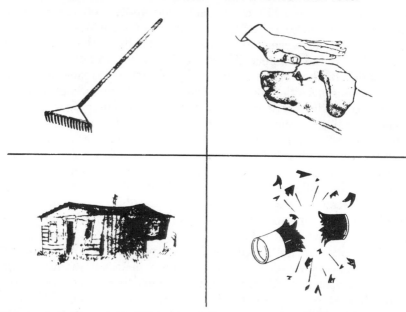

Reproduced with the permission of the American Guidance Service, Inc., Circle Pines, Minnesota.

There are four sections to the test. In the first, 15 four-item cards are used and the child is successively asked to point to two of the objects. The purpose here is to determine whether the child recognizes all the objects to be used throughout the test. Obviously, if the child does not know the meaning of the work *lock* when the taped voice says "lock," the child will not associate those particular sounds with the object *lock* and he will not respond correctly. A problem in linguistic development, then, may compromise the child's score. To avoid this potential contamination of the results, the first section enables the examiner to ascertain if the child does not know the meaning of some of the words and, if so, to teach the child what the word means. The test can be used for children as young as 3. Most of the words, however, are readily understood by most 3-year-olds (cat, key, rock, sack, shoe, back, etc.). The examiner is instructed to repeat the training procedure for any pages on which items have been missed. If after three trials, the child is still not familiar with all the words, the examiner is instructed to proceed with further testing with the caveat, "In this case, the interpretation of test performance must take into account the failure to train all word-picture associations." I consider this to be a defect in the test. I would have eliminated from the test any child who could not identify *all* items. To include children with incomplete recognition of the items, results in the examiner's not being able to differentiate between errors caused by impaired concentration and those that are the result of linguistic deficits.

Following the training session, the child and examiner proceed to the test which is divided into four sections. In the first, there is no background noise while the taped voice is presenting the words, in response to which the child is to point to the correct picture. Eleven words are presented and the child receives one point for each correct response. In the second section, a fanlike background noise is present and this becomes increasingly loud as the 32-item test proceeds. In this, as in the other two sections in which there is background noise, the spoken message is first much louder than the background noise. As the test progresses, the background noise becomes increasingly loud and tends to drown out the spoken instructions. By the end of the test section the background noise is so loud that the spoken message becomes almost inaudible to most subjects.

In the third section, the background distractions consist of cafeteria noise. The cafeteria sound was recorded in a noisy dining hall and then the sound was amplitude-compressed and rerecorded backward to remove any language content. Again, there are 32 items in the section. In the fourth section (also 32 items) the distraction is verbal: a verbally related story becomes progressively loud, making it increasingly difficult for the subject to attend to the instructions regarding which picture to point to.

Percentile ranks for each of the three noise subtests as well as for the total score on all four subtests are provided in the manual. Age-equivalent and stanine data are also provided.

The authors advise the examiner to administer the test with the child using earphones. (In order to monitor the test, then, the examiner also must use earphones so that he too can know when to turn the pages for the recorded instructions.) They warn that the child's score will be compromised by room noises if earphones are not used. I cannot emphasize this point strongly enough. Unless earphones are used the child's scores are likely to be significantly lowered.

In chapter 3, in my discussion of attention, I described tests that primarily measure visual attention. Here I have described a test of auditory attention. When we think of the attentional deficit in children with MBD we tend to view the problem as one of inner central-nervous-system mechanisms that are not functioning properly. Perhaps there are separate pathways governing attentional capacity for the different sensory modalities. If this is so, then it will behoove us to divide attentional deficits into various types and to assess them separately.

Further research is certainly necessary to help us decide whether such a division is necessary—whether we are justified in considering a single sensory deficit that exhibits itself with all sensory modalities or whether each modality can independently exhibit an attentional deficiency.

AUDITORY DISCRIMINATION

Once the child properly attends to the auditory stimulus, he must be able to differentiate among sounds if he is ultimately to understand auditory stimuli. I use the term *auditory discrimination* to refer to the capacity to *differentiate* between two auditory stimuli, that is, to be able to determine whether they are the same or different. Such capacity does not warrant the individual's *understanding* or giving meaning to the auditory stimuli. That is a higher order of functioning that I will discuss subsequently. The sounds could be in a language foreign to the testee, they could be nonsense words, or they could be nonlinguistic sounds. Some use the term *auditory perception* to refer to this capacity. Others reserve the term perception to refer to the capacity to provide meaning to a stimulus. Still others use the term to cover a variety of functions including discrimination, organization, selection, recognition, etc. Because of the confusion that may arise from the use of the term, I avoid it and prefer to identify the various processing elements as separate entities, regardless of whether a given function may or may not be included in someone's definition of perception.

The Auditory Discrimination Test

Wepman (1973) has designed what is probably the most widely used test of auditory discrimination (Figure 7.2). The examiner verbally presents 40 pairs of words to the child. In 10 of the pairs the words are identical (lack-lack) and in 30 the words differ only by a single phoneme (tub-tug). The child is asked to indicate whether the two presented words are the same or different. He can do this verbally, or he can communicate by gestures such as nodding or shaking the head. Trial words (man-man, house-pat) are first presented to ensure that the child understands the test. When presenting the words, the examiner does well to turn his face away from the child so that lip-reading visual cues are not provided. Otherwise, a child with an auditory discrimination defect might still obtain a normal score by compensating for his deficit with the visual information. As the test word pairs are presented the examiner places plus or minus signs in the unshaded box on the score sheet (Figure 7.2) in accordance with the child's correct or incorrect

Figure 7.2

Auditory Discrimination Test. Items 21–40 Not Reproduced.

			X	Y					X	Y
1.	tub	– tug		▓	11.	zest	– zest	▓	
2.	lack	– lack	▓		12.	wretch	– wretch	▓	
3.	web	– wed		▓	13.	thread	– shred		▓
4.	leg	– led		▓	14.	jam	– jam	▓	
5.	chap	– chap	▓		15.	bass	– bath		▓
6.	gum	– dumb		▓	16.	tin	– pin		▓
7.	bale	– gale		▓	17.	pat	– pack		▓
8.	sought	– fought		▓	18.	dim	– din		▓
9.	vow	– thou		▓	19.	coast	– toast		▓
10.	shake	– shape		▓	20.	thimble	– symbol		▓

Reproduced with the permission of Joseph M. Wepman and Language Research Assoc., Inc.

response. The score sheet is so structured that recording for scores for *different* words are placed in one column and recording for scores on *same* words are placed in a second column. In this way the examiner can more easily calculate a child's score.

After the 40 items have been administered, the examiner adds up the total number of correct items in each of the columns. If a child has more than 20 errors (out of a possible 30) in the *different* column and/or 7 or more errors (out of a possible 10) in the *same* column, his score is invalidated. Wepman believes that if either of these scores exists the test is not a true measure of discriminative ability. The implication is that so much more pathology is probably present that other factors must be considered before simply concluding that the child has an auditory discrimination impairment.

Normative data is presented for children ages 5–8. One can ascertain whether a child's score is in the upper 15% (good), sixty-fifth to eighty-fifth percentile (above average), thirty-fifth to sixty-fifth percentile (average), fifteenth to thirty-fifth percentile (below average), or in the lowest 15% (below the level of threshold adequacy). It has been Wepman's experience that there is no improvement in discriminative ability in normal development after the age of 8. Children above that age who do not score as well as the 8 year olds in Wepman's group are "most likely to have a specific auditory learning disability." Thompson's studies

(1963) support Wepman's findings regarding the development of auditory discrimination. He found that 24% of children have accurate auditory discrimination by the second grade.

One of the drawbacks of the Wepman test is that examiner's voices differ so that different children receive different tests. Because no two examiner's have the exact same voice, a given child might receive a different score if tested by a different examiner. There are even day-to-day differences in the same examiner's vocal pattern that could conceivably result in the child's obtaining different scores under these different testing conditions (Chalfant and Scheffelin, 1969). One could attempt to obviate this drawback of the test by providing recordings that would be used by all children. However, the particular dialect used by the recorded examiner would be more comprehensible to some children than to others. Accordingly, some children would be at a definite disadvantage with such a recording. All things considered, I think that the best arrangement is to use an examiner whose dialect is as close to the child's as possible. One removes, thereby, the more important contaminant and hopes that the aforementioned drawbacks will not significantly affect the child's score.

The Wepman test also assesses short-term auditory memory. The child is required to remember the two words in order to compare them. As is true of just about all of the tests described in this book, none is "pure." All test for a number of functions. The more the examiner is aware of the other functions being evaluated, the better will be the value of the instrument to the examiner. The test's primary value, however, is in detecting auditory discrimination deficits. Such deficits can be a significant handicap in the child's learning language via the auditory route. Letters such as b, p, t, and d may be hard to discriminate from one another. Similarly, letters such as m and n, as well as z and s are often confused with one another. Poor discrimination of phonemes then results in impaired reception of words. And this can contribute to reading and language deficiencies.

AUDITORY MEMORY

I believe that the concepts of short- and long-term memory are somewhat artificial because there is actually a continuum from extremely short-term memory to significantly long-term memory. There is no meaningful cut-off point that one can use to differentiate short-term from long-term memory. Should one use one hour, one day, one week, or one month as the point of demarcation to differentiate short-term from long-term memory capacity or impairment? The differentiation, however, is still commonly made even though most examiners appreciate the continuum. Generally, when the label short-term memory is applied, it refers to situations of immediate recall, or recall within a few seconds. Long-term memory generally refers to items that have been learned by the examinee days, weeks, months, or even years prior to the examination. The tests of auditory memory that I will discuss here, both short- and long-term, are primarily at the prerecognition level, that is, understanding is not a requirement of adequate performance. One need not know the meaning of the test items, such as the number and letters presented by the examiner. One is only being asked to recall them, their structure and their sounds.

The Digits Forward Section of the Digit Span Subtest of the WISC-R

In chapter 3 I made reference to the use of the Digit Span subtest of the WISC-R as a useful test of concentration. Although both parts of the test assess short-term auditory memory, the Digits Backward section also tests certain aspects of visual processing. In chapter 8 I will discuss the whole test in detail, with particular emphasis on the visual aspects. Here I will discuss only the Digits Forward section as a test of auditory sequential memory. In this section, the examiner presents the child with a three-digit number, given at the rate of one digit per second. If the child repeats the sequence correctly he is given a score of 1, if not he is scored zero. Then a second three-digit number is presented. Next two four-digit numbers are given and similarly scored. Each pair of sequences is one digit longer than its predecessor. Increasingly longer number sequences are presented until the child misses both series of the same length. The longest trial pair are two nine-digit numbers. The child's score on this part of the subtest is the total number of sequences recalled correctly. In the Digits Backward section (to be discussed in detail in chapter 8) the child is asked to repeat the number sequences backward rather than forward.

Wechsler (1958) did not consider the ability to recall rote material to contribute strongly to general intelligence. There are many people of average and below average intelligence who may exhibit very good memories for the repetition of rote material. He therefore designated Digit Span to be one of the two optional subtests (Mazes being the other). In addition, although recognizing that they did not measure the same functions, he combined them as one test in order to reduce their influence on the total IQ. Specifically, if he had included them as two separate tests they would have comprised 2/13 (15.38%) of the total IQ. However, by combining them into one, they contribute only 1/12 (8.33%)

of the total IQ. The examiner therefore must combine the raw scores of Digits Forward and Digits Backward before he or she can obtain a scaled score. The reader of the report gets no information about the breakdown, and even the person who administers the test has no way of quantitating any suspected irregularities in either of the two sections of the subtest. In order to provide such separate data, my assistants and I administered the Digit Span subtest of the WISC-R and collected *separate* Digits Forward and Digits Backward scores on 1,567 school children (782 boys and 785 girls) ages 5-0 through 15-11. (There were 2200 children used for standardization of the WISC-R.) The children were from schools in Bergen County, New Jersey (in suburban New York City). They came primarily from working class (blue collar and lower-to-middle-income white collar) families and were generally in the average range of intelligence. Their scores on standardized national achievement tests were primarily in the average range. Boys and girls in special classes, those with a history of grade repeat, or children who required special tutoring were excluded from the study.

Results

The subjects' scores were divided into 1/2-year age brackets. The average number of children for each of the 22 1/2-year age levels was approximately 35 (N range for boys 16–53, for girls 27–52). For Digits Forward, means, standard deviations, and percentiles for boys are presented in Table 7.1. Girls' data are presented in Table 7.2. With such data the examiner obtains information about auditory memory loss that is "purer" than that which is obtained from the total Digit Span subtest. An 8-year-9-month-old boy, for example, obtains a raw score of 11 (no scaled scores are used in this examiner's test). Referring to Table 7.1, we see that the average score for boys this child's age is 6.17 with a standard deviation of 2.32. His score then is over 2 standard deviations above the mean. We also see from Table 7.1 that his score is significantly above the ninetieth percentile (9.2). We can conclude then that this boy's auditory memory is very good and that such a deficit is not contributing to his presenting problems.

Digits Forward is a good test of auditory sequential memory. If the child recalls the correct digits but does not present them in the correct order, he is not given any credit. Differentiation is not made between the two groups of errors. The child who does well can be presumed to have intact auditory memory as well as auditory sequential memory. The child who does poorly, however, may have a defect in auditory memory in general, or may only have a deficiency in auditory sequential memory. Similarly, the Auditory Sequential Memory subtest of the Illinois Test of Psycholinguistic Abilities (Kirk, McCarthy, and Kirk,

Table 7.1
Digit Span—Digits Forward for Boys

Age	N	Mean	S.D.	Percentiles								
				10	20	30	40	50	60	70	80	90
5-0 to 5-5	26	3.27	1.31	2.0	2.0	2.0	2.8	3.0	3.2	4.0	4.6	5.3
5-6 to 5-11	29	4.03	1.70	2.0	3.0	3.0	3.0	3.0	4.0	4.0	6.0	7.0
6-0 to 6-5	33	4.67	1.93	3.0	3.0	4.0	4.0	4.0	5.0	5.0	6.0	7.6
6-6 to 6-11	43	4.88	1.73	3.0	3.0	4.0	4.0	5.0	5.0	6.0	7.0	7.0
7-0 to 7-5	45	5.18	1.86	3.0	4.0	4.0	5.0	5.0	5.6	6.0	7.0	8.0
7-6 to 7-11	53	5.47	1.99	3.0	4.0	4.0	4.0	5.0	6.0	6.8	8.0	9.0
8-0 to 8-5	36	5.81	2.05	3.7	4.0	4.1	5.0	6.0	6.0	7.0	7.0	8.0
8-6 to 8-11	47	6.17	2.32	4.0	4.0	4.4	5.0	6.0	6.8	7.0	8.0	9.2
9-0 to 9-5	38	6.21	1.77	3.9	4.0	5.7	6.0	6.5	7.0	7.0	8.0	8.1
9-6 to 9-11	34	6.85	2.22	4.0	5.0	6.0	6.0	7.0	7.0	7.5	9.0	10.0
10-0 to 10-5	29	5.97	1.78	4.0	4.0	4.0	6.0	6.0	7.0	7.0	8.0	8.0
10-6 to 10-11	22	7.18	2.02	4.3	5.0	6.0	6.2	7.0	7.8	9.0	9.0	10.0
11-0 to 11-5	34	7.00	2.10	4.0	5.0	6.0	7.0	7.0	8.0	8.5	9.0	9.5
11-6 to 11-11	35	7.06	1.91	4.0	5.2	6.0	7.0	8.0	8.0	8.2	9.0	9.0
12-0 to 12-5	35	7.80	1.94	5.0	6.0	6.0	7.0	8.0	9.0	9.0	9.8	10.0
12-6 to 12-11	40	7.88	2.04	6.0	6.0	6.3	7.0	8.0	8.0	9.0	9.9	10.0
13-0 to 13-5	51	7.71	2.12	4.0	6.0	7.0	7.0	8.0	8.0	9.0	10.0	10.0
13-6 to 13-11	38	8.29	2.00	6.0	7.0	8.0	8.0	8.0	8.4	9.0	10.0	10.1
14-0 to 14-5	35	7.89	2.04	5.0	6.0	6.8	7.0	8.0	8.6	9.0	9.8	10.4
14-6 to 14-11	36	7.56	1.98	5.0	5.4	6.0	7.0	8.0	9.0	9.0	9.0	10.0
15-0 to 15-5	27	7.26	2.49	3.0	5.0	6.4	7.0	8.0	8.0	8.6	9.0	10.0
15-6 to 15-11	16	7.06	2.02	4.0	5.0	6.0	6.8	7.0	7.2	8.9	9.0	9.6
	782											

Table 7.2
Digit Span—Digits Forward for Girls

Age	N	Mean	S.D.	Percentiles								
				10	20	30	40	50	60	70	80	90
5-0 to 5-5	27	3.48	1.19	2.0	2.0	3.0	3.0	4.0	4.0	4.0	4.0	5.2
5-6 to 5-11	22	4.86	1.70	3.0	4.0	4.0	4.0	4.0	4.8	6.0	6.0	7.7
6-0 to 6-5	30	4.60	1.43	3.0	3.0	4.0	4.0	4.0	5.0	6.0	6.0	6.9
6-6 to 6-11	36	4.97	1.84	3.0	3.0	4.0	4.0	5.0	5.0	6.0	6.0	7.3
7-0 to 7-5	43	5.26	1.65	3.0	4.0	4.0	4.0	5.0	5.4	6.8	7.0	8.0
7-6 to 7-11	42	5.86	1.76	3.0	4.0	5.0	6.0	6.0	6.0	7.0	7.0	8.0
8-0 to 8-5	37	6.19	1.93	3.0	5.0	5.0	6.0	6.0	7.0	7.0	8.0	8.2
8-6 to 8-11	51	6.61	1.80	4.0	5.0	5.6	6.0	6.0	7.0	8.0	8.0	9.0
9-0 to 9-5	38	6.42	2.09	4.0	4.0	5.0	5.6	6.0	7.0	7.0	9.0	10.0
9-6 to 9-11	28	7.54	2.96	2.9	4.8	5.7	7.0	8.0	9.0	9.0	10.0	11.2
10-0 to 10-5	30	7.10	1.69	4.0	6.0	6.0	7.0	8.0	8.0	8.0	8.0	9.0
10-6 to 10-11	29	7.00	1.85	4.0	6.0	6.0	7.0	7.0	8.0	8.0	9.0	9.0
11-0 to 11-5	52	6.77	1.95	4.0	5.0	6.0	6.0	7.0	8.0	8.0	8.0	9.0
11-6 to 11-11	36	7.17	1.93	5.0	6.0	6.0	6.0	7.0	7.0	8.0	9.0	9.3
12-0 to 12-5	37	7.43	1.88	5.0	6.0	7.0	7.0	7.0	8.0	8.0	8.4	9.2
12-6 to 12-11	47	7.85	1.90	5.0	6.0	7.0	7.2	8.0	8.8	9.0	9.0	10.2
13-0 to 13-5	42	8.12	2.27	5.3	6.0	6.9	7.2	8.0	8.0	9.0	10.0	11.0
13-6 to 13-11	36	8.61	2.18	5.7	7.0	7.1	8.0	9.0	9.0	10.0	10.6	11.3
14-0 to 14-5	36	7.25	1.93	4.0	6.0	6.0	7.0	7.5	8.0	8.9	9.0	10.0
14-6 to 14-11	34	7.88	1.53	6.0	7.0	7.0	8.0	8.0	8.0	9.0	9.0	10.0
15-0 to 15-5	25	8.08	2.27	4.6	6.2	7.0	8.0	8.0	8.0	9.0	9.8	11.4
15-6 to 15-11	27	7.56	1.99	4.0	6.0	6.0	7.0	8.0	8.0	8.6	9.4	10.2
	785											

1968) does not really make this differentiation either. When administering the test, the examiner may occasionally see a child who recalls many of the correct numbers from a sequence but is not given credit because he repeats the numbers out of order. Such children should be suspect for auditory sequencing problems, but I know of no test at present that quantifies this function. The WISC-R would lend itself well as a tool for collecting such data. All the examiner need do is to divide response errors into two groups: (1) those in which the numbers, *per se*, are correctly recalled but related in incorrect sequence, and (2) those in which the child does not recall all the numbers accurately. A test of auditory sequential memory should not use stimuli that relate to one another. For example, if sentences were used instead of numbers it would not be as likely that the child would repeat the words in incorrect order as he will when numbers or rote sounds are utilized. The meaning, rhythm, and syntactical structure of the sentence as a whole provide valuable hints regarding word order.

The Sound Blending Subtest of the ITPA

The Digits Forward section of the Digit Span subtest is primarily a test of short-term auditory memory. I say primarily because there is a long-term memory element still involved. The numbers are generally familiar to the examinee and he recognizes them to be identical to others that are stored in memory and can be retrieved rapidly enough to enhance the subject's performance in the test. I strongly suspect that if an English-speaking subject was readministered the test in a language that was totally foreign to him (for example, in Chinese), the patient would exhibit a much poorer performance in the oriental language. We are interested, however, in ascertaining the patient's long-term memory capacity because this tells us something about storage capacity, especially with regard to the duration of such capacity. To put it in other words, we want to know how long things can "stick" in the child's brain. Unfortunately, it is almost impossible to ascertain such storage capacity without bringing into play *retrieval* capacity. Until we have devised instruments that can get into the brain and determine what is stored there in memory, we have to rely on the patient's retrieving the information and communicating it to us. Such tests also involve the apparatus by which the patient communicates (usually verbally) what has been retrieved.

In order to separate auditory memory from the capacity to understand an auditory stimulus (the latter being a higher and more complex function) the tests described in this section (Sound Blending) and the next (Auditory Closure) are those that could conceivably be passed by someone who may not necessarily understand the meaning of the word that is being recalled. For example, a child might be able to take the word presented in the form of its phonetic components and fuse them into the word without knowing the meaning of the word. In fact, there is a section of the Sound Blending test that uses nonsense words for this purpose. Or a child might provide the missing s from *a tronaut* without knowing what the word *astronaut* means (see Auditory Closure Test, below).

The Sound Blending subtest of the ITPA (Kirk et al., 1968) consists of three parts. The first section is for children under the age of six. The child is presented with a sample picture of a dog, and while the examiner is pointing to the dog the child is asked to say "dog." This is repeated with the picture of the man. The examiner then says "d-og," breaking the word down into its phonetic components. He then asks the child, "Which one am I talking about?" The child then has to point to the picture of the dog. Following this demonstration the child is presented with seven such words, broken down into their phonetic components (Figure 7.3). For the test items the examiner is not permitted to repeat the word or otherwise provide the child with help. He merely says, for example, "f-oot" and asks the child, to whom he presents the array of pictures, "Which one am I talking about?" The child is given one point for each correct answer.

In the second section, no pictures are provided. The words begin at two phonemes length (ea-t) and end with seven (t-e-l-e-ph-o-ne). Whereas in the first section the child is given the assistance of a visual stimulus, no such help is given in the second section. The second section, therefore, is a "purer" test of auditory memory. One can speculate that the auditory stimuli presented in section two bring about the formation of some kind of model of what the word should be. There must have been previous experience with the word or previous auditory input regarding its correct form. There must have been some storage of information necessary for the formation of this correct model (or engram) and there must be the capacity to retrieve this model word from memory and compare it to the incoming auditory stimuli. (One can accomplish this without necessarily knowing the *meaning* of the word. We are all familiar with words that we recognize to be part of our language but words of whose meaning we are ignorant.) Presumably if an incorrect engram is retrieved, it is compared, recognized as incorrect, and rejected. This section of the test, therefore, assesses long-term auditory memory. It also evaluates the ability to retrieve (as mentioned, this may be impossible to differentiate from memory) and to compare (discriminate) auditory stimuli (the internal stored engram with the external pattern that has just been received).

In the third section, nonsense words (a-f-e, t-e-k-o) are used. These vary from three (l-e-k) to six (o-p-a-s-t-o) phonemes in length.

Figure 7.3
Sound Blending Subtest of the ITPA.

SOUND BLENDING

BASAL: SEE DIRECTIONS
CEILING: SEE DIRECTIONS

SCORE

Section A
Words with pictures

DEMONSTRATION I
d – og

1. f – oot
2. m – an
3. sh – oe
4. c – ap
5. c – ar
6. c – u – p
7. sh – i – p

Section B
Words without pictures

DEMONSTRATION II
d – og

8. ea – t
9. e – gg
10. u – p
11. c – ow
12. m – e
13. f – i – sh
14. c – a – t
15. b – i – g
16. s – a – d
17. b – oa – t
18. n – o – se
19. d – i – nn – er
20. f – ea – th – er
21. l – i – tt – le
22. k – e – tch – u – p
23. b – a – b – ie – s
24. t – e – l – e – ph – o – ne

Section C
Nonsense words

DEMONSTRATION III
ō – g
z – ē

25. l – ĕ – k
26. ā – f – ē
27. v – ŭ – m
28. r – ā – s – t
29. t – ē – k – ō
30. t – ā – p – ī – k
31. r – ŭ – s – ō – p
32. ō – p – ā – s – t – ō

Whereas the second section is essentially a test in long-term memory, this section tests short-term memory.

Although the patient receives one point for each item answered correctly, there is a somewhat complex system for determining when to shift to the next section, either forward or backward. The raw score is determined by adding the sum of scores on each of the three sections. This is converted to an age-equivalent score by referring to the proper chart. The age-equivalents range from 2-4 to 8-7. Whereas all the other tests in the ITPA cover ages 2 through 10 + , for reasons not given by the authors the highest age-equivalent level on this subtest is only 8-4. One can also convert the raw score to a scaled score by referring to the proper chart for the child's age. As is true for all of the subtests of the ITPA, the mean scaled score is 36 with a standard deviation of 6. An 8½-year-old child, for example, gets a raw score of 24 points. This corresponds to a scaled score of 40 which is less than 1 standard deviation above the average. One can conclude that this child's score on this test is in the normal range.

A superficial consideration of this subtest might give the examiner the notion that the subtest merely presents tasks of increasing complexity in the area of sound blending. In fact, Paraskevopoulos and Kirk (1969) state that the first and third sections of the test were introduced to extend the test's usefulness "downward to age two and upward to age 10." Actually, it is three separate subtests, each measuring different functions. Although there is some overlap, the differences among the three sections are so great that I believe that the authors were in error to have presented this as one subtest. I use the test, however, because it does provide some information about whether there is adequate storage and retrieval capacity for internal engrams corresponding to auditory stimuli, both linguistic (sections one and two) and quasi-linguistic (section three). (Although letters are used in section three, it cannot justifiably be called a *linguistic* test because language capacity is not really being assessed. Language uses a symbol to stand for an entity; no true entity is being symbolized in section three.) When a child performs significantly below age level, then the test has served as a clue that something is wrong. Because of the variety of possible impairments that can result in a low score (impairments that may be present in one or more of the three sections), I must resort to other instruments to help me determine (or speculate about) the nature of the deficit(s). Scores on other tests in the auditory battery being presented in this chapter may be helpful.

When a child's score is average for his age, I consider two possibilities: (1) that he is normal on all three sections, and (2) that he may be above average on one or more and below average on one or more and that things have so compensated that the resultant score is in the average range. Because separate normative data for each of the three sections are not available, one is not likely to be able to determine which of the two possibilities is the more likely. So I am left with the conclusion that *severe* problems in one of the areas assessed in this subtest are probably not present. If a child's total score is quite high, then I am more confident that pathology in the many areas covered by the three sections is probably not present. However, even here there may be some of the aforementioned cancelling out (or "burying") of low socres by high ones, but it is not as likely.

Another drawback of this test is the problem of the examiner presenting the same auditory stimuli as those given to the group from which the normative data was obtained. In order to avoid the problems resulting from such variation among examiners, the authors suggest that "those examiners who are not trained in sound blending should be checked by someone who is familiar with the system." The statement leaves me wondering how many examiners have gone to the trouble of finding such a person. I would suspect that very few have. A phonograph record is also provided that gives the test as it was administered during standardization. Even if the examiner were able to imitate exactly the dialect of the person on the record, he might be introducing accents that are so unfamiliar to the child that his score would be artificially lowered.

In conclusion then, I generally consider this test a poor one. However, I still include it in my battery when an auditory impairment is suspected, because it may, on occasion, provide some useful information if one thinks carefully about one's findings.

The Auditory Closure Subtest of the ITPA

Fortunately, the authors (Kirk et al., 1968) have not divided this subtest into further subsections and so it is "purer" and more useful than the Sound Blending subtest with which it has some points in common. In this test the examiner presents words with one to three phonemes omitted (Figure 7.4). The child is asked to verbalize the complete correct word, supplying the omitted phoneme(s). There are two practice words, Da / y (Daddy) and bo / le (bottle), and then 30 words that range from simple words like airpla / (airplane) to difficult ones such as / ype / iter (typewriter). The child receives one point for each correct response and the examiner is not permitted to repeat a test item. The child's raw score is converted to an age-equivalent by referring to the proper chart. The raw score can also be converted to a scaled score. As mentioned, the mean scaled score for all subtests of the ITPA is 36 ± 6. An 8-year-

Figure 7.4
Auditory Closure Subtest of the ITPA.

AUDITORY CLOSURE

BASAL: NONE
CEILING: 6 CONSECUTIVE FAILURES

DEMONSTRATION

a. Da / y (Daddy)_____

b. bo / le (bottle)_____

1. airpla / (airplane)_____

2. sunshi / (sunshine)_____

3. banan / (banana)_____

4. tele / one (telephone)_____

5. tele / ision (television)_____

6. / acaroni (macaroni)_____

7. tricyc / (tricycle)_____

8. / ingernail (fingernail)_____

9. ele / ant (elephant)_____

10. peanut / utter (peanut butter)_____

11. / aseball (baseball)_____

12. co / eepot (coffeepot)_____

13. cho / /late (chocolate)_____

14. side / alk (sidewalk)_____

15. / uffalo (buffalo)_____

16. auto / o / ile (automobile)_____

17. / uper / arket (supermarket)_____

18. es / / lator (escalator)_____

19. / isher / an (fisherman)_____

20. / a / er / elon (watermelon)_____

21. / an / a / aus (Santa Claus)_____

22. a / tronau / (astronaut)_____

23. / ovie / tar (movie star)_____

24. re / ig / / ator (refrigerator)_____

25. new / pa / er (newspaper)_____

26. ho / pita / (hospital)_____

27. Ea / ter / unny (Easter bunny)_____

28. / andy / ar (candy bar)_____

29. ta / le / oon (tablespoon)_____

30. / ype / iter (typewriter)_____

SCORE

1-month old child, for example, gets a raw score of 15. This corresponds to a scaled score of 23, which is more than 2 standard deviations below the mean. One can conclude that this child's performance on this subtest is significantly poor.

In order to perform successfully on this test the child must have previously been exposed to the word and have some kind of a stored model of it (or at least information that can readily formulate such a model). The engram so formed (retrieved) is then compared to the presented partial word and the child must then be capable of supplying the missing phoneme(s). Long-term storage is clearly being assessed here. In addition, retrieval capacity and comparison ability is also being measured. I consider this to be a good test of auditory memory capacity and a relatively "pure" test for this function.

Again, there is the drawback (so often the case with tests of auditory functioning) that the examiner's accents will serve as a contaminant. The authors provide a phonograph record to enable the tester to attempt to reproduce the words as they were presented to the group used for standardization. As mentioned, this may introduce the problem of the child's not understanding the dialect used by the initial examiners.

AUDITORY LANGUAGE

For the purposes of this discussion, I will use the definition of language used by Benton (1966) who states that "language consists of the use of symbols for purposes of communication." In expressive language, one *encodes*, i.e., one "uses conventional symbols to communicate one's perceptions, ideas, feelings or intentions to other persons or to oneself." Here the mental content evokes the symbol. In receptive language, one *decodes*, i.e., one utilizes "symbols to apprehend the perceptions, ideas, feelings of intentions of other persons or oneself." Here the symbol evokes the mental content. It is the latter aspect of language that we are concerned with here. More specifically, we are interested in the process by which an auditory symbol (a spoken word) evokes an internal image of an entity. For example, there is no intrinsic relationship between the spoken word "chair" and the object *chair*. By social convention we have agreed that the constellation of sounds that we utilize to utter the word chair shall be used to denote that particular object. There is absolutely no intrinsic relationship between the particular sounds a society chooses to use to denote an object and the object itself (with the exception of rare onomatopoetic words). Before there can be language there must be the capacity to form this link. The individual must reach the point where a particular sound constellation evokes an internal mental image or idea that corresponds specifically to it. Chalfant and Scheffelin (1969), in their discussion of language, state that the child must be able to "establish a reciprocal association between the auditory-vocal sound units and objects or events." Such appreciation of receptive language occurs within the first few months of life and precedes spoken language. It is one of the more complex functions to have developed on the evolutionary scale and it is most highly developed in man, who can be distinguished from lower animals, in part, by his superiorirty regarding this function.

The Language Subtest of the Denver Developmental Screening Test [DDST]

The Language subtest of the DDST (Frankenburg and Dodds, 1969) provides the examiner with an opportunity to assess objectively the earliest phases of language development. If the child exhibits the capacity to say "Dada" or "Mama" and the examiner is convinced that the words are being used with specific reference to one of the parents, the child is given a "pass" on this item. Referring to their table, one sees that 25% of children accomplish this by 9 months, 50% by 10 months, 75% by 12 months, and 90% by 13 months. In one section of this part of the DDST, the child is shown five pictures (cat, bird, horse, dog, and man) and asked to name them. Twenty-five percent of 16-month-old children will name at least one correctly, 50% will do so by 20 months, 75% by 24 months, and 90% by 30 months. The normative data for all items is expressed in this way. Other areas covered in the language subsection include tests that assess the child's comprehension of plurals, prepositions (on, under, in front), opposite analogies (hot vs. cold, big vs. small), and word definitions (ball, lake, desk, house). The recognition-of-colors test is somewhat vague in that it does not differentiate between asking the child to state what a particular color is ("What color is this?") and asking him to point to a color among many presented by the examiner ("Which of these is red?"). Although both capacities are related to language (appreciating the link between the particular color red and the word used to denote this entity), verbalizing the word red is a more complex task than merely pointing to the color. (In chapter 9 I will discuss in greater detail various aspects of "naming.")

Peabody Picture Vocabulary Test [PPVT]

The Peabody Picture Vocabular Test (Dunn, 1965) was introduced primarily to serve as a test of general intelligence that could be administered in 10–15 minutes. Terman and Merrill (1937) considered the vocabulary section to be the most valuable test in the *Revised Stanford-Binet Test of Intelligence* and Wechsler (1949) found the vocabulary subtest of the *Wechsler Intelligence Scale for Children* to correlate more highly with the Full Scale IQ than any other subtest. It is because of the high correlation between vocabulary, IQ, and school success that the PPVT was introduced as a quick method of ascertaining a child's IQ. Dunn recognizes that measuring vocabulary by picture selection is not the same as asking the subject to define a word orally. But both methods of vocabulary evaluation assess the subject's comprehension of the spoken word. And it is this aspect of the test that I wish to focus on here, namely, the test's capacity to evaluate a child's ability to recognize the meaning of a word presented orally by the examiner.

The test is quite simple to administer. The child is presented with a page on which are printed four pictures (Figure 7.5 is a composite of two different pages). The examiner reads a word from the test booklet and the child is asked to point to the picture that depicts the word. Children under 8 may be instructed as follows: "Put your finger on _____." "Can you find _____?" "Point to _____" "Where is _____?" Each picture has a number. Older children can be instructed as follows: "There are four pictures on this page. Each one is numbered. I will say a word, then I want you to tell me the number (or point to) the picture which best tells me the meaning of the word." The words proceed from the simplest to the most difficult. For each age bracket there is a suggested word with which to begin. Eight consecutive correct responses establish the basal level. If the child is not sure which picture best corresponds to the word presented by the examiner, he is allowed to guess and no inquiry is conducted to determine whether the child really knows the words whose meaning he has correctly guessed. The examination is discontinued when the child has made six errors in eight consecutive responses. The sixth error in this final sequence is defined as the ceiling level. The raw score is obtained by subtracting the errors from the ceiling item. Percentile rank, mental age, and IQ can be obtained by reference to the proper tables.

Although I do use the PPVT as a rough test of intelligence, I have found that children who come from homes in which the parents are highly educated and/or verbally sophisticated will sometimes score high on this test and give the impression of being more intelligent than they really are. Accordingly, for a short-form test of intelligence, I prefer the Slosson Intelligence Test (Slosson, 1963) which assesses a variety of areas similar to the WISC-R. I find the PPVT more valuable as a test of auditory language capacity. However, like the first section of the Sound Blending subtest of the ITPA, the visual cues lessen the "purity" of the instrument as a test for auditory language comprehension. Also, accepting correct guesses as correct answers enables "lucky" children to score higher than the "less fortunate."

Figure 7.5
Peabody Picture Vocabulary Test.

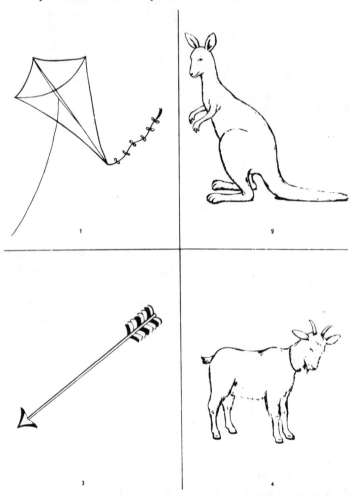

The Receptive Language Test
of the Physician's Handbook:
Screening for MBD

Peters et al. (1973) include a 53 item receptive language section in their MBD screening battery. The test utilized is actually the Blair Language Evaluation Scales (Blair, date not given). Items have been selected from a variety of tests and scales (Gesell, Vineland, Catell, Terman, etc.)

from ages 6 months to 7 years. By ascertaining whether the child understands a series of instructions and requests made by the examiner
(Figure 7.6) one can determine the child's approximate level of receptive
language development. However, the items are quite varied and test

Figure 7.6
Receptive Language Test of the Physician's Handbook: Screening
for MBD.

Item	Language Age	Language Behavior	Normative Source
45.	5 years	Can identify four colors.	Gesell
46.	5 years	Carries out, in order, a command containing three parts, e.g., "Pick up the ball, put it on the table, and bring me the book."	Gesell
47.	5 years	Definitions. a) "What is a ball?" b) "What is a hat?" c) "What is a stove?"	Terman
48.	5 years (2+)	Memory for sentences. "I want you to say something for me. Say, 'big boy (or girl).' Now say, 'I am a big boy (or girl).' Now say . . . a) 'Jane wants to build a big castle in her playhouse.' b) 'Tom has lots of fun playing ball with his sister."	Terman
49.	5 years (2+)	Counting four objects. Present the objects in a row in following series: a) 4 blocks b) 4 beads c) 4 pennies Ask, "How many?" for each series.	Terman
50.	6 years	Knows right and left.	Gesell
51.	6 years	Number concept to 10. Responds correctly to 3 out of 4 requests as: "Give me three blocks; give me nine blocks, etc." (when twelve are available).	Terman
52.	6 years	Understands the following concepts: a) more and less b) a pair c) many and few d) across e) morning and afternoon	Hausserman
53.	6 - 7 years	Reads on pre-primer level. Is able to read a pre-primer book and recognizes the majority of the words without having to refer to the pictures in the books.	Mecham

many different functions as well. The request to define certain words (item 47) involves expressive language functioning. Item 48 assesses auditory memory. Items 49 and 51 require counting ability. And item 50 tests right-left discrimination capacity. Item 52, in which the examiner ascertains whether the child comprehends such concepts as *more and less, a pair, many and few,* is a "purer" test of auditory language development in that other functions are not so heavily involved in determining the child's response. If a child does "pass" the item, one can conclude that he has understood the examiner's request or instructions, and so auditory language (among other things) at that level is intact. If the child does not pass an item, one is not sure whether there was an impairment in auditory language appreciation or whether other functions necessary for a correct response were deficient.

The Listening Comprehension Section of the Standard Reading Inventory (SRI)

McCracken (1966) includes in his Standard Reading Inventory (SRI) a Listening Comprehension Test that assesses a child's level of auditory language development. The SRI is a complex and comprehensive test of reading ability in which a wide variety of reading functions (written word recognition, oral reading comprehension, silent reading comprehension, etc.) are assessed. In the Listening Comprehension section the examiner reads a short story to the child who is then asked 10 questions about what has been read. Six levels, from the second to the seventh grade, can be used. Figure 7.7 presents the sixth-grade-level story and questions. The test is the most comprehensive of auditory language comprehension of all those presented in this chapter. Rather than testing the child's capacity to understand isolated words or phrases, it assesses his ability to understand complex linguistic material. Accordingly, it comes closest to the ideal test of auditory language capacity in that it assesses the child's capacity to comprehend the kind of auditory language material to which he will generally be exposed in life. A child is considered to pass a particular level if, of the 10 questions asked, he meets *all* of the following criteria:

1. Four or more questions are answered correctly in the unaided response.
2. Seven or more questions are answered correctly in unaided and aided response.
3. The unaided response is in sentences.

Although I was originally enthusiastic about the test in principle, my experience with it has been somewhat disappointing. My experience

Figure 7.7
Standard Reading Inventory. Listening Comprehension Test.

The Sound Stage   (sixth level)

A southern California sound stage is an amazing place. From the outside it looks like a huge airplane hangar, entirely without windows. To get in you use ordinary doors. Over each door is a red electric bulb. On each door is a sign which says: "Do not enter while red light is on. Recording." If the red light is on, you have to wait for it means that the cameras are turning and the sound recorders operating. No outside noise whatsoever is allowed. Even the most important people have to wait until the red light is turned off before entering the sound stage. Those red lights really mean "stop."

If the red light isn't burning, you open the door and find yourself in a little foyer or hallway. The inner door usually will not open until the outside door is closed. This is an added protection against outside noises.

1. What does the sound stage look like from outside?
2. What does the sign say?
3. If the red light is on what is happening?
4. How effective is the "do not enter" rule?
5. Why do they have two doors?
6. What is being made in the sound stage?
7. Why don't they have windows to let light in?
8. What does the word *recording* mean in the sentences, "Do not enter while red light is on. Recording?"
9. What does the word *operating* mean in the sentence, "The sound recorders are operating?"
10. What does the word *foyer* mean in the sentence, "You find yourself in a little foyer or hallway?"

Reproduced with the permission of Klamath Printing Co., 320 Lowell St., Klamath Falls, Oregon 97601.

has been (admittedly, not on numbers of children large enough to validate statistically) that the second level test is more difficult than the third level. In addition, a few of the questions do not relate to material given in the paragraph read by the examiner. For example, one of the questions for the second level test asks whether Joey, the protagonist of the story, lives in the city or the country. At no point in the three paragraph story is any mention made of where Joey lives. Two questions of the fourth level paragraph can only be answered by the child's speculating about or extrapolating from the story. I am sure there would not be much agreement among examiners regarding whether responses to these two questions were correct. These drawbacks notwithstanding, I find the test a useful one in giving the examiner a general idea of the child's level of auditory language comprehension.

The test also measures auditory attention in that the child must attend well to the story if he is to correctly answer the questions. Auditory memory and verbal expression capacity are also measured. Accordingly, these possible contributing factors must be considered when interpreting a child's score. If a child does well at a given level, one knows that auditory language comprehension has advanced at least to that level. If he does poorly at a given level, one is not certain whether there is a primary auditory language problem that has reduced the score or whether some of the other functions that are involved are defective.

AUDIO-VISUAL INTEGRATION

Birch and Lefford (1964) agree with Sherrington (1951) who theorizes that the evolutionary development from lower to higher animals is not characterized by an increase in the number of sensory modalities. Rather, the greater complexity and sophistication of the higher forms is the result of their greatest *integration* of the basic sensory modalities. A frog, for example, is presented with a board of closely set spikes, on one of which is impaled a struggling fly. The frog sees the fly and his tongue immediately darts out in an attempt to ingest it. The spikes are so closely set, however, that each time the frog's tongue lashes out it is injured by the spikes (presumably the frog feels pain as well). Following the initial reflex withdrawal of its tongue, the frog again attempts to capture the fly. It is as if the frog does not associate the fly he sees with the shredding of his tongue (Abbott, 1882). Information from the frog's tactual sensory system does not seem to be getting to the visual centers. Pathways that connect the two modalities are either absent or only minimally functioning.

Birch and Lefford (1964) believe that the MBD child does not have the same degree of development of such integration and association pathways as the normal child. In their studies they have found that children with neurological learning impairments have deficient haptic (cutaneous pain, temperature, and light touch sensation), haptic-kinesthetic, visual, and visual-kinesthetic integration when compared to normals. A good way to view their findings is to consider that in the child with a visual-haptic impairement, for example, the defect is less likely to be in the "visual" or in the "haptic" areas than in the "-," that is, in the *hyphen* that refers to the fibers that connect the two modalities. Adequate capacity to integrate different sensory modalities is crucial to adaptive functioning. We not only hear the words of the speaker but learn much from the gestures and facial expressions that we see. The teacher spells a word as she writes it, providing the child with both auditory and visual inputs, each of which enhances the other.

The Audio-Visual Integration Test

Kahn and Birch (1968) have introduced a test that attempts to objectively measure audio-visual integrative capacity. Some of the tests already described in this chapter measure such capacity. For example, in the Goldman-Fristoe-Woodcock Selective Attention Test and in the Peabody Picture Vocabulary Test the child is asked to match an auditory stimulus (a word) with a visual stimulus (a picture). The Digits Backward section of the Digit Span test also requires audio-visual integration because the child will usually form a visual image of the presented auditory sequence in order to repeat it backwards. Although sensory integrative capacity is involved in the successful performance of the aforementioned tests, their primary focus is to measure other functions. In the test devised by Kahn and Birch, the primary purpose is to measure objectively integrative capacity, because they view such impairment as a central problem for many children with MBD.

The equipment (Figure 7.8) consists of a standard telegraph key (which is most conveniently operated by batteries) and a set of 23 visual stimulus cards. Each card depicts three sets of dot patterns as shown

Figure 7.8
The Audio-Visual Integration Test Equipment.

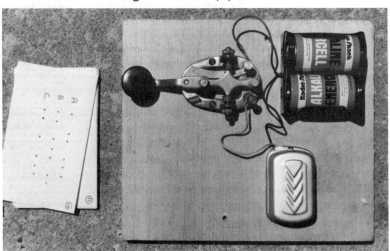

on the right side of Figure 7.9. (The examiner who wishes to utilize this test can readily make up stimulus cards from the information provided here.) The examiner taps an auditory pattern by following the sequences shown on the right side of Figure 7.9 and then shows the child the card that depicts three possible visual patterns, one of which corresponds to the auditory sequence. It is important that the examiner not show the child the card until *after* the tapped sequence has been completed. Otherwise the test becomes too easy and will not be in conformance with the methods used by the authors in collecting their normative data. Three sample sequences are first presented (A–C) and then the 20 test items. The child received one point for every correct selection. Normative data are presented in Table 7.3. The reader will note that mean scores are recorded for both age and grade simultaneously. I

Figure 7.9

Auditory Tap Patterns and Visual Stimuli of the Audio-Visual Integration Test.

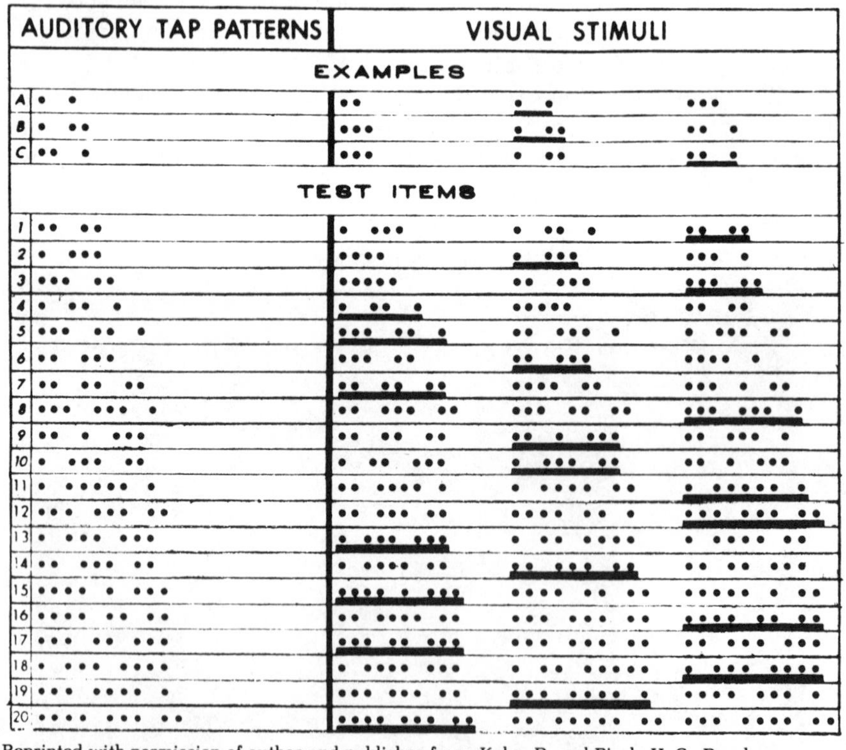

AUDITORY TAP PATTERNS	VISUAL STIMULI		
EXAMPLES			
A • •	• •	• ·	• • •
B • ••	•••	• ••	•• •
C •• •	•••	• ••	•• •
TEST ITEMS			
1 •• ••	• •••	• •• •	•• ••
2 • •••	••••	• •••	••• •
3 ••• ••	•••••	•• •••	••• ••
4 • •• •	•• •	••••••	•• ••
5 ••• •• •	••• •• •	•• ••• •	• ••• ••
6 •• •••	••• ••	•• •••	•••• •
7 •• •• ••	•• •• ••	•••• ••	••• • ••
8 ••• ••• •	•• ••• ••	••• •• ••	••• ••• •
9 •• • •••	•• •• ••	•• • •••	•• ••• •
10 • ••• ••	• •• •••	• ••• ••	•• • •••
11 • ••••• •	•• ••••• •	• ••••• ••	• •••••• •
12 ••• ••• ••	•• ••• ••	•••• •• •	••• ••• ••
13 • ••• •••	• ••• •••	• •• •••••	• ••••• •
14 •• ••• ••	• ••••• ••	•• ••• ••	•• •• •••
15 ••• • •••	•••• • •••	•••• •• ••	••••• • ••
16 •••• •• ••	•• ••••• ••	••• ••• ••	•••• •• ••
17 ••• •• •••	••• •• •••	••• ••• ••	•• ••• •••
18 • ••• ••••	• ••••• •••	• •• •••••	• ••• ••••
19 ••• •••• •	••• ••• ••	••• •••••	•••• •••• •
20 •••• ••• ••	•••• ••• ••	•• ••••• ••	••• •••• ••

Reprinted with permission of author and publisher from: Kahn, D. and Birch, H. G., Development of Auditory-Visual Integration and Reading Achievement. PERCEPTUAL AND MOTOR SKILLS, 27:459–468, 1968.

Table 7.3

Normative Data for the Audio-Visual Integration Test [N = 70 Per Grade]

Grade	Auditory-visual Integration			Age		
	Mean	S.D.	Range	Mean	S.D.	Range
2	9.6	4.0	2–17	8-4	5.1 mo.	7- 7 to 9-5
3	13.5	3.8	5–20	9-3	4.1 mo.	8- 7 to 10-4
4	15.1	2.9	7–20	10-1	5.7 mo.	9- 5 to 11-6
5	15.8	3.5	6–20	11-2	6.0 mo.	9-10 to 12-5
6	17.0	2.7	7–20	12-2	4.6 mo.	11- 5 to 13-3

Reprinted with permission of author and publisher from: Kahn, Dale and Birch, Herbert G. Development of auditory-visual integration and reading achievement. PERCEPTUAL AND MOTOR SKILLS, 1968, 27, 459–468.

believe that the examiner does well to ignore the grade level column and to use only the age column in evaluating a child's score. The average age of children in a given grade varies with the school system. In Kahn and Birch's group, the average second grader was 8-4 years of age. In many school systems, the third graders would not be this old. The authors' data cover mean ages from 7-7 to 13-3 and no asymptote was reached.

One problem confronting the examiner who is trying to evaluate the meaning of a child's poor score is that of differentiating between poor performance that is the result of a defect in either of the sensory modalities from a defect in their integration. A defect along any point along the pathway may result in impaired performance and it may be difficult to ascertain whether either of the sensory pathways was impaired or whether it was a deficient integrative mechanism that resulted in the child's defective performance. Rudel, Denckla, and Spalten (1976) and Rudel and Denckla (1976) suggest that such deficiency is less likely to be the result of integrative difficulty and more likely to be related to impaired functioning in one of the sensory pathways, refuting thereby Birch and Lefford's theory. I consider it reasonable that association pathways can become neurologically impaired. Clearly, further research should clarify this issue.

DICHOTIC AUDITORY COMPARISON TESTS

In recent years an area of research has developed that promises to provide new insights into the mechanisms of auditory functioning as well as the nature of auditory processing defects. Central to such research is the recognition that the right and left auditory systems work independently as well as in integration and that *comparing* the auditory functioning of the two sides can provide valuable information about both normal and pathological audition. Although some of the auditory fibers of the cochlear nerve transmit messages to the homolateral temporal lobe, via connections in the ipsilateral nucleus of the lateral lemniscus, inferior colliculus, and medial geniculate body, most transmit their impulses via decussation to the opposite superior olivary nucleus and then upward along tracts through the contralateral nucleus of the lateral lemniscus, inferior colliculus, and medial geniculate body to the opposite temporal lobe. Auditory impulses entering the right ear, then, are mainly received in the left temporal lobe; and auditory stimuli received by the left ear are primarily transmitted to the right temporal lobe. Because the left hemisphere is more specialized than the right for linguistic processing, the right ear-left brain complex is superior for such functioning (Studdert-Kennedy and Shankweiler, 1970). Because the right hemisphere is more specialized for spatial functions, the left ear-right brain complex appears to be superior for such nonspeech auditory functions as music, tones, and noises (Kimura, 1964; Curry, 1967). The brain stem, however, where many of the aforementioned auditory centers lie, is viewed as the site of *integration* of auditory stimuli.

Based on these concepts of auditory processing, a number of tests have been developed that utilize dichotic (both ears) comparison to localize auditory processing pathology. The tests are based on the principle that, the aforementioned differential functioning notwithstanding, the normal person should have bilaterally equal capacity for processing auditory stimuli. This is considered to be true for both *peripheral* processing (from the external ear to the cochlear nerve cell bodies in the pons) and *central* processing (involving all the aforementioned tracts and nuclei internal to the cochlear nuclei that ultimately end up in the temporal lobe cortex).

Before administering any of these tests, the patient should be carefully checked to be certain that there are no deficiencies in peripheral auditory functioning. If the standard autometric examination is normal and auditory acuity is completely intact bilaterally, then these special tests for *central auditory dysfunction* can be given. If such peripheral defects are present, then the results are much more difficult to interpret. The kinds of tests that will be discussed here are those that attempt to ascertain the location and nature of central auditory processing impairments by comparing the functioning of ears with normal auditory acuity on these special tests. They are tests that generally require the expertise of an audiologist or other similarly trained professional. They are discussed here because of their theoretical interest to those involved in MBD diagnosis. In addition, the person evaluating a child for MBD might wish to refer the child to a person trained to administer these tests. However, the examiner does well to appreciate fully the limitations of these tests (to be discussed below) before making such referral.

Dichotic Competing Sentences Test

Competing stimuli are simultaneously introduced bilaterally into the earphones. Verbal messages are introduced in a soft voice in one ear and a loud voice in the other. The subject is asked to identify the message relayed by the softer voice. The normal person should be able to ignore the louder voice and concentrate well enough on the softer voice to repeat it. The test detects temporal lobe lesions. If the soft voice is on the left and the patient cannot identify it, this suggests a right temporal lobe lesion. Clinically, children with such problems would have trouble differentiating the teacher's softer voice from the louder voices of children in the milieu.

Rapidly Alternating Speech

A sentence is divided in half and the first half is transmitted into one ear and the second half into the other. The sentence is presented rapidly so that approximately 300 msec of message goes into each ear. The brain stem is responsible for placing these messages in the proper time sequence, i.e., it has the capacity to put the impulses in the correct sequence. The normal person should be able to accomplish this task, and the patient who cannot presumably has some defect in brain stem integrative capacity. Clinically, a child with such a problem would have trouble understanding auditory messages in a large gymnasium where sounds may be echoed. Another situation where there might be trouble is the one where the child is listening to a lecture where the microphone is echoing.

Binaural Fusion Test

Vowels are of low frequency and consonants are high frequency. In this test (Ivey, 1969) the high frequency parts of the word are transmitted into one ear and the low frequency parts come into the other ear. The brain stem fuses and integrates the two parts. The normal person should be able to recognize words so presented. Impairment in the capacity to do so suggests brain stem dysfunction.

The Staggered Spondaic Word Test

All the words used in the test are two syllable in length and equal stress is placed on both syllables during presentation. However, when the second part of a word is being introduced into one ear, the first part of another word is being introduced into the other ear. For example, the right ear may receive the word *upstairs* and the left ear the word *downtown*. However, while *stairs* is coming into the right ear, *down* is simultaneously coming into the left ear. Accordingly, *up* is heard without competition in the right ear and *town* is heard alone in the left ear. *Stairs* and *down* are heard while competing with one another, *stairs* in the right ear and *down* in the left ear. There are 40 items in the test and the ears are alternated with regard to receiving the first syllable of the first word. The healthy person should be able to say the word *stairs-down*. Impairment here suggests temporal lobe lesions. Katz (1977) has done extensive work with this test, including the collection of normative data. Unfortunately, he has much more data on adults than children.

The Filtered Speech Test

Here speech is degraded so that it is slurred and presented with poor articulation. This is done by selectively attenuating sounds above 500 Hz. Each ear is tested separately and then both ears are compared with regard to the percentage of errors. If one does significantly more poorly in one ear, it can suggest temporal lobe lesions contralateral to the ear that is impaired.

Synthetic Sentence Identification

In this test, first introduced by Speaks and Jerger (1965), the child is given a card on which is written a series of *synthetic* sentences. Because "real" sentences could be recognized by recall of one or two words, synthetic (meaningless) sentences are utilized, e.g., "Do mind instead edge drop quickly till" and "Laugh along name my French woman laugh." In the first part of the test the right ear is presented a story (a distraction) and the left ear is presented the message: 'Point to ...'" followed by verbalization of the sentence that the child is to point to on the card. The verbally presented sentences are not presented in the same sequence as they appear on the card. In the second part of the test things are switched so that the left ear now receives the story and the right the sentences. This is another test of temporal lobe functioning. The intact temporal lobe should be able to identify the sentence and drown out the competing story.

Discussion

Most will agree that these tests are extremely clever and show promise of providing us with useful information about auditory processing. Unfortunately, extensive normative data collected on large numbers of subjects has not yet been collected. This is especially the case for children, both normal and those with MBD. Examiners commonly utilize the tests using as their base line their relatively subjective experiences with other patients or data with small numbers of subjects. It is important that we ascertain the exact percentage of errors that normal children exhibit on each of these tests. For any of these tests younger children are going to make errors. Where is the cut-off point for each age that separates the normal from the pathological? We cannot simply use preferential functioning of one ear over the other as a criterion for pathology. First, the brain is not symmetrical and, as mentioned, it is certainly asymmetrical regarding centers for language and spatial functions. And for developing children, such asymmetries may be greater. Accordingly, we cannot simply equate asymmetry with pathology; we must know the extent of the differences between the two sides that warrants the conclusion that pathology is present. We also need to compare the performance of normal children with those with MBD. Until we have such good data, one must be very cautious about interpreting the results of these tests.

There is the additional complicating factor of asymmetrical brain development, which probably occurs in the normal child. Kimura (1963) and Satz et al. (1975) describe right-ear advantage of normal children on some of these tests, children from ages 4 through 11. They believe that this relates to the superiority of the left hemisphere for language functioning and these tests are primarily linguistic. Porter and Berlin (1975) consider a failure of such right ear superiority to reflect a defect in the establishment of healthy left cerebral hemisphere dominance. If this is the case, if normal children do indeed have such superiority, then it would be even more difficult to interpret the meaning of asymmetries. There is much controversy among workers in the field regarding these issues and only further research can clarify some of these questions. The reader interested in a good statement of the present status of research in the field does well to refer to Keith's book (1977) on the subject.

Research in central auditory dysfunction has important implications for most of the tests discussed in this chapter. With the exception of the audiometric examination, in all other tests the auditory stimuli were presented simultaneously to both ears. It is possible that a child may have had a deficiency in one ear that was compensated for by the other and so the defect was not detected. A person could be blind in one eye and yet appear to read adequately, the intact eye performing the function being assessed. In taking the Goldman-Fristoe-Woodcock test, for example, a child might have a unilateral impairment in focusing on the verbal stimulus ("Point to ...") and ignoring the background distracting story (part 4). However, the intact ear might so compensate that the child might score in the normal range. This deficit, however, could be detected on the Dichotic Competing Sentences Test or The Synthetic Sentence Identification Test. One could argue that for clinical purposes this is irrevelant. The child got the right answer so what difference does it make if one ear (and its auditory pathways) was doing most of the work? The best argument against this reasoning is that the child may not be getting along as well as one might think. The tests may not be picking up the clinical difficulties that might be interfering with functioning—difficulties possibly amenable to remediation. The child, for example, might have done better in school if he had sat on the side of the room where his "good" ear was getting most of the teacher's messages. Or the child's capacity to learn in a setting where there are distracting auditory stimuli may be particularly difficult. Some children might profit from intermittent use of one ear plug to occlude input into the side that is malfunctioning and compromising the efficiency of the intact side. Or echo situations may make it particularly difficult for the child to learn. One could say, then, that normative data for all the tests described in this section should have been collected in each ear separately. This seems reasonable, but it has not yet been done. Accordingly, we have to work with the data we have. We should recognize, however, that this potential drawback is present and that the compensation of one side by the other may be providing us with a false sense of security about a child's auditory normality.

8

Visual Processing

THE LEVELS OF VISUAL PROCESSING

If the reader is to understand the various visual processing deficits the MBD child can manifest, a detailed excursion into the various levels of visual processing is necessary. Terminology in this area is especially vague and the problem is worsened by the common failure of authors to define the words they use. Accordingly, I will present here my concept of *visual* processing (auditory, haptic, and other forms of sensory processing will not be focused upon here unless particularly pertinent to the issue under consideration) and describe what I mean by each of the terms I utilize.

The eye is a *receiver* of visual stimuli and the ganglion cell pathways are the transmitters *(transducers)* of visual impulses. The retinal rod and cone cells are connected to a network of interconnecting cells (bipolar, horizontal, and amacrine), which in turn are connected to many of the ganglion cells that transmit retinal impulses to the occipital cortex. Accordingly, a light stimulus to a specific point on the retina is spread to many parts of both occipital lobes in no simple pattern. States Haber (1974): "It is from these kinds of interconnections that it is impossible to think of the eye as sending anything like a copy of the pattern in the optic array to the brain." Elsewhere he states: "An individual cortical cell is sensitive to patterns in the retinal projection covering an area of retina much larger than a single retinal receptor." There is *general* transmission but not *specific*. Light from the right will fall on the left side of each retina and will generally be transmitted back to certain specific regions of the occipital cortex. But within the regions there is no point-by-point specificity. The impulses for a particular image get projected throughout these areas on both sides of the brain. For example, light from the right visual field passes through the lens of each eye and is projected onto the nasal half of the right retina and the lateral half of the left retina. Axons from the ganglion cells of the left lateral retinal field pass through the optic chiasm to the lateral geniculate body. There they connect to ganglion cells of the optic radiations which carry visual impulses directly back to the left occipital cortex; however axons from the ganglion cells of the right nasal retinal field cross to the left in the optic chiasm and end up in the left occipital cortex as well.

Such an arrangement is quite adaptive. With multiple field overlap, damage to an isolated area of the occipital cortex does not produce impairment in the visual image transmitted to the cortex. And constant saccadic (minor involuntary) movements of the eye continually shift the point at which an image is projected on the retina. Retinal cells quickly fatigue and an image projecting more than 2–3 seconds on a retinal cell is no longer perceived. The saccadic movements insure that "fresh" receptor cells will continually be present to receive visual stimuli. Accordingly, a person with a small occipital-cortical or retinal lesion does not have a "hole" in the visual image. Much more extensive retinal and/or cortical damage is necessary to produce an observable defect in the visual field. In addition, there is good evidence (Corballis and Beale, 1976) that the cerebral commissures transfer visual stimuli to the opposite hemisphere, providing a further pathway for "spread" of incoming visual impulses.

We have followed the impulses to the point where they are spread over the occipital cortices. They are no longer simple visual projections, but are in some electrical-chemical form (henceforth to be called *coded information* or merely *information*). The brain has the capacity to use this information in a variety of ways that we are just beginning to understand.

The brain has the capacity to form *engrams*, i.e., visual images similar to those that Ireland, Orton, and others (see below) thought were actually projected. The coded information is converted to an internal display in topographic form analogous (but certainly not identical) to the way in which a TV set converts its incoming signals into a picture. We do not see television pictures flying through the air.

Rather they are transmitted via coded electronic signals that are converted into pictures by our home receivers. Similarly, we cannot see little pictures on videotapes. The tapes store information that is transformed by the videotape recorder and monitor into visual images. But these images that the brain reconstitutes are *not* identical to what may have been projected onto the retina. The brain takes the slightly different views of the world provided by eyes that observe the same object from slightly different angles (producing thereby slightly different images on each of the retinas) and provides us with a sensation of *depth* and *distance*.

The retinal projections may not accurately portray reality and the brain makes the necessary corrections. For example, doors and windows usually appear rectangular to us, regardless of the visual angle at which they are viewed. Unless we are observing such objects straight on, the retinal projection of them is trapezoidal. Yet the brain is able to make the necessary corrections that enable us to maintain our images of them as rectangles. Depth perception is not simply the result of the stereoscopic vision provided by two eyes viewing an object from a slightly different angle. Even one eye can provide us with an appreciation of depth even though a two dimensional image is being projected on the retina. A picture of a cube printed on a page is certainly projected in two dimensions on the retina. Yet we see it as three dimensional. By utilizing such factors as texture gradients, shadow, interposition of one object in front of another, and size perspective, we are able to provide ourselves with a sense of depth in spite of the two dimensional retinal image (Haber, 1974).

The brain enables us to appreciate *spatial relationships* between objects: above-below, in front-behind, right-left, right side up-upside down, within me-out there, next to-at a distance from, etc. It has discriminative ability, enabling us to apprehend whether two visualized entities are different or identical *(visual discrimination)*. It selects the salient features of a visual array by distinguishing foreground from background *(figure-ground discrimination)* enabling us thereby to focus on the important and attend less to the unimportant stimuli.

I use the term *visual memory* to refer to the capacity to *store* or *retain* visual information. But simple retention of coded information is of little value without the capacity to *retrieve* selectively what has been stored. Although two independent processes are present here, it may be difficult to differentiate clinically between them. If a stroke patient is asked to provide the name of an object, a book for example, and cannot, there are primarily two possible explanations. Either the memory of the name of the object has been obliterated or the ability to retrieve the name from the "memory bank" is impaired. Differentiation is often made between *short-* and *long-term memory*. The ability to reproduce geometric forms 10 seconds after viewing them would test short-term memory. Recalling the place of one's birth requires long-term memory. I wonder about the usefulness of these concepts. The more often one thinks about something, the more deeply it will be embedded in the psychic structure and the more readily will it be recalled. There is really no sharp cut-off point between short- and long-term memory, and one does better, I believe, to view such memory as being on a continuum.

We also have the capacity to compare new stimuli with remembered old ones, a capacity that is quite useful in helping us determine what kind of action to take. For example, we have stored images of cats and panthers. We also have stored associated information about how we can expect each of these two animals to behave (some of this is also visual in the form of snarling, purring, cuddling, attacking, etc.). When confronted with one of these animals we compare what we see with stored and retrieved visual images of other animals in the same category, and act accordingly. This comparison process is different from visual discrimination. In visual discrimination one merely determines whether two *external* visual stimuli are the same or different. They may even be stimuli that we have never encountered before. Here the comparison is between an external stimulus (familiar or not) and an internal visual image that has been retrieved from memory. If the external stimulus is totally novel, then there will be no exact stored image to compare it with, and new information will have to be obtained if one is to decide upon appropriate action.

Taking the comparison process one step further, the brain has the capacity to identify the whole from parts (this is a central element in conceptualization). The child, for example, who is shown a picture of a dog with only one ear is asked, "What's missing?" retrieves an image of a whole dog, makes a comparison, and answers, "The ear." The child who is shown a picture of a rubber tire and a steering wheel and asked, "What does this make you think of?" retrieves an image of a total automobile and says, "A car."

Another process that depends upon visual memory, retrieval, and comparison is that of visual organization. Given a doll house and a pile of toy furniture, the child places the correct furniture in the appropriate room and within each room places the furniture in its proper position (chairs around the table, plates on the table, TV set facing viewing chairs, etc.). Block design tests in which the child is asked to reproduce with colored blocks a visual pattern depicted on a card also requires visual organizational ability.

Language requires the highest, most complex, and most difficult utilization of sensory processing. Central to the development of language is the capacity to appreciate the relationship between an object and the linguistic symbol that by convention has been devised to denote it. There is nothing intrinsic to the letters c-u-p that should warrant their being used to denote the object we call a cup. Each language has its own symbols (both written and verbal) to denote this particular object. Such conventions are crucial to communication; without them there would be chaos since no one would be able to transmit to another what was going on in his or her mind. Because there is no *intrinsic* association between an object and the word used to identify it, appreciating the link or the association may be difficult for many children. And dyslexics may find it a formidable, if not impossible, task.

The term *decoding* is used to refer to the process by which the individual associates the linguistic symbol with the entity it has been designed to denote. If one sees the written word *house*, one has successfully decoded it if one forms in one's mind the visual image of a house. The decoding process gives meaning to an intrinsically meaningless symbol. *Encoding* refers to the opposite process. A child, for example, is shown a house (picture or an actual house) and asked what it is. If he says "house" then he has demonstrated the capacity to encode, to form the conventional linguistic symbol utilized to denote this entity. But the word here has been verbalized; therefore, only auditory and verbalization processes are manifesting themselves. If the child can write and/or spell *house*, then visual encoding ability has been demonstrated. As mentioned, it is the visual processes that I am primarily focusing upon here.

To go further into the *decoding* process, let us consider a child who has seen many houses and has been taught by parents and teachers both the verbal and written symbols to denote this entity. Such a child is then shown the written word *house* and asked what it means. To successfully answer the question the child must first have successfully stored accurately coded information regarding a house's particular attributes. The child must then be able to retrieve selectively this information—and only this information—from storage. This information must then be converted into a visual image of a house. The three operations crucial to successful association between the written word and its image are *storage, selective retrieval,* and *engrammatic display*. The written word *house* should bring about a selection *only* of that information necessary to form the specific image of a house. The child with a decodng impairment may have a memory problem: the basic coded information regarding a house's particular attributes are not efficiently or accurately stored, and/or the child may have difficulty in retrieval, in selecting the proper information requisite to the formation of an accurate visual image, and/or the child may not be able to organize or synthesize the information into a meaningful *engram*. If the child does perform this task successfully we say that he has understood the meaning of the word, that the capacity of interpretation is intact. The visualized word house usually brings forth from auditory memory the sounds of the verbalized word as well. When the child was first shown the word *house*, the teacher said "house" and may have also shown the child a picture of a house. This capacity to bring together, in a meaningful way, information from two or more sensory modalities is called *integration*. (The automatic utilization of auditory processes in silent reading will be discussed in chapter 9).

Now to a more detailed inquiry into the *encoding* process. The child with previous experience in linking the written word house with an engram of a house is shown a house and asked to write the word for what is being shown. To successfully accomplish this the child must have stored proper coded information about the letters h-o-u-s-e. By proper, I mean the correct form and orientation of each letter. He or she must then selectively retrieve these five letters from many others and then form a visual image of the word with the letters in correct sequence. This engrammatic display is then used as a model for writing the word. The brain must be able to give the hand proper instructions to enable it to perform the task of writing the word. And the hand must be able to execute the instructions. At least six operations are necessary for the successful completion of this task: *storage, selective retrieval, organization, engrammatic display, brain-hand instructions,* and *hand execution.* If the information is not properly coded and/or is not accurately stored (regarding form and orientation) the child will obviously not be able to spell the word. If the retrieval process is not successful in selecting the correct coded information, then the task will not be accomplished. Children with trouble in this area are sometimes referred to as having problems in *word finding* or *naming.* The letters must then be correctly formed and oriented and then properly *organized,* i.e., placed in proper sequence. These steps are required for proper encoding. The child whose brain forms the proper word and visualizes it accurately but somehow cannot transmit the proper instructions to the hand is said to suffer with *dysgraphia* or *agraphia* (if severe), a form of *dyspraxia* or *apraxia* (if severe). And/or if the child has a coordination problem, motor weakness, spasticity, tremors, chorea, or other neuromuscular impairment, the correct instructions may not be successfully executed.

The decoding and encoding processes are central to language. The key word, basic to both processes, is linkage or association. The child must be able to link an entity with an intrinsically meaningless symbol. The child who gets "the hang of" this association is said to exhibit *reading readiness,* the child who does not is *dyslexic,* or in severe cases *alexic.* In my experience, it is this impairment, more than anything else, that is central to the dyslexia problem.

The reader may have noted that I have not defined the term *visual perception* in the above discussion. This omission was not by chance. The term has been used in so many different ways (often, as mentioned, without definition) that it has become almost meaningless. Some use it narrowly to refer to visual differentiation. Others use it as synonymous with the ability to ascribe meaning to a visual sensation (red light means stop; *dog* means a specific kind of animal). Others use it as a rubric under which is subsumed a variety of visual phenomenon: discrimination, organization, integration, decoding, etc. To avoid the communication problems inherent in such use of the term, I avoid it and use the rubric *visual processing* under which are included the variety of visual operations described above, which originate in the eye and end in various parts of the brain (especially the occipital lobes). I also have not found the terms *visual analysis* and *visual synthesis* too useful, for the same reasons that *visual perception* no longer has specific meaning to me.

It is important for the reader to appreciate that the various steps described above are executed ever more rapidly as the child grows older. Many are never consciously broken down or thought about, e.g. forming an engram from stored coded information. Others are first done in stepwise fashion and then become more automatic. For example, we associate a picture of a dog when the word is read only in the earliest phases of reading. Later we *know* what is being communicated by the word without necessarily having to form the visual image.

Although it is obvious that many of the aforementioned visual phenomena are not isolated entities, it is useful to try to ascertain in the clinical evaluation which functions are compromised. The instruments described below are divided into categories in accordance with the primary function being assessed. None of them is "pure" as a test for any single aspect of visual processing. In the discussion of each, an attempt will be made to describe other functions that are being evaluated when the test is administered. The examiner who does not consider these additional contributing factors is likely to come to simplistic and erroneous conclusions regarding a child's impairments.

I have invited Dr. Melvin Schrier, an optometrist, to write the section on ocular dysfunction. The role of certain types of ocular disorder in MBD is presently a subject of much controversy. Many in the field of medicine (including neurology, pediatrics, and ophthalmology) hold that the kinds of learning disorders that are typical of children with MBD are the result of pathological processes in the brain and that ocular pathology is rarely, if ever, the cause of the kinds of learning disability one sees in MBD children. At the other extreme are those (primarily in the field of optometry) who take the position that one reads with one's eyes and if one has trouble reading the place to direct one's attention is the eyes. Between these two extremes are all degrees of conviction regarding the role of ocular deficits in neurologically based learning disabillities. Those at the extreme ends hardly talk to one another and each dismisses the other as ignorant and not to be taken seriously. Some routinely refer all children with learning disabilities to an optometrist and consider any other type of evaluation or treatment unwarranted. Others never make such a referral.

My own position at this point (pending better studies) is that there are probably some MBD children who have some kind of ocular difficulty. I would guess that about 5%–10% of all children whom I would consider to have MBD have ocular disability. I have no good statistics on the subject (and I don't know of any either); this is just my guess. Embryologically, anatomically, and neurologically the eyes are direct extentions of (and can be considered to be an intrinsic part of) the brain. It is reasonable to suspect that the same factors that can be detrimental to the brain can affect the eyes as well. I believe that one is just as likely to find mild neurophysiological abnormalities in the eyes as in other parts of the brain. As I will discuss in chapter 12, there are studies that demonstrate a higher incidence of strabismus, epicanthal folds, and hypertelorism in MBD children than normals. It is hard to imagine that other ocular and periocular disorders are not to be found in MBD children as well. In addition, MBD children, like normal children, are subject to the same kinds of ocular problems that may interfere with their reading and learning.

The standard visual screening examination with the Snellen chart only tests one small aspect of visual functioning, namely, it is a screening test for myopia. To say that a child's eyes are completely normal if he has 20/20 vision, is to make an unwarranted generalization. It is like saying that a person is completely normal because his height is average, or because his weight is average, or because his temperature is normal. All children deserve a more sophisticated ocular evaluation. And MBD children, because of the greater likelihood of their having ocular disorders, are even more entitled to such an evaluation.

The person who is administering an MBD battery should know something about the kinds of ocular disorders that can interfere with children's learning. Some of these may be intrinsically related to MBD; others may not. In either case it is important that they be detected because not to do so is likely to deprive such children of what may be extremely useful therapy (corrective lenses, orthoptics, etc.). Dr. Schrier's article provides the MBD evaluator with just such information. In addition, Dr. Schrier describes an instrument he has devised that can serve as a screening device for detecting the most common kinds of ocular-visual difficulties seen in children (both with or without MBD). This instrument can be used by any examiner who is willing to go to the small amount of effort required to learn how to use it. The examination itself only takes a few minutes. In a short time, then, one is in an excellent position to decide whether ocular problems are present and whether referral for further optometric and/or ophthalmologic evaluation is warranted.

One final, and important, point. One of the crucial issues of difference between optometrists and ophthalmologists concerns the question of whether the neurophysiological abnormalities described by the optometrists are bona fide disorders or merely mild abnormalities that are still within the normal range of human variation. The central question is: Where does normality end and pathology begin when one is considering neurophysiological phenomena? The analogy I prefer to use here relates to height. Consider the distribution of heights to be found in a normal population. One will observe a range from the shortest to the tallest person. At what point does one say that a person is *short* and at what point do we define *tall*? Clearly, examiners will vary regarding the cut-off points that they would utilize. One is safer using terms like *percentile rank* and *standard deviation from the mean*. The individual who receives such data can then decide what label he or she wants to provide and what to do with the information. We do not yet have enough data on normal children to help us make important decisions about whether the optometrists or the ophthalmologists are right here. The optometrists claim that the proof of their theories lies in the therapeutic benefit their patients enjoy from their treatments. No one can deny that glasses help the myopic child see the blackboard more easily. But it is difficult to prove the efficacy of optometric treatment measures that require a long time to prove their worth. One could always argue that the child would have gotten better anyway, and that the improvement was due to normal development and little, if anything, else. Similarly, for this reason there is no proof that psychotherapy works. We may never be able to prove that psychotherapy works. With further well-controlled research studies we probably will be able to prove whether or not many of the optometric theories and treatments are efficacious. Until such evidence is in, I believe that it behooves the MBD examiner to take a receptive (but not gullible) attitude toward what the optometrists are telling us about ocular dysfunction in children with learning disabilities.

OCULAR DYSFUNCTION IN MBD

Melvin Schrier, O.D.

There is a dichotomy of attitudes toward the role of ocular skill impairments in the child with MBD. Just how important they are seems to depend greatly on the criteria used by each researcher. Those who conclude that vision plays no part in MBD base their conclusions on gross visual tests such as visual acuity. Researchers who conclude that vision does play an important part in MBD base their conclusions on more subtle measures of visual skills that test performance.

The two eye professions, optometry and ophthalmology, have different opinions about the importance of many visual functions. This difference of opinion sometimes clouds the understanding of related professionals who work in the field of MBD. If the educator, psychologist, or school nurse is medically oriented, he or she will tend to believe the medical literature that states that vision is minimally related to learning problems. If he or she is optometrically oriented, more credence will be put into the importance of vision on learning. This difference of opinion has left some professionals and many parents confused about the actual visual needs of the learning-disabled child.

The difference in opinion stems from the differences in training of ophthalmologists and optometrists. The ophthalmologist, a physician by training, begins to concentrate on the eyes in his residency. His four years of medical school training is based on general medicine, and includes instruction on the eye. Only when he becomes a resident does the ophthalmologist begin to specialize. His specialty involves pathology and surgery, with less emphasis on visual function. Consequently, his practice is geared to surgical procedures and therapy of unhealthy eyes. Many ophthalmologists consider the eyes "fine" when the patient's visual acuity is 20/20 and there is no pathology.

The training of the optometrist pursues a rather different path. The four years of optometry school are devoted to studies in every aspect of vision and vision care. Although he is carefully trained to examine the inner and outer tissues of the eye for pathology, he does not undertake drug therapy (although very recently some states have allowed minor incursions into medication). The optometrists' education concentrates on the efficiency and comfort of vision, that is, the ability to see clearly, binocularly, and with a minimum of stress. Consequently, emphasis is placed on healthy eyes that do not function well. Because of this training, after the optometrist decides that the patient's eyes are healthy and seeing clearly, he concerns himself with visual stress and discomfort. The optometrist then is more likely to be trained to explore the finer nuances of visual efficiency than the ophthalmologist, hence the difference of opinion regarding role of ocular dysfunction in MBD.

I confine myself here to the role of the optometric examination in MBD diagnosis. (Other tests that the optometrist might include in his diagnostic workup of an MBD child will be discussed elsewhere in this chapter and book). For example, after all of the routine vision tests, the optometrist might obtain data on visual motor skills, visualization skills, visual memory, visual perception skills, posture, and directionality.

The interest of the optometrist in those visually related skills was brought about by the void of information in the field of learning disorders in the 1950s and 1960s, when many optometrists active in the field of visual training found that they were involved with children with learning problems. When conventional optometric methods didn't go far enough, and other professions, at the time, did not fill the gap, concerned optometrists expanded the scope of their practices and became involved with visually related skills. A great impetus was given to this movement by the work of Gesell (1950) and his optometric colleagues at the Gesell Institute, and the teachings of Skeffington through the Optometric Extension Program based in Duncan, Oklahoma. Both Gesell and Skeffington described vision as a total complex, much more complicated than the previous acceptance of good vision as the ability to see "20/20." Rather, visual acuity is only one of many skills that are part of total visual competence. Gesell said, "Vision is ... a prime constituent in the development of the *total child*." Skeffington created this model of visual development in an infant (only those aspects of his concept applicable to this discussion are presented here):

1. Awareness of space: eyes must coordinate with inputs of muscles, limbs, body movement, and labyrinths.
2. Centering: aligning the eyes so that the child knows where he is in relation to his environment. Using both eyes together easily and skillfully leads to adequate binocularity. Imagine a child feeling one toy and seeing two. He will be frustrated, confused, insecure, and use significant energy trying to resolve this problem. Also, proper recognition of visual space assures awareness of differences between p, q, b and d.

3. Identification: correlation of all senses and memory in the learning process, e.g., the word *onion* is a group of squiggles to the uninitiated. By properly reading the five letters, and having the memory of experience with an onion, the reader can conjure up the size, feel, smell, taste, and color of the onion from the printed word.

Skeffington says, "Vision is the learned ability to see for information and performance ... I see, truly means, I know, I understand." With these definitions in mind, optometry went beyond the conventional practice of measuring eyes, with appreciation of the fact that vision is not total until the brain interprets what we see. Therefore, examining the eyeball alone will not test for the adequacy of vision. It is on the assumption that vision is learned and is a brain-involved system, that all of the following is based.

Extent of the Problem

Jens (1970) reported that "visual deficiencies have a higher incidence among underachieving children." The National Advisory Committee on Dyslexia and Reading Disorders (1969) stated that "8,000,000 children experienced difficulty in learning to read, although they seemed to have adequate intelligence and emotional stability. These children come from all segments of society." However, the president's commission on dyslexia in the early 1970s estimated that the number of reading disabled children varied from 2% to 35% of the school population, depending on how one defines it (Rosner et al., 1974).

It seems rather obvious that a great discrepancy exists in the minds of various people and related organizations about the extent of the problem. Statistics aside, anyone involved with MBD children will agree that a large population is in need of diagnosis and therapy. If we take the eight million number as a guide, and if we agree that vision correction and/or therapy can conservatively rehabilitate even 10% to 15% of these patients, then we will have contributed significantly to the aid of about one million children.

From the vision specialist's point of view, it is the most direct and least time-consuming task to visually check a child who is having a learning problem. In the one to two hour complete diagnostic examination, we can determine whether vision is a component of the child's problems, or eliminate it as a cause, thereby allowing efforts to be expended in other directions.

Ocular Defects and MBD

When a variety of ocular defects that are generally considered by optometrists to be associated with reading disability are listed, it is probable that problems that some professionals deem important will be omitted, and others that might be controversial will be included. It must be emphasized that this whole subject is open to personal, professional, and clinical differences of opinion. Because this book is written to be as comprehensive as possible, all aspects of diagnostic testing will be included. Some defects are well researched and there are data on the pros and cons of their involvement with reading disability. Others are unquestionably not involved with learning disorders. The great majority, however, are still objects of interprofessional controversy. It is important to emphasize that subtle signs are more important than gross visual defects (Betts, 1946; Gates, 1949). Gross defects are obvious under all types of testing, but subtle defects can only be detected by refined, specific testing procedures.

In my opinion, any of the following may be found in MBD and therefore warrant evaluation in the MBD diagnostic battery:

1. Visual-Acuity Deficits
   a. Myopia
   b. Hyperopia
   c. Astigmatism
2. Anisometropia
3. Aniseikonia
4. Accommodation/Convergence Inefficiency or Insufficiency
5. Binocularity
6. Phorias
   a. Lateral Eye Posture
   b. Vertical Eye Posture
7. Fixation Abilities
   a. Direct fixation
   b. Pursuit ability
   c. Saccadic ability

All of the above visual problems have their proponents for their validity and importance in the overall learning problem. It is extremely important to remember that the degree of the problem is the key to its involvement in the patient's difficulties. Therefore, the criteria used to determine the importance of each skill must be understood. Unfortunately, many papers do not list these criteria and much may have to be accepted without refined scientific studies. When dealing with individuals on a clinical, office-based level, it is difficult, if not impossible, to create control groups to present impeccable scientific facts. On the basis of my clinical experiences I am convinced that the criteria presented here are valid. However, I recognize that future controlled studies might warrant some modification of what is presented here. Here I describe the various ocular problems that may be seen in MBD children. Subsequently I will discuss the ways in which these deficits can be detected with the Schrier Vision Screening Test.

Visual Acuity Deficits

Myopia—[Nearsightedness]

A condition where the visual acuity of the patient (normally tested at 20 ft, which is considered optical infinity) is below the prescribed norm of 20/20. 20/20 means only that the patient can see a $^3/_8$-in. block letter at 20 ft. For example,

> 20/20 means that the person sees letters at 20 ft that one should be able to see at 20 ft.
>
> 20/40 means that the patient sees letters at 20 ft that one should be able to see at 40 ft.
>
> 20/100 means that the patient sees letters at 20 ft that one should be able to see at 100 ft.

Myopia results from the focus of light at a point in front of the retina. Minus (concave) lenses correct this defect by causing light to properly focus on the retina.

The concept of 20/20 vision was devised by Hermann Snellen in the latter part of the nineteenth century. He devised a standardized letter chart to test the visual acuity of patients based on the notion that the "average" eye could read a block letter $^3/_8$-in. high at 20 ft. The Snellen chart is traditionally composed of eleven lines of varying sized letters. It is hung on a wall 20 ft from the patient or a slide of the chart is projected 20 ft away. School personnel and pediatricians usually use the traditional cardboard chart. It may be clean or dirty, it may be well lit or poorly lit, and usually the third child in line will have memorized the letters in order not to fail the test. Consequently it is difficult to make this a foolproof test of visual ability. Yet it is still used as the major test of visual skills. It tells us nothing of near-point vision (the place where we read and write), or of binocular visual skills.

The size of the letters on a Snellen chart range from the $3/8$-in. "20/20" letters to the $3\frac{1}{2}$-in. 20/200 letters. By Snellen's definition the $3/8$-in. letters should be read at 20 ft and the $3\frac{1}{2}$-in. letters should be read at 200 ft. Therefore, a patient who sees 20/200 can only see a letter at 20 ft that he should be able to see at 200 ft. That is all that it means.

Snellen decided that 20/20 acuity was the "norm" for the population at that time. Unfortunately, this has become the sole criterion for many test situations and has been accepted as such by a great number of professionals and vision-related groups. It is this finding that creates the greatest controversy between the various professionals. If 20/20 is accepted as "perfect vision," then other visual findings are often considered unimportant, and the child might be assumed to be visually competent. If, on the other hand, acuity is considered just one of many functions, then it takes its proper place in the evaluation of the total accumulation of information.

There are varying degrees of myopia, from the mild to the very severe. Those who are mildly or moderately myopic have trouble seeing things clearly at a distance. Said deficit is most often easily corrected with glasses or contact lenses. Moderately myopic people (better than 20/400 visual acuity) can usually function very well without visual correction at the person's usual reading distance. High degrees of myopia (worse than 20/400 visual acuity) can create difficulties with vision both at the far point (20 ft and beyond) and also at the usual reading distance. Patients with vision this poor can read without correction, but they must hold the reading material closer than 12 in. from their eyes. The more myopic, the closer they must hold the material. This creates binocular visual stress, and should be avoided.

Because most myopic individuals can function at the near point, without stress, just about all studies (Gates and Bond, 1936; Dalton, 1943; Jackson and Schye, 1945; Robinson, 1968; Leisman, 1976) showed "no relationship between visual acuity and reading ability." As a matter of fact, it is clinically known that myopic students may be the best readers in a group. Severe myopia, however, may become a psychological problem. Because such patients' clear visual world is limited to their arms' length, they may avoid social relationships. Many myopic children have been labeled "dumb" because of their poor academic achievement. Such children can literally not see clearly more than an arm's length away. Blackboards are a complete blur instead of a source of information.

Myopic children will usually be detected by any type of simple distance visual acuity test (such as the commonly used Snellen test) and/or by parent or teacher observation. These are the children who squint at the board, and show general discomfort when looking at distance objects.

When a patient does not exhibit clear distance vision (usually considered to be beyond 20 ft), minus lenses are prescribed to produce clear visual acuity. The least amount of lens power that gives the greatest amount of acuity is prescribed. Most practitioners adhere to this approach. However, some doctors hold back on the amount of minus lens power "so the eyes will have work to do." This approach, in my opinion, robs the patient of clear vision and may impede a student's progress in school because he does not clearly see the blackboard. In addition, I am dubious about the therapeutic value of such "work." Consider, for example, the student who misreads a number. Even the most brilliant math student will get the wrong answer. Will the teacher know that it was a vision error and not a lack of understanding?

There are times, however, when the proper visual correction for distance is stronger than the patient needs for reading. This is determined after taking and evaluating a thorough case history and conducting the eye-muscle tests. On many occasions a student (even one in the lower grades) will be given a separate pair of reading glasses that is weaker than the distance prescription or a pair of bifocal lenses. The bifocals assure the doctor that the student will use the proper prescription when he is doing close work. If the bifocal is designed properly, the student will automatically look through the reading portion of the lenses and avoid reading through the stronger distance portion. These are the cases where reading through the distance part would cause visual stress. The reading segment of the lens enables the child to avoid this. If the doctor could be sure that the patient would change glasses whenever he read, then two pairs of glasses would be appropriate. Unfortunately, most youngsters cannot be relied upon to use the proper lenses for the proper task. Most will not change their glasses in a classroom each time they must read from a book and then from the blackboard. With a bifocal, this become automatic. Children rarely complain once they have worn their bifocals for a short period of time. They adapt to them very well and are generally pleased with the visual relief they get while wearing them. Bifocals should not be prescribed routinely. The total visual system must be evaluated before this decision is made.

Bifocal lenses, or plus lenses for near vision, can also be used preventively. Many believe (and I consider myself among them) that judicious prescribing can slow up the advancement of myopia, or at least minimize a stressful visual situation. The optometric literature abounds with articles devoted to this subject (Burian, 1946; Feinberg, 1959; Melkin, 1960; Roberts and Banford, 1967; Harris, 1974; Nolan, 1974), while the ophthalmological literature is quite devoid of them.

This is a condition in which distance vision appears to be unimpaired, even without correction. Hyperopia results from the focusing of light behind the retina. Plus (convex) lenses correct this defect by causing light to properly focus on the retina. However, the *amount* of hyperopia is a key consideration. High degrees of farsightedness cause as poor visual acuity as high amounts of myopia. Hyperopia may not be detected in children because they have a built-in defense against hyperopia. Muscles supporting the lens (ciliary muscles) automatically alter the lens curvature so that light properly focuses on the retina. (Children are much more capable of accomplishing this than older people.) Most young people are not aware of the energy that is being used to clear the blur. Because they see clearly, they may not be aware that the headaches, fatigue, sleepiness, or avoidance of near-point work is a manifestation of their farsightedness.

To compound the problem, many eye professionals still quote the Donders Table (also promulgated in the latter years of the nineteenth century) that assumes a large amount of reserve accommodative eye muscle strength in the young person, e.g., a 10-year-old should be able to overcome 14 diopters [A diopter (D) is a measure of a lens' converging or diverging power] of farsightedness; a 15-year-old should be able to overcome 12 diopters of farsightedness.

Unfortunately, despite the theoretical validity of the table, the doctors who use it as gospel, overlook the important fact that energy is being used to compensate for *any* amount of farsightedness. The higher the amount of hyperopia, the greater the use of energy. Many healthy, well-functioning children can, and do, overcome this problem with a minimum of difficulty. They see well at distance, they appear to read well with comfort, and show no signs of stress when they study. Other children, with equal amounts of hyperopia, have a lower threshold of comfort and cannot sustain prolonged periods of near-point tasks, such as reading, without some discomfort. Hyperopia may not manifest itself as an obvious vision problem, but we must consider the possibility of hyperopia in patients who cannot read for long periods of time, who may avoid any near-point task completely, or who rub their eyes and complain of visual or general fatigue after using their eyes. These children may involuntarily mask their condition by becoming the class clown, the class nuisance, or the day-dreamer, using any means to avoid reading or any extended near-point task.

To point up the importance of hyperopia in the reading disability population, Nielson (1962) reported that in a class of 157 Danish children, aged 8–14, in a remedial reading class, 67% had "perfect" vision or were slightly hyperopic, 26% were moderately hyperopic, 5% were highly hyperopic, and only 2% were myopic. Other examiners as well (Farris, 1936; Eames, 1955; Young, 1963; Robinson, 1968) have also described a significant frequency of hyperopia among children with learning disabilities.

If farsighted students who can see 20/20 on a Snellen chart are overlooked in a vision screening program, any possibility of help will be delayed until someone aware of the importance of hyperopia in its relationship to reading difficulties begins a proper therapeutic regimen. For screening purposes, two diopters of hyperopia is the maximum allowable. Any more would suggest potential strees. Some manifestation of hyperopia should alert the practitioner that a potential reading problem may exist. Proper testing that combines the patients' eye muscle performance with their refractive problem will go a long way in picking up a student with a potential learning problem.

It is also important to point out that students who may have excellent visual acuity both at distance and near, may still benefit from a reading prescription to overcome stress from prolonged near-point visual tasks. This clinical approach is being utilized by many vision specialists as a preventive method to avoid stress. Clinical evidence shows definite positive results (Dunphey, 1968; Birnbaum, 1973).

There is no set approach to the care of patients who are farsighted. Correction of hyperopia is most important for reading. The age of the person, the amount of his hyperopia, and his visual needs determine the prescription. Young people with moderate amounts of hyperopia (up to + 2.00 D) can generally compensate for the problem by using their focusing (accommodative) muscles to see clearly without stress. Others, with the same amount of hyperopia, but who are esophoric, (to be discussed below) may not be able to function easily. It is only after professional evaluation of all the visual data that a proper prescription can be written. Some doctors overlook large amounts of farsightedness, others prescribe for small amounts. However, the prime needs of the patient should be the determining factor in prescribing.

Astigmatism

Astigmatism is a problem where images entering the eye focus in different planes. In myopia light is focused in front of the retina. In hyperopia light is focused behind the retina. In astigmatism, because of lens, corneal, and other ocular abnormalities, light is focused in two different planes either in front of, behind, or both in front of and behind the retina. Most people have some degree of astigmatism. If the visual acuity is poor enough, this problem will usually be found and corrected.

Uncorrected astigmatism may make the number 8 look like the number 3. However, astigmatism itself doesn't appear to cause reading difficulties, unless moderately severe and uncorrected. Small amounts (less than 1.00 D) of astigmatism may be overlooked if no other visual problem exists. Larger amounts will contribute to some degree of blur. It must be the decision of the examining doctor. Other than a massive blur from a large uncorrected degree of astigmatism, this problem does not specifically affect MBD patients. Normal or regular astigmatism is easily correctable with glasses. Irregular astigmatism, where the cornea is irregularly distorted, is best corrected with contact lenses.

Anisometropia

When the visual defect of one eye is significantly different from the defect in the other eye, the condition is called anisometropia. The disorder can take a number of forms: one eye being much more myopic than the other; one eye being myopic and the other eye being hyperopic; one eye being visually perfect and the other eye being astigmatic, myopic, or hyperopic or a combination of two of these problems. Despite the large number of possibilities, clinically we find that only a small percentage of the population has an anisometropic problem. Lebensohn (1957) reports that 10% of refractive problems are anisometropic. Eames (1964) stated, "It appears probable that if the eyes each send to the brain a different image of the text, the added neuropsychological load of attempting to make a single cortical image from the two dissimilar stimulus patterns can militate against good reading performance." He suggested that anisometropia was more important in reading failure than equal refractive problems, no matter what type. To the clinician, this makes sense. If we assumed that visual stress is a valid cause of reading difficulty, a child trying to overcome uncorrected anisometropia is a prime candidate for a reading problem.

The correction of anisometropia can be handled in many ways. Contact lenses are the therapy of choice because they provide the best optical solution. Contact lenses create the most equal sized images in the brain when both eyes are properly corrected. This allows the best possibility of binocular vision. Some eye specialists do not take this course and may prescribe spectacles, which could be as effective. However, depending on the visual acuity available in each eye, some doctors may elect to prescribe for one eye alone and allow the other eye to suppress vision. Obviously this approach is open to question, but it is done many times. It is my philosophy to do all that I can to create binocular visual skills, so that allowing suppression would be the last choice. It must be remembered that patients with monocular vision may report less visual discomfort because there is no conflict between their eyes. However, if it is possible to create comfortable binocular vision, I believe it should be attempted.

Aniseikonia

Aniseikonia is a rare [3%–4% of the population (Burian et al., 1946)] visual disorder that can be quite debilitating. Normal images are of equal size and shape. This allows the brain to fuse them and project the visual image as a binocular, three-dimensional one. With aniseikonia the two optical images (one from each eye) record themselves on the brain as similar objects, but of different size and/or shape. Attempting to overcome the problem of trying to fuse unequal images, causes the patient visual stress, usually at the reading or working distance. The problem may be suspected when the patient presents with headaches and an inability to read comfortably and efficiently. Diagnosis can be made with an instrument called an eikonometer. The condition can be corrected with proper lenses designed to magnify one image to match the image size of the other eye; so that both images will then be able to fuse in the brain. Many "hopeless" reading problems have been corrected by judicious use of iseikonic lenses.

Dearborn and Anderson (1938) found that in a group of one hundred subjects, 51% of the reading disability group showed 1% or more of aniseikonia, while 23% of the control group had significant aniseikonic findings. Burian, Walsh, and Bannon (1946) hold that a difference of at least 0.75% size difference between ocular images is clinically significant. Dearborn and Anderson concluded that "aniseikonia is one of the many factors that may contribute to the causation and persistence of difficulty in reading." This interference with the ability to fuse may cause visual or general fatigue, leading to avoidance of reading tasks or seriously curtailing periods of concentration."

All studies have not come to the came conclusion. Imus, Rothney, and Bear (1938) in a survey at Dartmouth College, concluded that ocular defects, including aniseikonia, were no more common among deficient readers than the rest of the group. Rosenbloom (1968) in a study of 80 school children concluded that "aniseikonia could not be regarded as a major inhibiting factor to reading achievement." Spache (1940) concluded, however, that "aniseikonia seemed to hinder reading ability of younger students, but adults seemed to compensate for the difficulty." Personal clinical observations have led me to the conclusion that not all adults compensate for this disability. We have many patients that rely on proper eiseikonic lenses as the only means to comfortable reading.

Aniseikonia is a very specialized field of vision care. Few doctors work at this specialty and their expertise should be honored. A specialized instrument called an eikonometer is used for aniseikonia testing. Poor readers can be helped by wearing eiseikonic lenses when nothing else works. These lenses are difficult to design but may be the only solution to some patients' visual discomfort. When other visual tests fail to disclose a reason for discomfort, an aniseikonic examination could be useful.

Accommodation/Convergence Inefficiency or Insufficiency

There are four ocular-motor problems that are potential causes of reading disability. *Accommodation* enables the eyes to focus, i.e. to produce a clear image or correct a blurred image. Specifically, by contraction or relaxation of the ciliary body (a ring of muscle surrounding the perimeter of the crystalline lens), the lens' convexity can be varied to produce a clearer image on the retina. Young, healthy, properly functioning eyes are able to focus from 6 in. (or closer) to optical infinity (20 ft and beyond) with little or no effort. Of course, factors such as proper light and adequate size of print must be taken into account, but theoretically the focusing ability of eyes is limitless for people up until their early 20s. Afterwards there is slow but progressive reduction in focusing efficiency.

In addition, properly functioning eyes should be able to converge with little or no effort on an object as close as two or three inches in front of the nose. Convergence is the rotation of the eyes inwardly to point to an object. Convergence is accomplished by the extraocular muscles. The ability to read easily depends on the proper functioning of accomodation and convergence, working together. Physiologically, when accomodation is stimulated (when reading material is held close to the eyes), convergence is automatically enhanced. Conversely, if an object is held close to the eyes, the accommodation reflex will try to clear the image. All of this happens automatically so that one is rarely aware that many adjustments take place during all visual tasks. Only when accommodation and/or convergence is impaired, will symptoms appear that may be related to faulty visual skills. Headaches, fatigue (general or visual), inability to concentrate for long periods of time, holding the head close to the working surface, losing one's place while reading, and doubling of vision may be noticed and blamed on lack of interest. Obviously, a proper visual examination would determine whether these symptoms were physiological or psychological in nature.

From a practical point of view, whether the patient has insufficient accommodation or convergence or whether he is using his visual assets inefficiently is a moot point. Either way, the patient is not performing well and should be given proper therapy. This may be in the form of glasses to aid accommodation (readers over the age of 45 will understand the difficulty of reading easily without the need of longer arms to hold their reading matter), or eye exercises to enhance convergence abilities.

Some authors divide accommodative skills into three other specific categories. Woolf (1969) defines *accommodative accuracy* (aiming) as "the ability to focus eyes close to the point of regard." Inability to do this will cause the patient to hold his book either too close or too far, and to tend to move the book closer on new words. The eyes might tear, or he may report blurring of the print after a while. *Accommodative facility* (focusing) is defined as "the ability to control focus for all distances and when changing distances." A patient whose accommodative facility is impaired will report that he has to "make the vision clear" when looking from near to far, or from far to near. Woolf found that 80% of his sample of 100 children with reading problems had poor "aiming" and 70% had poor "focusing." Sherman (1973) reports that 76% of his sample of 50 children with "learning disability" had difficulty with *focus ability* and 88% had difficulty with *focus facility*.

Dynamic Accommodative Facility is a specific skill described by Taylor and Solan (1957) as the ability to clear reading material within four seconds for each presentation when a pair of + 2.00 and then a pair of -2.00 diopter lenses are placed before the eyes. This tests that ability of the eyes to quickly refocus when relaxing lenses (+ 2.00) and stimulating lenses (-2.00) are presented. Properly functioning young eyes (under the age of 35) should be able to pass this test. Patients who cannot do this will probably have difficulty in a classroom where they normally have to look up from a book to the blackboard and vice-versa. If they have trouble clearing either visual target, fatigue and avoidance may very well occur.

Ophthalmologists and optometrists differ regarding the importance of accommodation/convergence deficits in reading disabilities. Ophthalmological opinion is based on the strict interpretation of the Donders table and on the fact that eye muscles are usually 100 times "stronger" than they need to be to perform their normal function. Based on the theoretical norm, the ophthalmological view makes sense. However, little account is taken of individual differences, visual tasks normal to each individual, and most important, the use of excess energy, and subsequent stress, to achieve the theoretical norm. Wold (1971) concludes that " ... inefficient near-point binocular accommodative convergence relationship may cause undue stress and result in avoidance" of visual tasks.

Many ophthalmologists still routinely use the cycloplegic (a drug that paralyzes the accommodation of the eye) method of refraction for children. Yet, Sir W. Stewart Duke-Elder (1935), perhaps the most prestigious opthalmological spokesman stated, "The eye with its accommodation paralyzed is a pathological eye, and cannot be legitimately compared with the normal organ."

Clinical observation leaves little doubt about the importance of stress-free accommodation and convergence for the comfortably functioning student. To this end, many optometrists, following the lead of the above-mentioned Optometric Extension Program, and the clinical reports from the Gesell Institute (1950), routinely prescribe low-power plus lenses to students for near-point use. Such lenses aid the accommodative process and thereby lessen the likelihood of stress. Patient acceptance is extremely positive by both achievers and underachievers, both noting that they are able to read more comfortably for longer periods of time. Carter (1967) has reported that many underachievers show significant scholastic gains after receiving a low-power plus lens prescription for near use. Pierce (1968) reported that "prescribing low-powered (plus) lenses allows the child to pull accommodation in and effect an efficient binocular accommodative convergence relationship."

All of the accommodation or convergence problems described in this section may lead to visual discomfort. Accommodative or convergence problems may cause visual or general fatigue, inability to concentrate for long periods of time, avoidance of visual tasks, headaches, eyestrain, seeing double, or seeing blurred. There are three ways of dealing with such a syndrome: (1) It can be ignored with the position that it has nothing to do with reading difficulty. (2) One may prescribe appropriate lenses to stimulate or relax accommodation and/or convergence. (3) One may prescribe proper eye exercises (orthoptics) to specifically help the problem. In my experience approaches 2 and/or 3 are the ones most likely to produce alleviation of these difficulties. Orthoptics has been overplayed, misunderstood, or undervalued as an approach to correcting reading problems. The proper utilization of orthoptics is to create a vision climate that enables the patient to use his eyes comfortably and efficiently. Orthoptic techniques can be prescribed to overcome any accommodative and/or convergence problem and good patient cooperation can change a nonfunctioning visual patient into a comfortable functioning one.

Misunderstandings often arose from the presumption by many educators and other professionals that orthoptics alone would change a poor reader into a good one. In fact, orthoptics can only change the visual efficiency of the patient and, when it is done well, allow the patient to overcome his reading problems without visual stress. Of

course, the reading problems must be handled specifically by a specialist in that field. The vision therapy sharpens the tools of reading.

It is beyond the scope of this book to describe in detail the various
approaches to orthoptic training. When a patient is diagnosed as
having a possible orthoptic problem, the referral should be made to an
optometrist who concentrates on this specialty. He will be able to
determine the most judicious therapeutic approach to the specific
problems unearthed in diagnostic process. All of the accomodative
and convergence problems discussed in this section are amenable to
orthoptics.

Binocularity

There are three stages that make up the theoretical norm of visual
binocularity, which is the ability to use both eyes comfortably and efficiently as a team. The first stage is called *simultaneous binocular
vision*. This means that both eyes are seeing at the same time. The next,
fusion, describes the stage when both eyes lock onto a target and fuse
both images in the brain. The ultimate binocular visual skill, *stereopsis*,
is the state of three-dimensional vision, where the eyes and brain perceive depth. This can only be achieved when both eyes work properly
as a team.

Binocularity problems can be intermittent or continual. Continual
problems are easily observed by the parent or teacher without refined
diagnostic acumen. These visual anomolies are called *strabismus*,
squint, or, to the layman, crossed-eyes or wall-eyes. If the eyes, in fact,
do not point to the same point in space, the patient will not have fusion
and stereopsis, but may still have simultaneous binocular vision (SBV).
Unfortunately, this individual would see double. Normally, the brain
does not allow a person to see double; it suppresses (turns off) vision in
one eye and allows some relief from double vision. This can lead to
amblyopia, a condition in which in the extreme an eye's acuity may be
irreparably damaged, because it has been suppressed for so long.
Functioning as a one-eyed person may be less stressful than seeing
double. But if one eye stops working, nothing is left to yoke both eyes
together in the brain. Thus, there is the probability that one eye will
wander off center and create the cosmetic distress of crossed-eyes.
These are the children who are noticed and cared for. If there is no
visual therapy, at least nature takes a hand, suppresses the vision in
one eye, and allows the patient to function adequately.

The patient with simultaneous binocular vision but only *intermittent fusion* has the most potential for learning and reading problems. This is the child who may show excellent visual acuity and, to the

unsophisticated observer, appears to have "perfect" eyes. By probing with dynamic visual tests the eye specialist will uncover findings that point to a stress situation. If the binocularity is very tenuous, the patient may be a nonreader, completely avoiding any near-point visual tasks. If the binocularity is fragile, the patient may be able to function for a short period of time before the stress is too great to overcome. At this point he will quit, and may become known as a student who never finishes work or is lazy. Proper visual tests will uncover these problems. Appropriate visual therapy provides a good possibility to overcome or ameliorate these problems. At least, a potential reason for learning difficulty will be uncovered.

Despite the logic of this approach, the role of binocularity in reading disability is still in dispute. Again, the optometric literature has much discussion of the importance of binocularity, and ophthalmological publications tend to put down its importance. Swanson (1972) describes some students who are good spellers and good readers "especially on a short paragraph test, but cannot complete a one or a two hour examination. The visual skills, such as fusion, fixation, convergence, and focus (accommodation) simply give out." He cites a study of 100 children with learning problems. Among the problems uncovered, the following pertain to this discussion:

30% had convergence excess (a tendency of the eyes to turn inward)

17% had divergence excess (a tendency of the eyes to turn outward)

25% had fusion anomalies (inadequate fusion, suppressions)

37% had low fusional reserves (the ability to maintain single vision (SBV) under stress)

27% had oculomotor problems (usually unstable control of the eyes)

25% had accommodative insufficiency (difficulty maintaining a clear image, or lack of flexibility)

Shorr and Svagr (1966) concluded that, "The present research indicates that the one perceptual-motor skill group which cannot be compensated for, is the ability to make smooth conjunctive use of the two eyes in the reading act." Friedman (1971) concurs by saying, "My own experience has been that most of us suppress images because of the discomfort and visual annoyance, however slight at times, which we commonly experience during binocular fixation. If we have to strive and struggle visually to any degree to bring the two images of an object into ... [functional] unity, we surely try reflex[ive]ly to rescue the eyes from the fusional annoyance by removing or suppressing one or a part of one of the images out of the fusional picture." Smith (1971) adds to this philosophy by saying, "While constant suppression or amblyopia are not culpable factors, intermittent suppression and intermittent diplopia and intermittent low angle strabismus or high heterophorias can be contributing factors in disabilities of reading and learning." Woolf (1969), in describing the profile of the dyschriescopic child (a child with awkward, or "hard to use" vision) shows that, among other problems, 80% had a "poor aiming" problem, 70% had a "poor focus-ing" problem, and 80% had a "poor teaming" problem. Despite the overwhelming evidence from the optometric point of view that binocu-larity problems are an important cause of reading disability, ophthal-mologists, in general, still cling to the traditional 20/20 concept of "perfect vision." The importance of functions other than visual acuity, as they relate to dyslexia, was denied formally in a joint statement of the American Academy of Ophthalmology and the American Academy of Pediatrics in "The Eye and Learning Disabilities" (1972).

Intermittent problems of binocularity are particularly suited to orthoptic intervention. Strabismus, however, is not easily handled. The approach depends on the amount of eye turn found, the direction, and the visual acuity available in the turned eye. More sophisticated testing is necessary to determine the best way to handle the individual problem. When the eye turn is extreme surgical intervention is pre-ferred. However, with the right kind of orthoptic care, time, patience, and parental and patient cooperation, surgery may not be necessary. Ludlam (1961) reports on 149 cases of varied types of strabismics cared for orthoptically alone. The results show that 76% of the sample were *functionally* cured, that is, the eyes were straight cosmetically and they were binocular 95% of the time or better. Surgical interven-tion may result in immediate cosmetic improvement, but unless the eyes are trained to function as a team, most patients lose their good cosmetic appearance and return for further surgery. I have seen some patients who have had up to four surgical interventions over a period of years and have ended up with no binocularity, poor vision in one eye, poor cosmesis, and scar tissue around the extraocular eye muscles.

Krimsky (1948) states that, "Eye muscle surgery may be safely performed at all ages, provided surgery is really necessary to help sight or to straighten the eyes.... One aims to avoid too much surgery at any age even if the cross-eye cannot be completely corrected." He goes on to say, however, that "Reeducation of the eyes, know as binocular training (orthoptics), frequently proves extremely valuable and suc-cessful in selected cases. The true aim of such training is not to strengthen the eye muscles, as some believe, but to educate the eyes to cooperate more intimately with the brain. Through such training both eyes become alive to each other and learn to focus in unison." Despite this statement by a highly respected surgeon many ophthalmologists consider surgery the only "cure" for strabismus. Parents, torn between two opposing points of view, may need some knowledgeable advice from the MBD counselor.

Surgery or orthoptics are not the only approach to the care of strabismus. Proper eyeglasses, including bifocals, or specific drugs have been used in dealing with crossed eyes. If we understand that the eyes are controlled by the brain, then a lasting, functional "cure" must include retraining the brain to utilize the eyes properly. If the results are only cosmetic, the patient will still have uncomfortable, stressful vision, certainly not the kind that will function well in a learning situation.

Phorias

Phorias are tendencies of eyes to turn relative to each other under a test situation and are measured in prism-diopters. They may range anywhere from orthophoria, where the eyes are exactly straight, to large amounts of turn. Most findings are within 10 prism-diopters. Measurements can be made to ½ prism-diopter, but this fine a gradation is more theoretical than clinical. Phorias can be measured by many different tests. Basic findings should be generally the same no matter which technique is used. Phorias should be evaluated both at distance (20 ft) and near point (16 in.). The findings are subjective (because the examiner must rely on the patient's responses), and may vary from time to time, but in general we find that the results of testing are quite stable from year to year. What one does with the findings is the key to their use in the visual diagnosis of MBD.

Lateral Eye Postures

Exophoria is the tendency for the eyes to turn outward. Clinically, I would accept 2 to 6 prism-diopters of exophoria as the norm at a distance, and 4 to 10 prism-diopters at the near point. Patients who manifest these degrees of exophoria rarely complain of visual discomfort. Higher amounts of exophoria would be suspect and further questions might be posed to be certain that the patient is not accepting some discomfort or inefficiency unnecessarily. I would want to know of any eye or general fatigue, any tendency to stop reading sooner than the patient would want to or need to, and headaches that might not be attributable to the eyes.

Anapolle (1971), in a study of 482 dyslexic students, found that 48.5% exhibited exophoria for distance, and 43.6% for near-point tests. He does not give his criteria for the amount of exophoria that he considers significant. Kelly (1957) does not consider exophoria a problem, but considers esophoria a significant cause of reading problems. Eames (1938) found all distance phoria findings inconclusive, but he stated that any variation from orthophoria at near point is significant. Shearer (1938) found exophoria in about 10% of children with reading difficulties at the near point.

Esophoria is a tendency for the eyes to turn inward. Clinically, this is a most significant finding. Patients who show even small amounts of esophoria at distance, but especially at near point, are suspect in terms of visual stress. These are the patients who will report inability to concentrate for long periods of time. They will manifest their problem to the skilled observer by holding their reading material close to their eyes (less than 12 in.) or "putting their noses into their work." It must be pointed out, however, that the normal reading distance also depends on the arm length of the individual. A tall adult with long arms will more likely read beyond a "normal" 16-in., while a short adult may normally hold the print 13 in. from his eyes. Of course, a child will generally hold his book relatively close. The rule of thumb that we use is that the reading distance should be at, or farther than, the distance equal to the length between the child's elbow and knuckle. Anyone holding reading material closer than that is in a visually stressful situation and probably will show esophoria in testing. This makes physiological sense. If the eyes turn inward more than the normal amount necessary to converge on a printed word, the patient will subconsciously bring the reading material to where the eyes are pointed, instead of pointing the eyes to where the reading material should be.

As with all visual skills, one cannot be isolated from the others. Phoria measurements alone, without consideration of the patients' refractive status (myopic or hyperopic), would not be significant. Esophoria combined with hyperopia may be controlled simply by prescribing plus lenses to correct the farsightedness, thereby minimizing the esophoric effect. Minus lenses correcting a myope would maximize an esophoric problem and possibly cause discomfort for reading. Conversely, a myopic exophore would probably function well with his distance glasses, but a myopic esophore might be uncomfortable if he read with his distance glasses. All of this theory relates to the previous discussion on the intimate relationship between accommodation and convergence, where plus lenses, used for hyperopic patients, relax accommodation, and minus lenses, used for myopic patients, stimulate accommodation. Stimulation of accommodation automatically stimu-

lates convergence, and relaxation of accommodation relaxes convergence. There seems to be a fascinating parallel between esophoria and
the development of myopia. Statistics accumulated at Annapolis
(Hayden, 1941) and other schools (Dunphy, 1968) showed an increase
in nearsightedness after four years of extensive studying. Midshipmen
who were accepted because of superior physical attributes, including
eyesight, left the Naval Academy with acquired myopia. In my own
practice, dozens of senior law students have reported the same history:
excellent vision until their extensive reading for exams and the bar.
Then, all showed changes towards myopia. There seems to be enough
clinical evidence to suggest the importance of near-point visual stress.
Esophoria seems to be the clinical warning sign. I want to reemphasize
that these findings alone do not cause learning disability, but they can
contribute to stress and discomfort, which in turn create a poor, or
nonreader.

The intervention of the eye specialist in either exophoria or esophoria is generally dependent on the amount of eye turn shown in a
diagnostic workup and the needs of the individual. For instance, a
student with high degrees of exophoria or esophoria would more likely
be visually uncomfortable than a farmer with the same findings. Specific visual needs will determine the type of treatment. Proper eyeglass
prescription, in single lens, or bifocal form, will generally alleviate
most phoria problems. On occasion, orthoptics may be prescribed on a
short-term or long-term basis in office or at home, to retrain the eyes to
function comfortably. The key to proper care is to diagnose the problem as a component of reading disability and choose the method best
suited to relieve it.

Vertical Eye Posture

Of all the visual functions, I believe that vertical muscle posture
(hyperphoria for one of the eyes tending to point up) is the most important, and probably the most controversial. For some reason that
clinical experience belies, vertical phorias are generally glossed over
in the professional training of eye practitioners. However, I would
judge that 25–30% of my patients have a clinically significant degree
of hyperphoria.

Roy (1954), Jacques (1957), and Denton et al. (1954), discuss the
importance of hyperphoria from a clinical point of view and acknowl-
edge the fact that this subject receives slight attention in the literature. Fink (1953) offers a scholarly paper on the etiological considerations
of hyperphoria, but fails to present the clinical importance of the
problem. He does, however, state that " ... major defects are readily
recognized because of the binocular problem which is usually present.

Slight defects are frequently not evident and are discovered only on careful examination. However, minor defects are of considerable importance because they may be a factor in the development of squint at a later date, if for some reason binocularity fails to function."

Hyperphoria can, and does exist with binocularity. However, while trying to keep the eyes working together, the visual system is under constant stress adjusting for a vertical muscle discrepancy. This, in turn, leads to symptoms of discomfort and avoidance that the patient may not attribute to his eyes. Only careful diagnostic procedures followed by therapy will alleviate hyperphoric problems. These are the signs to look for: Head tilt to any observable degree, loss of place from line to line on a printed page, nausea while reading in a moving vehicle, neck and shoulder strain, photophobia (light sensitivity), vague but disturbing visual discomfort in a crowded environment such as a supermarket or department store. These patients function, but not comfortably and efficiently. Many times the symptoms persist for so long that they become a way of life and are accepted as "normal." On occasion I have had patients report daily headaches, accept them, and take 12 aspirins a day regularly, with no thought that something was unusual. I do not suggest that all headaches and "vague" symptoms are due to hyperphoria. I do suggest, however, that when these symptoms occur, a careful evaluation for hyperphoria is warranted. An interesting way to corroborate one's suspicion of vertical phoria is to look at old snapshots of the patient. It is likely that a head tilt will be evident in many of the pictures.

If there is disagreement over the importance of hyperphoria, there is even more question about the amount that is significant enough to correct. Although a small amount of hyperphoria (½ prism diopter) can create untold visual discomfort in some sensitive patients, others will shrug off 7 prism-diopters. However, there is logic to this. With the small amount, the brain will attempt to compensate for the problem by tilting the head, by pulling the eyes level (with expenditure of energy), causing symptoms of discomfort. With a large amount, perhaps 5 prism diopters or more, it is impossible for the brain to compensate. Therefore one eye will be suppressed, avoiding the binocular conflict that creates discomfort. Rarely will the brain allow the patient to see double. The brain will suppress the vision in one eye or attempt to fuse the two disparate images in order to avoid diplopia (seeing double). All of this occurs with great use of energy, eventually leading to avoidance of the visual task. It is conceivable that small, undetected amounts of hyperphoria play a decided role in the visual aspects of reading disabilities. It would be wrong to presume that a patient with a reading disability passed a vision examination, without carefully exploring the possibility of a latent problem of hyperphoria.

When hyperphoria is disclosed, the problem can be alleviated by the proper prescription of prism lenses. The prism is designed to counteract the muscle posture of the eyes. A prism is prescribed, usually in spectacle form, to bend the incoming image in one eye to match the incoming image to the other eye. For instance, if 2 prism-diopters with its base up is prescribed so that it bends the higher image of the right eye a distance of 2 prism-diopters in order to match the image of the left eye. This will level both images and avoid the need for the brain to do the same work.

The amount of hyperphoria may not be static. Careful follow-up care is essential to make sure that the patient maintains comfortable vision. My experience has been that once a prescribed amount of prism is worn for a period of one to two months, latent amounts of additional hyperphoria may emerge. Theoretically, the eyes, freed from some amount of stress, relax more and show some residual hyperphoria. This is easily corrected by adjusting the amount of prism prescribed. Once the eyes achieve a final balance, the situation remains stable for long periods of time. It is important to emphasize that the prisms must be worn when visual needs are critical. My experience has shown that the relief obtained with prisms allows many patients to function at a level that they never thought possible.

Fixation Abilities

Fixation enables the eye to aim precisely and easily. Although the fixation functions are generally taken for granted, they may not be easily accomplished and may contribute to reading inefficiency. When we look at an object, we turn our eyes so that the macula of the eye is pointing directly at the object. The macula, or fovea, is a tiny area in the retina that allows us our most precise visual acuity. If our eyes shift even a millimeter off the macula, our visual acuity drops precipitously. Therefore, in all visual tasks the macula is the focal point of seeing. It is relatively rare, other than by accident, that a macula is damaged in a young person. In older people, pathological problems can make a macula nonfunctional. There is interference with macular function in children with amblyopia (lazy-eye). If the problem is diagnosed at an early age, preferably by the age of four, therapeutic measures can hopefully retrain the macular area to function normally. Without normal macular function, fixation cannot be precise. Fixation ability may be broken down into three distinct categories.

Direct Fixation

Direct fixation is the ability to aim the eyes at a specific point anywhere in space. If we look 20 ft and beyond (optical infinity) the eyes should be lined up parallel to each other. If we fixate at a word in a book, the eyes (in reality, the maculae) should point inward to that word. Both maculae pointing at that spot will provide the person with single, binocular vision. If one eye is deviated, even slightly, the brain will receive two disparate images and will be under stress to fuse them or will suppress one image.

Pursuit Fixation

Pursuit fixation is the ability of the eyes to smoothly follow a moving object. This skill is generally taken for granted, but it requires complex use of the eyes. Each eye is moved by six muscles. In order to turn the eyes to the right, the outer lateral muscle of the right eye must contract while the inner laterial muscle relaxes. At the same time, the left inner lateral muscle must contract, while the left outer lateral muscle relaxes. Even a simple eye movement such as looking to the right requires smooth and efficient movements of four eye muscles. Turning our eyes upward, downward, and diagonally is much more complex. Following a moving object is a very complicated orchestration of 12 eye muscles constantly relaxing and contracting in proper sequence. In most persons these motions occur thousands of times a day automatically. When a patient has eye coordination problems, all the muscle movements we take for granted become a chore, use untold amounts of energy, and may lead to avoidance of visual tasks that require regular coordinated movement. Of course, reading is a task that utilizes pursuit movements.

Saccadic Fixation

Saccadic fixation is the ability to move the eyes accurately and smoothly from one point to another and stop precisely at each point. This ability, best of all, describes the act of reading. In order to read (English) we start at the left side of the page, sweep our eyes to the right, stop at the end of the line, sweep back to the left side and one line down, stop precisely at the beginning of the first word, sweep across the page to the right, stop, etc. The good reader will do this automatically, precisely, and with a minimum of effort.

Consider the reader with problems of saccadic fixation. If every time his eyes have to stop, they overshoot or undershoot that point, the measures taken by the brain to correct the problem uses excessive amounts of energy. After reading a page of print in this manner, it is conceivable that the student will quit, fatigued and disgusted, and avoid the next bout with the book.

Poor, or inadequate fixation abilities are usually easily solved with vision training. Most of the time, simple home training techniques will alleviate any poor fixation abilities. Enjoyable games can be prescribed by the eye specialist to improve fixation. If the patient and the parent are cooperative, this problem is short-lived and can be eliminated as a cause of visual discomfort.

Since all fixation abilities are important in vision comfort and are usually learned spontaneously early in development, many good nursery and elementary schools include fixation ability exercises as part of their program.

Summary

To summarize this section on visual problems affecting learning:

1. If the student has healthy eyes, good visual acuity for both far and near, has properly functioning binocular vision, the probability is that his eyes are not contributing to a reading or learning problem.
2. If a student has gross visual defects such as poor vision, especially at the far point, obvious strabismus, or other signs of difficulty, the probability is that someone will be alerted and attempt to correct the gross problem. If it was a major contributing factor to a learning disorder then the correction of the problem facilitates educational retraining.
3. If the student has good visual acuity, especially at distance, but poor binocular skills, the visual problem may be overlooked. Subtle, but constant stress will debilitate this patient, and until the visual component of his problem is found and corrected, other means of rehabilitation may be frustrated.

Evaluation of Visual Abilities

Complete Vision Examinations

If all children could have professional vision examinations by the age of 5, and then be routinely reexamined every couple of years, few would be troubled by visual stress. A well-designed examination that assesses all of the skills that have been discussed would detect a visual problem early and allow for proper therapy. Preventive prescriptions, spectacles, and/or vision training are plausible when one can anticipate the visual needs of a patient during the next year. The prescription is designed to prevent visual stress.

Parents' Observations

An alert and aware parent is the best line of defense against early visual problems. Parents must be educated to be suspicious of signs that children show at home: rubbing their eyes frequently, blinking excessively, frowning, scowling, squinting, tilting their heads, covering or closing one eye, reddened eyes or lids, repeated headaches, unusual posture when reading or writing, and others that will be listed later in this chapter.

Many parents who have had visual problems themselves will usually be more aware than others of the early signs of visual difficulties. Most seem to depend on the pediatrician or school nurse to alert them to their child's vision difficulties.

Teachers' Observations

Teachers have to be educated to notice students with visual problems. In addition to the symptoms listed above, the teacher should be alert to the students who skip words or sentences, use a finger or marker when reading, move their heads while reading, avoid close work, complain of blur while reading or writing, write crookedly or space poorly, or have difficulty copying from the blackboard.

With proper training, teachers would be more suspicious of students exhibiting the aforementioned symptoms and would be less likely to assume that these manifestations were only bad habits to be ignored. The teacher should be responsible to alert parents and/or the school nurse that the student might have a vision problem.

The School Nurse

The school nurse should be aware of the symptoms that we have discussed so far. If students with such difficulties are not brought to her attention she cannot be expected to discover them. Many schools have vision screening programs and place the responsibility on the school nurse to administer them properly. This is where her specific training and judgment come into play. If she is eyesight oriented, she may be content to use the Snellen chart as the sole testing device. If she is vision oriented, she can create a more extensive vision screening program. Once a child is found to have one or more visual skills defects, the nurse can only recommend that the parents take the child for more comprehensive eye care. It will then be up to the examining doctor to determine the mode of treatment.

One of the serious problems that has arisen over the last 15 years is the question of "over-referral." School nurses using sophisticated screening equipment uncovered many children with vision difficulties other than distance-vision deficiency. When such a child saw an eye practitioner who only tested distance vision, the parents were told that the child's eyes were "perfect." This kind of frustration causes school nurses to simplify their testing and only refer the very obvious problems for further care. Consequently, the children who need care the most are bypassed. It is important for nurses to understand the criteria used to refer students and to have enough conviction in their screening to stand up to the erring practitioner and demand further testing.

The Pediatrician

Most parents are dependent on the pediatrician to alert them to their children's eye problems. They assume that the pediatrician routinely checks the eyes and will be aware of the need for referral to an eye practitioner. This is certainly true of many pediatricians. It is not the rule for all. Some pediatricians have elaborate vision screening devices, but most depend on the Snellen chart. Therefore, their criteria for referral may be inadequate. Meanwhile the parents presume that all is well with their child's vision and neglect to program routinely a professional vision evaluation.

Vision Screening

Over 50 years ago, the Parents Teachers Association began to recommend vision screening programs (Price, 1969). In 1934 the National Society for the Prevention of Blindness added emphasis to the PTA vision program (McKee, 1972). School systems throughout the country embarked on vision screening programs utilizing standardized testing equipment, or creating programs of their own. In 1961 the Euclid, Ohio public schools published the "Blueprint for Vision Screening." Prince George's County, Maryland reported on a vision screening program for preschool children (Burman, 1959). Leverett (1955) described a Danbury, Connecticut school vision health study. Perhaps the most accepted study is the one designed for the Orinda, California school system in 1958 (Peters et al., 1959). These programs vary from the primitive to the most sophisticated.

It is the purpose of a good vision screening program to find children with vision problems that might interfere with their learning. A good program should be quick and accurate, should assess important vision skills, and should be inexpensive. It must be emphasized that a screening program is not a thorough vision examination. Therefore, some children will be properly referred for further testing, but others might not have the visual difficulties that the screening is designed to detect. Professional monitoring of the program should maintain a high degree of accurate referral.

About a half-dozen professional screening devices have found their way into the market and some of these are to be found in school programs. The available screening devices most familiar to the vision community are the Titmus Optical Tester, the Keystone Telebinocular, the Bausch & Lomb Orthorator, the American Optical Sight-Screener, and the American Optical Massachusetts Vision Test. All of these instruments sell for several hundred dollars and provide preprinted answer sheets. When these instruments are used, the pass/fail criteria established by the manufacturer must be accepted. However, it is quite possible that a professional committee involved in a vision screening program could establish pass/fail criteria of its own. Either way, deciding on this crucial point is paramount when creating a useful screening program. These instruments assess up to a dozen visual skills and referrals are determined by the parts of the test that are failed. The examiner must decide where the line is drawn for referral. A well-run screening program may utilize lay personnel for the actual testing. If tight guidelines are drawn for pass/fail, there is little question of interpretation.

Table 8.1 compares the pass/fail criteria designed into the aforementioned systems. It is important to reemphasize that defining the criteria used in any of the screening systems is of prime importance. Many children with potential visual problems will be bypassed with loose criteria or by eliminating some of the tests. Keeping criteria too tight will defeat the purpose of screening: to discover students with *potential* visual problems without requiring a complete visual analysis for all children.

The Schrier Vision Screening Test

In my many talks with pediatricians and school nurses, the conclusion I generally came away with was that they would appreciate a simple, inexpensive, but comprehensive vision screening device for routine use. Most schools would not invest $500–$600 for a sophisticated vision screening instrument, and most pediatricians wanted a device that their nurses could use quickly and routinely with all their young patients. Keeping these requests in mind, I designed a test that simply designated "pass/fail" using criteria that generally conformed to current screening devices and to my own clinical observations. The device had to give much more information than the simple $2 Snellen test chart, furnish the data that the expensive systems provide, and cost considerably less than $550.

Table 8.1
Fail Criteria of Vision Screening Instruments.

Test Performed	Schrier Vision Screening Test	NSPB & ASHA[a]	Titmus Tester	Keystone Telebinocular	B & L Orthorater	A.O. Sightscreener	Massachusetts Test
Distance visual acuity (right eye) 20 ft	< 20/30	K–3 20/40 or less 4 and up 20/30 or less	< 20/30	< 20/30	< 20/20	< 20/20	< 20/20
Distance visual acuity (left eye) 20 ft	< 20/30	K–3 20/40 or less 4 and up 20/30 or less	< 20/30	< 20/30	< 20/20	< 20/20	< 20/20
Distance visual acuity through + 2.00 lenses 20 ft	> 20/30	K–3 + 2.25 (20/20) 4 and up + 1.75 (20/20)	20/20	Not applicable	Not applicable	Not applicable	20/20
Lateral phoria 20 ft	> 4$^{\Delta}$[b] esophoria > 8$^{\Delta}$ exophoria	> 6$^{\Delta}$ esophoria > 4$^{\Delta}$ exophoria	> 6$^{\Delta}$ esophoria > 4$^{\Delta}$ exophoria	> 4$^{\Delta}$ esophoria > 6$^{\Delta}$ exophoria	> 7$^{\Delta}$ esophoria > 5$^{\Delta}$ exophoria	> 7$^{\Delta}$ esophoria > 5$^{\Delta}$ exophoria	> 6$^{\Delta}$ esophoria > 4$^{\Delta}$ exophoria
Vertical phoria 20 ft	> 1$^{\Delta}$	> 1$^{\Delta}$	> 1¼$^{\Delta}$	> 1$^{\Delta}$	> 1$^{\Delta}$	> 1$^{\Delta}$	> 1¼$^{\Delta}$
Near-point visual acuity (right eye) 16 in.	< 20/30	Not applicable	Examiner's decision	< 20/25	< 20/20	< 20/20	Not applicable
Near-point visual acuity (left eye) 16 in.	< 20/30	Not applicable	Examiner's decision	< 20/25	< 20/20	< 20/20	Not applicable
Lateral phoria 16 in.	> 2$^{\Delta}$ esophoria > 10$^{\Delta}$ exophoria	> 6$^{\Delta}$ esophoria > 8$^{\Delta}$ exophoria	> 6$^{\Delta}$ esophoria > 8$^{\Delta}$ exophoria	> 6$^{\Delta}$ esophoria > 8$^{\Delta}$ exophoria	> 7½$^{\Delta}$ esophoria > 9$^{\Delta}$ exophoria	> 8$^{\Delta}$ esophoria > 9$^{\Delta}$ exophoria	> 6$^{\Delta}$ esophoria > 8$^{\Delta}$ exophoria

[a] National Society for the Prevention of Blindness and the American School Health Association
[b] Δ = prism-diopter

In order to standardize the data, all variables are built into the instrument including lighting and a 20 ft measuring tape. However, since many offices will not have 20 ft for testing, a 10-ft chart is available. The test charts are designed to be easily cleaned or changed.

The Schrier Vision Screening Test is a two-part instrument. One part is provided for distance vision testing (at 10 or 20 ft), (Figure 8.1), and the other part is hand-held for near-point testing (Figure 8.2). The distance chart is self-illuminated, while the near-point chart is used with illumination generally available in a school or doctor's office. A gooseneck lamp with a 75-watt bulb will provide proper illumination for the near-point test.

Accessories are included in the screening kit: A clear Maddox rod (a lens etched with parallel lines), an occluder, a pair of + 2D lenses in a holder, and a Worth 4-Dot Test (built into a hand-held flashlight) with accompanying red-green glasses. Test sheets (Table 8.2) are included.

The test sheet is designed to provide the examiner with clear-cut criteria for referral, which is based in failure of any portion of the screening. If the Schrier Vision Screening Test is used in school screenings, lay people can administer the test.

The pass/fail criteria are generally accepted by the ophthalmic community (Table 8.1). The only major deviation is the lateral phoria criteria. I have found clinically, as I have discussed earlier, that visual discomfort will occur more readily with esophoric findings than with moderate exophoric findings. Thus, the fail criteria are more weighed in the esophoric direction.

Figure 8.1
Distance Vision Chart for the Schrier Vision Screening Test.

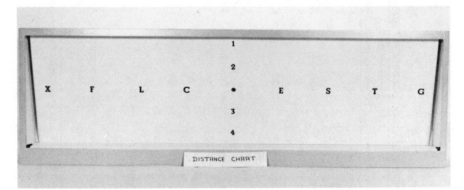

Figure 8.2
Near-Point Chart and Accessories for the Schrier Vision Screening Test.

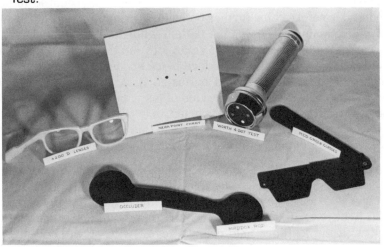

Table 8.2
Schrier Vision Screening Test.

Name:		Age:		Grade:
School:		Date:		
		Wearing Glasses:	Yes___	No___

	Pass	Fail	Comments
Distance visual acuity (20/30)			
Right eye (6 letters correct—pass)			
Left eye (6 letters correct—pass)			
Plus lens test			
Both eyes (all letters blurred—pass)			
Vertical white-line test (between S and X—pass)			
Horizontal white-line test (between 2 and 3—pass)			
Near visual acuity			
Right eye (6 letters correct—pass)			
Left eye (6 letters correct—pass)			
Vertical white-line test (between S and X—pass)			
Worth 4-dot test (4 dots—pass)			
Total evaluation			

Using the Instrument

The test for distance visual acuity. This test utilizes the line of eight 20/30 letters on the distance visual target. The patient is positioned (either sitting or standing) 10 or 20 ft from the chart. (The instrument is designed to be used at either 10 or 20 ft depending on the amount of space available.) If the patient can see at least six of the letters with his right *and* left eyes, with his normal vision (with or without glasses), he passes this part of the test. If he cannot he is considered to have failed and is referred for further optometric or ophthalmologic evaluation. The examiner observes the patient while he reads the chart and notes whether he works hard or squints to see the target. Each eye is occluded separately with a standard black occluder provided with the screener. The right eye should be tested first, then the left eye. Because children hate to "fail" any kind of test, and because only one line of letters is presented, it is suggested that one patient at a time be present for the testing, otherwise those in line will have memorized the letters and negate the validity of this section of the test.

Distance Visual Acuity Through Plus Lenses. This is a most important screening test to detect farsightedness (hyperopia). After the patient has been asked to read the distance line of letters with his normal vision (with or without glasses) a pair of + 2.00 diopter lenses (provided with the test) are held over the eyes (with or without glasses). If the patient *can* read the letters one can conclude that he is using excess energy to focus and he may be under visual stress. Accordingly, he is considered to have failed the test and should be referred. Lenses of + 2.00 diopter power were chosen because most studies and present screening devices utilize this lens as the maximum power that can be cleared by the patient before excess stress is used to see clearly.

Distance Lateral Phoria. This is tested with the red light on the distance visual target and the Maddox rod. The lines in a Maddox rod (a lens with parallel lines etched into it) are lined up horizontally in front of the subject's right eye as he looks at the light. This will create a situation where the right eye sees a vertical white line while his left eye sees the small red light. The subject is asked where he sees the vertical line. If he sees it directly through the light his eyes are parallel to each other. If he sees the line to the right of the light he is esophoric; the further to the right, the more esophoric. If he sees the line to the left of the light, he is exophoric. The placement of the target letters is designed to measure the amount of phoria. Specifically, if the line is at the letter S or beyond, referrable esophoria is present. If it is at the letter X or beyond, referrable exophoria is present.

Distance Vertical Phoria. This is tested by shifting the Maddox rod 90° in front of the right eye so that the parallel lines are in the vertical position. The patient will then see a horizontal white line and the red light. He is to report where he sees the line in relation to the red light. If the line is seen passing directly through the light, or anywhere between the numbers 2 and 3, referrable phoria is not present. If the line appears above the number 2 or below the number 3, a hyperphoric condition exists and the patient should be referred. Clinical observation has shown that the vertical finding using the near-point target will generally be the same as for the distant target. Therefore, for the purposes of screening, vertical phoria is only tested at the far point. This approach is utilized by all of the aforementioned screening devices.

Near-point Visual Acuity Tests.   These tests are performed with the subject holding the reading target 16 in. from his eyes. Young subjects may normally hold the reading target closer. If they hold it closer than 12 in., this should be noted on the test sheet. Otherwise, a few inches closer than the prescribed 16 in. is not significant. Subjects should be able to read 8 of the 10 letters of the 20/30 near-point size target with or without normal glasses under a 75-watt lamp. If they do not, or if they assume an unusual posture while reading the letters, they should be referred for professional evaluation.

Near-point Lateral Phoria.   Testing is similar to distance testing. The parallel lines of the Maddox rod are held horizontally in front of the right eye and the patient is asked to look at the light in his reading target at his normal reading posture. When the vertical white line is seen directly through the red light, there is no phoria. When the vertical white line seen to the right, at the letter S or beyond, referrable esophoric is present. When the white line is seen to the left of the red light at the letter X or beyond, referrable exophoria is present.

Binocularity.   Binocularity is tested with the Worth 4-Dot Test. If both eyes are not functioning together, the test will show which eye is suppressing vision. This is a rather gross determination of binocularity, but it is adequate for screening purposes.

The examiner holds the flashlight (the face of the flashlight shows four dots: two green, one red, and one white) about 3 ft from the subject, at eye level, and points the face of the flashlight towards the subject's eyes. The subject holds the red-green glasses in front of his eyes, with the red over the right eye. The subject reports how many dots he sees through the red-green glasses. If he sees four, both eyes are functioning together and binocularity is present. If he reports seeing two red dots his right eye is seeing, but his left eye is suppressing. If he reports three green dots, his left eye is working and his right eye is suppressing.

The examiner need only mark "pass" or "fail" on the data sheet (Table 8.2) for each part of the test. If there is one failure, the subject should be referred for professional confirmation and treatment.

In summary, it is important to understand the reasoning behind the design of any visual screening device. If the importance of *all* the visual skills are accepted as significant in the evaluation of reading disability problems, then a coherent program (no matter which one) of vision testing should be included in any total evaluation. In order not to overlook any visual problem as a component of reading disability, none of the described tests should be eliminated.

Dr. Schrier's section was included by me to acquaint the reader with present optometric views regarding ocular-visual disorders in MBD. The controversy surrounding the role of such deficits in MBD will only be resolved by well-controlled studies. Until such experiments are done the reader should consider the possibility that ocular-visual problems are contributing to his patient's difficulties and include in his MBD battery the kind of examination described by Dr. Schrier.

VISUAL DISCRIMINATION

By visual discrimination, I refer to those processes that enable the individual to differentiate between two visual stimuli, to ascertain whether they are the same or different. There are some who prefer to use the term visual perception for this function. One advantage of this use of the term is that it might lessen confusion about what *perception* means. Operationally, visual differentiation is relatively easy to define and evaluate. It is not difficult to be objective about whether or not an individual recognizes visual stimuli to be the same or different. However, because this relatively narrow definition of perception has not enjoyed widespread use and because many use it to include other phenomena such as organization capacity and comprehension, I prefer to avoid using the term perception entirely and use visual differentiation or visual discrimination.

The Colored Progressive Matrices

In 1947 Raven introduced the test that is commonly referred to as Raven's Colored Progressive Matrices. My discussion here is based on the 1956 revision (Raven, 1956). The test consists of 36 plates divided into 3 series of 12. In each series the questions progress from the simplest to the most difficult. Basically, each plate consists of a pattern with a defect. Below each pattern are 6 segments, 1 of which correctly fills the defect in the larger pattern (Figure 8.3). When administering the test the child is told: "Look at this. A bit of this pattern," moving his finger across the design and pausing in the space, "has been cut out. We want to find it and put it back in position. It has been put with these." The examiner then points to the 6 segments below the pattern. "Now you point to the one that best fits into the hole."

Figure 8.3
Raven's Colored Progressive Matrices.

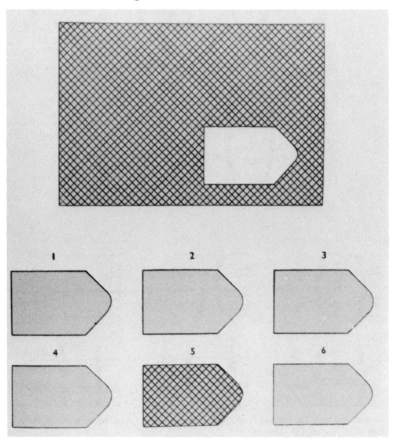

Unfortunately, the more difficult items (those near the end of each series of 12) not only test visual discrimination, but visual conceptualization as well. As can be seen in Figure 8.4, the child must consider three factors: (1) thick line pattern, (2) double thin line pattern, and (3) curve direction. The child must extrapolate from the adjacent curves and try to determine the directions that the lines will take as they pass through the defect area. Actually, the conceptualization capacity required for successful completion of the plate depicted in Figure 8.4 is relatively easy compared to some of the more complex patterns presented to the child near the end of the third set of 12 plates. Visual differentiation capacity in these final plates is a minor

Figure 8.4
Raven's Colored Progressive Matrices.

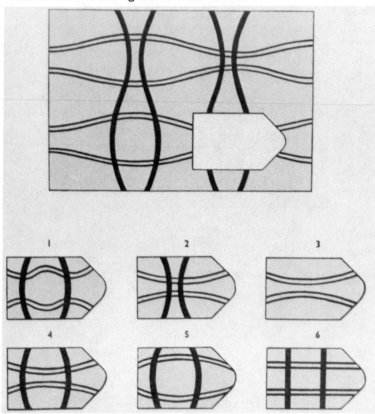

Reproduced from *The Colored Progressive Matrices* by Dr. John C. Raven with the permission of J.C. Raven, Ltd., London.

consideration compared to the complex kinds of conceptualization being assessed. This contamination, notwithstanding, I find the test a useful one. Most children enjoy doing the test and rise to the challenge. The child who does well can be said to be adequate in both visual differentiation and visual conceptualization. The child who does poorly, however, may do so because of impairment(s) in one or both of these functions. Only by examining such a child's score on other visual tests of differentiation and conceptualization, will the examiner be in a position to determine which of these deficits are present.

Normative data are provided for children ages 5½ to 11, at ½-year levels. The child's total raw score (maximum score is 36) is converted to a percentile rank by reference to the proper chart. For example, an 8½-year-old boy obtains a raw score of 21. We note from the chart of normative data that a score of 20 is at the fiftieth percentile rank for children his age and a score of 23 is at the seventy-fifth percentile rank. Accordingly, we can say that this child's score is slightly above average. A girl of 10½ also obtains a raw score of 21 points. We note that a score of 20 corresponds to the tenth percentile level for children her age and a score of 22 is at the twenty-fifth percentile level. We can conclude that this girl's performance is significantly below average. But we cannot, on the basis of this test alone, ascertain the exact nature of her visual processing problem. We can say that a problem in visual differentiation and/or conceptualization is present. Her performance on other tests described in this chapter should help the examiner ascertain more accurately the nature of her deficit.

The Form Constancy Subtest [III] of the Developmental Test of Visual Perception

The Form Constancy subtest of the Developmental Test of Visual Perception (Frostig, 1961) is a good test of visual differentiation. The child is shown an array of complex geometric forms (Figure 8.5). Among the

Figure 8.5
The Form Constancy Subtest [III] of the Developmental Test of Visual Perception.

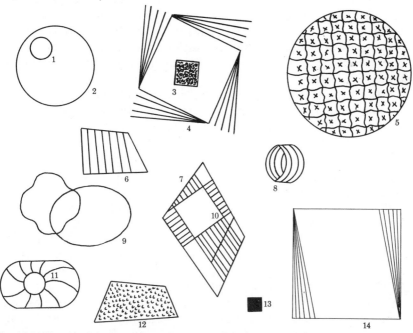

various forms depicted are circles as well as forms that are similar, but not exactly identical, to circles (ovals, ellipses, etc.). Also to be found are squares and forms that are similar (rectangles, trapezoids, etc.). The child is first given a green pencil. The examiner presents the child with demonstration cards showing a circle and an oval and says, "This is a round ball (circle). This is an egg (oval). On this page are some round balls (circles). Find as many balls (circles) as you can. Take your green pencil and outline (put a line around the edge of) all the balls (circles) you can find. Do not color them in. Do not mark anything that is not a ball (circle) like this (examiner points to a circle on the test sheet). Now you go ahead. Remember, don't mark the egg-shaped ones (ovals), just the round balls." There is no time limit on the test and if the child stops after he has outlined only 1 or 2 circles, he is encouraged to look for more.

After the child has outlined as many circles as he can find, he is given a brown pencil and the examiner, while holding up the demonstration square and rectangle says, "This is a square. See, all the sides are just the same. This is a long box (rectangle). On this page (pointing to test booklet) there are some squares and also other things that look like long boxes (rectangles). Now look at your book. Find all the squares you can and outline them. Do not mark anything that is not a square. Do not mark the long boxes (rectangles) or wiggly lines or anything else. Mark only the squares. See *how many* squares you can find. Now take your brown pencil and do it." After the child has finished, the examiner turns to a second page on which is a different array of geometric forms. Again the child is instructed to circle only the circles in green and the squares in brown.

The child is given 1 point credit for each circle and square that has been correctly outlined and a point is deducted for each figure that has been incorrectly marked (ovals, rectangles, etc.). The maximum raw score for the subtest is 17 points. By referring to the proper table, one can convert the child's raw score to an age-equivalent. For example, a 7-year-1-month-old girl obtains a raw score (correct responses minus errors) of 13. This corresponds to an age-equivalent of 9 years 0 months. Referring to the table that converts raw scores to scaled scores for children her age, we find that her scaled score is 13. The average scaled score is 10. We can conclude that this child does not have a problem in visual differentiation because she is functioning significantly above her age level on this test. Although manual operations are also involved in this test (the child must outline the figures), no points are lost if the outlining is poorly executed. All the child need do is adequately demonstrate that he is outlining the correct figure. Therefore, it is a poor test for manual dexterity, fine motor coordination, or dyspraxia. The examiner should be wary of coming to the conclusion that a child has a visual discrimination deficit merely from the results of this one test. He or she does well to utilize the other tests of visual differentiation described here to either confirm or refute this finding. As mentioned, I do not find the "perceptual quotient" that is obtained from the sum of the scaled scores on all 5 Frostig tests to be particularly useful. It is an average that "buries" significant information.

The Geometric Forms Subtest of
Cancellation of Rapidly Recurring Target Figures

In chapter 3, I discussed the Cancellation of Rapidly Recurring Target Figures test (Rudel et al., 1978) as useful in detecting problems in concentration. As the reader may recall, the child is presented with a sample figure (diamond or 592) below which is an array of figures some of which are identical to the target and many of which are similar but not exactly like the target. The child is asked to put a line through each identical figure as rapidly as he can. Normative data are provided for children ages 4 through 13. The geometric form subtest of this instrument (Figure 3.2) is useful as a test of visual discrimination. The child who does not differentiate the diamond from the other geometric forms on the page may have a problem in visual discrimination. Whereas the aforementioned Raven's and Frostig tests are untimed, this test is timed. As is often the case, a timed test may detect mild forms of deficit that would not be picked up when the child is given unlimited time to check his responses. The examiner must keep in mind that some children will do poorly on this test because of impulsivity, while their visual processing may be intact. Typically such children's test time is short and their error score is high.

An 8½-year-old boy, for example, makes 3 errors on the diamond test and takes 70 sec to complete the page. Referring to the normative data (Table 3.2) we note that the normal child his age makes 4 ± 3 errors and takes an average of 66.26 ± 21.63 sec. This boy's score then is in the average range for both number of errors and the time he took to complete the test. A 10-year-old girl makes 7 errors and takes 103 sec to finish the test. We note that the average child her age makes 3 ± 3 errors and takes 70.10 ± 24.55 sec. Her scores are over 1 standard deviation above the mean for both the number of errors and the time it took her to complete the test. One can suspect that this child has a problem in visual differentiation. However, a concentration problem must also be considered. A 7¼-year-old boy makes 10 errors and takes 53 sec to complete the test. Referring to the normative data, we see that the average number of errors for children his age is 5 ± 3 and that the average time is 103.43 ± 46.30 sec. This child made significantly more errors than the average child his age but also did the test much more rapidly than most children. Although a visual differentiation problem may be present here, impulsivity and/or a concentration problem may have caused this child's poor performance. In such cases, the examiner does well to let the child review his paper more carefully, without time limit, to see if he can detect his errors. By observing the manner in which the child approaches the test and finding out whether he can detect his errors, the examiner may be able to learn which of the three possible factors (impaired visual differentiation, impulsivity, or poor concentration) has caused the child's high error score.

The Matching Section [III] of the Reversals Frequency Test

Section III of my Reversals Frequency Test (Gardner, 1978) can be used to assess visual discrimination. This is the third of a three-part test designed to ascertain reversals frequency. The other two parts of this instrument will be discussed later in this chapter and the test's value in providing information about the causes of reversal errors will also be described.

The child is presented the test sheet (Figure 8.6), and while pointing to the triangle in the upper left-hand corner, the examiner says, "Here is a picture. On the other side of the line are four pictures." (Examiner's index finger sweeps across the four geometric figures to the right of the dividing line.) "One of these four is the same as this one here" (again pointing to the original triangle) "and the other three are different. With your pencil put a circle around the one that is the same." If the child is capable of understanding and correctly executing this task, he is given the remainder of the test. If he is not, then the test should not be given.

The examiner then continues: "On this side of the line, on your left (examiner points to the column to the left of the dividing line), is a number or letter. On the other side of the line, on your right" (examiner sweeps index finger across figures to the right of the dividing line) "are four letters or numbers. One of the four is the same, and the other three are different from the one on your left, over here. Put a circle around the letter or number here" (examiner points to the series of four) "that is the same as the letter or number here" (examiner points to the isolated number or letter). "You may take as much time as you like. If you

Figure 8.6

The Matching Section [III] of the Reversals Frequency Test.

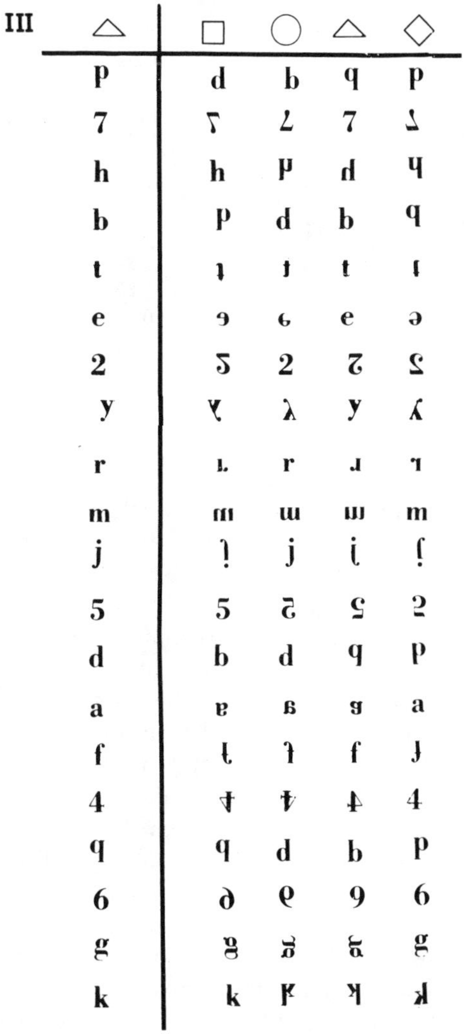

III △	□	○	△	◇
p	d	b	q	p
7	┌	∠	7	⅃
h	h	ʮ	ʮ	physical
b	p	d	b	q
t	ɿ	ɿ	t	ſ
e	ɘ	ɞ	e	ɘ
2	ƻ	2	ƻ	ƨ
y	ʏ	ʎ	y	ʎ
r	ʟ	r	⅃	˥
m	ɱ	ɯ	ɰ	m
j	ʇ	j	ɿ	ʄ
5	5	ƹ	ƹ	ƹ
d	b	d	q	ᑫ
a	ɐ	ɒ	ɒ	a
f	ʇ	ʇ	f	ʃ
4	↴	↳	↳	4
q	q	d	b	p
6	ɘ	ǫ	9	6
g	ɓ	ƌ	ƃ	g
k	k	ʞ	ʞ	⅄

change your mind and want to change an answer, you can do so by erasing the circle and putting another circle around your new answer."

The test is an easy one for most children and they generally enjoy doing it. Normative data was collected on 139 boys and 115 girls by me and my assistants (Table 8.3). All children were within the normal IQ range (90–110) or scored in the average range on national standardized achievement tests. As can be seen, the drop-off for errors after the

Table 8.3

The Matching Section [III] of the Reversals Frequency Test: Normative Data.

Age	Normal Boys		
	N	Mean	S.D.
5-0 to 5-11	23	4.61	3.81
6-0 to 6-11	33	1.42	3.12
7-0 to 7-11	40	0.25	0.44
8-0 to 8-11	43	0.33	0.69
	139		

Age	Normal Girls		
	N	Mean	S.D.
5-0 to 5-11	26	4.19	3.52
6-0 to 6-11	23	1.65	3.41
7-0 to 7-11	37	0.19	0.46
8-0 to 8-11	29	0.24	0.57
	115		

age of 6 is marked, so much so that 7- and 8-year-olds hardly make any errors. Because of this, no data was collected on children 9 years of age and above. It is important for the examiner to appreciate that successful performance on this test does not require a child to be familiar with English letters and Arabic numerals. Conceivably, an oriental child would do just as well, because all the child is being asked to do is to select and encircle the figure that matches the sample and leave alone the figures that do not. A 5½-year-old boy, for example, makes 12 errors. We note from Table 8.3 that the average child his age makes 4.61 ± 3.81 errors. This child's number of errors, then, is about 2 standard deviations above the normal. One must consider the possibility here that a visual discrimination problem is present. However, one would want to have observed this child while taking the test to be sure he was concentrating properly and that he wasn't impulsively racing through the test. A 6-year-old girl makes 2 errors. We note that normal girls her age make 1.65 ± 3.41 errors. Her score is in the normal range, and a visual discrimination problem is probably not present.

The instrument was found to be of limited value in the MBD diagnostic battery. The main reason for this limitation is that most MBD children, in my experience, do not have a primary problem in visual discrimination; rather, they are more likely to have a problem with visual memory. Accordingly, many children who do poorly on the execution and recognition sections of the Reversals Frequency Test perform normally on the matching section. The test, however, may occasionally detect a visual discrimination problem. The test is more useful as a research tool. Later in this chapter, in my discussion of the theories of reversals etiology, I will describe its use in this regard.

FIGURE-GROUND DISCRIMINATION

The term figure-ground discrimination is used to describe the function by which an individual differentiates between foreground and background, between the salient feature that is supposed to be selectively recognized and the less important elements that are to be somewhat ignored. The term is generally used to refer to visual, and to a lesser degree auditory, stimuli. When looking at a portrait, for example, we generally tend to focus on the person depicted in the center and not pay as much attention to background features such as clouds or trees. Strauss and Lehtinen (1947) and Strauss and Kephart (1955) considered figure-ground deficits to be a central problem for children with "brain injury." In recent years, we have been hearing less about figure-ground impairments in these children. Focus has shifted to the attentional deficits (chapter 3) and many (for example, Conners, 1974, 1976; Douglas, 1974a, 1974b) would consider the figure-ground impairment to be an artifact. Their view is that if the child concentrated better he would focus on the more salient feature. The child, for example, who does poorly on the traditional "hidden picture" game, in which the child is asked to find the hidden animals and objects in a complex scene, would have been considered by Strauss et al. to have a primary deficit in differentiating figure from ground. The aforementioned recent workers would consider the MBD child's poor performance on this test to be the result of his problem of focusing for long on any one part of the picture. Were he to be able to do so, he would be able to detect the hidden figures and objects. The question then is whether the problem is "perceptual" or attentional. My own opinion is that most (but probably not all) MBD children who appear to exhibit figure-ground difficulties do so because of an attentional deficit. But there are some (a minority, I believe) who have genuine deficits in the perceptual (discriminatory) area. My main reason for taking this position is that psychostimulant medication appears to improve children's functioning on figure-ground tests (such as those to be described below). I use the word *appears*, however, because I have not conducted studies to ascertain the effects of such medication on children's performance on these particular instruments.

Southern California Figure-Ground Visual Perception Test

The Southern California Figure-Ground Visual Perception Test (SCFGV-PT) (Ayres, 1968) is an excellent test for objectively assessing impaired ability to differentiate figure from ground. The test was standardized on 1,164 children (578 boys and 586 girls) ages 4-0 to 10-11. In the first test plate, the child is shown a sample box in which are drawn a shoe, a spoon, and a stool. They partially overlap one another and the areas of overlap are transparent. Below are six objects: a stool, a truck, a spoon, a knife, a boot, and a shoe. The examiner says to the child, "Three of these pictures" (pointing to the multiple choice plate below) "are up here" (pointing to the sample box above). "Which three are they?" The examiner then assists the child if necessary to ensure that he understands what is being asked of him and to determine if the child has the basic capacity to identify the three pictures that are depicted in the sample and the three that are not.

The child is then given eight more such tasks, one of which is shown in Figure 8.7. For each plate, there are three correct responses from the six possibilities shown. There is a one-minute time limit for each page, at the end of which the examiner turns to the next page. After the eighth plate has been completed, the child is shown another

Figure 8.7
Southern California Figure-Ground Visual Perception Test.

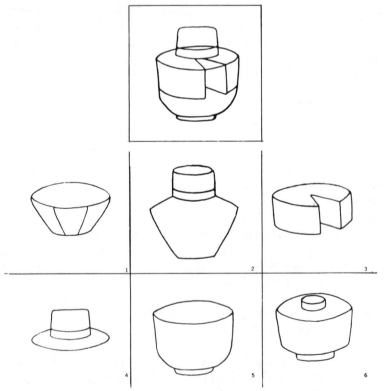

demonstration plate. This time geometric designs rather than objects are depicted. Again there are three and only three correct responses from the six possibilities shown. Also, the one-minute time limit still applies. The test is discontinued when a total of five errors have been made. Errors need not be consecutive and it is possible to make three errors on one plate. An omission is considered an error. A child may make all of his errors in the first series of eight (objects); in such cases, the second series of eight (designs) is not administered. No points are deducted for incorrect answers. The maximum possible score (rarely obtained by children) is 48 (16 charts with a possibility of 3 points for each chart).

Means and standard deviations are provided at 1/2-year levels for ages 4-0 through 10-1. A 5-year-10-month-old boy, for example, obtains a score of 15. Referring to the proper table we note that the mean score for children in the 5-6 to 5-11 age bracket is 12.3 ± 2.8. This child's score is approximately 1 standard deviation above the average. Accordingly, it is unlikely that a figure-ground differentiation problem is present. An 8-year-3-month-old girl obtains a score of 10. The normal score for children her age is 16.0 ± 3.0. Therefore, this child's score is 2 standard deviations below average. In fact, she is at the 4-6 to 4-11 level. One can conclude that this child probably has a figure-ground differentiation problem. In such cases one does well to observe the child carefully during the administration of the test to ascertain whether the child appears to be concentrating. Other tests of concentration should also be given (such as those described in chapter 3) in order to determine whether the child's problem is visual or attentional. Other tests of visual processing should also be given (such as those described in this chapter). If a child does well on all the other tests of visual processing and the SCFGVPT is the only one on which the child did poorly, I would tend to discount the likelihood that a basic visual processing problem is present. I would be more likely to conclude that a concentration deficit was responsible for the child's poor performance, especially if tests from chapter 3 also indicated that an attentional deficit was present.

The Figure-Ground Discrimination Subtest [II] of the Developmental Test of Visual Perception

The Figure-Ground Discrimination subtest of the Developmental Test of Visual Perception (DTVP) (Frostig, 1961) is also a useful test of figure-ground differentiation. There are eight items in the test. In each item, a target figure is embedded in a constellation of other geometric forms (Figure 8.8). The examiner holds up a picture of the target figure and

Figure 8.8

The Figure-Ground Discrimination Subtest (II) of the Developmental Test of Visual Perception.

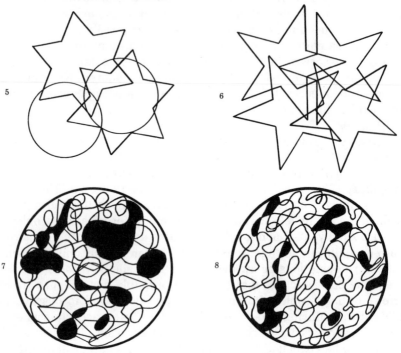

Reproduced by special permission from the Developmental Test of Visual Perception by Marianne Frostig, Ph.D. Copyright 1961. Published by Consulting Psychologists Press, Inc.

asks the child to outline each and every one of that particular form that may be present in the constellation under consideration. During the process of outlining, the child may be "pulled" off course by lines that are parts of other designs that are overlapping the one he is focusing on. When this happens, the child does not get credit for the outline. The total possible score for this subtest is 20.

Age-equivalents and scaled scores are provided. The scaled scores are useful if one wishes to obtain a child's "perceptual quotient" for all 5 subtests together. As mentioned, I do not calculate such a number. I am more interested in the child's score on each of the subtests. A 6½-year-old boy, for example, gets a raw score of 17. Referring to the age-equivalent table, one ascertains that a score of 17 is average for the child of age 6–6. Accordingly, this child probably does not have a figure-ground differentiation problem. A 5-year-2-month-old boy obtains a raw score of 6. This we find corresponds to an age-equivalent of 4–3. Such a child, then, is about 1 year behind and may have a figure-ground discrimination problem. However, as described in my discussion of the SCFGVPT, one does well to do other tests for concentration and visual processing impairments before coming to any conclusions regarding the presence of a figure-ground deficit.

VISUAL MEMORY

As discussed in chapter 7, the differentiation between short- and long-term visual memory is somewhat artificial in that the cut-off point between the two must be arbitrary. Actually, there is a continuum and any memory task lies on some point along the range. When I use the term memory in the discussion below, I will be referring to the capacity to store visually derived information and to selectively retrieve such data as is warranted for the situation.

The Administration A Subtest of the Revised Visual Retention Test

Benton's (1955) Revised Visual Retention Test is a useful test of relatively short-term visual memory. Benton describes it as a test of "visual perception, visual memory, and visuoconstructive abilities." It is a test of visual perception because the child is required to recognize, differentiate, and organize visual stimuli presented as geometric patterns. It is a test of visual memory because the child is asked to recall the observed patterns after a specific passage of time. And it is a test of visuoconstructive abilities because the child is asked to reproduce the patterns by drawing them to the best of his recollection. Benton describes four modes of administration.

> Administration A: Each design is exposed for 10 sec followed by immediate reproduction from memory.
> Administration B: Each design is exposed for 5 sec followed by immediate reproduction from memory.
> Administration C: Each design is copied by the subject, with the design remaining in the subject's view.
> Administration D: Each design is exposed for 10 sec, followed by reproduction from memory after a delay of 15 sec.

Normative data were not collected on children for administrations B and D. Normative data were collected on administration C; however, it is not, in my opinion, a good test of visual memory because the design remains within the subject's view while he is copying it. Therefore, I only use administration A in assessing visual memory problems in children. I use administration C in evaluating a child for constructional dyspraxia (I will discuss this in chapter 9).

The child is told that he will be shown some pictures and that he should try to remember what he is looking at because each card will be taken away after he has had the chance to look at it for 10 sec. The examiner times each card exposure with a stopwatch. There are a total of 10 plates, the first 2 of which contain only 1 item, and each of the remaining cards contains 3 items. A sample of the latter category is shown in Figure 8.9. Before introducing the third card, the child is told, "Do not forget to draw everything you see." Three different, but comparable, sets of the 10 cards are available, enabling the examiner to retest without concern for practice effect.

Figure 8.9
Revised Visual Retention Test.

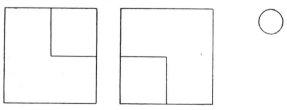

Two types of scores are utilized. The number of *correct* reproductions are determined by giving the child a score of 0 or 1 depending upon whether or not the *whole* card was correctly copied. No partial credit is given here, so a child's score can range from 0 to 10. The number of *errors* is also scored. Benton provides very specific criteria for scoring errors, which fall into the following categories: omissions, distortions, perseverations, rotations, misplacements, and size errors. Descriptions as well as drawings of both the common correct and incorrect renditions are provided. It is theoretically possible for a drawing to have as many as 4 or 5 errors. However, in Benton's experience, about 24 errors has been the usual upper limit.

Normative data are provided for children aged 8–14. The data are presented as the expected scores for children of different ages at various levels of intelligence. Separate tables are provided for correct responses and number of errors. The levels of intelligence breakdown is: 105 and above, (high average and superior), 94–104 (average), 80–94 (low average), 70–79 (borderline), and 69 and below (defective). A score that is 3 points above the expected level "raises the question" of a disability. A score of 4 or more points above the expected level "suggests" a disability. I personally appreciate Benton's caution here because I believe that the examiner does well not to rely too heavily on any one test. It is preferable to administer a number of tests in an area of suspected disability before coming to any conclusions regarding the presence of a particular disorder. A 10½-year-old girl with a 103 IQ gets 5 points for correct responses and 7 errors. Referring to the tables of normative data, we find that the expected number of correct responses for 10-year-old children of average intelligence is 5 and that the expected number of errors for average children at that age is 7–8. Accordingly, we can conclude that this child's score is average for both correct responses and errors and that visual memory and visuoconstructive deficits are probably not present. In addition, one could say that pathology in certain areas, traditionally referred to visual-perceptive, is not present. A 9-year-old boy with an IQ of 108 obtains 2 points for correct responses and gets 13 errors. Referring to the tables, we see that the expected number of correct responses for children of this age and IQ is 5 and the expected number of errors is 7–8. This boy has gotten 3 fewer correct responses than expected (a score that "raises the question" of pathology) and 5–6 more errors than expected ("suggestive" of pathology). It is reasonable to conclude that this child most likely has some difficulty in visual processing, either "perception," memory, or construction. To ascertain whether the problem is primarily visuoconstructive, administration C might be utilized. Also, the tests of fine motor coordination, described in chapter 5, and those for dyspraxia, to be discussed in chapter 9, could provide additional information on this issue. Regarding "perceptual" deficits, one would have to utilize a variety of the tests described in this chapter to determine the particular kind of visual processing deficit that might be contributing.

The Picture Completion Subtest of the WISC-R

The Picture Completion subtest of the WISC-R is a good test of long-term visual memory. The child is presented with a series of 26 pictures, each of which has an essential part missing. (Figure 8.10 is a facsimile of one of the pictures.) The child is told: "I am going to show you some pictures in which there is a part missing. Look at the picture carefully and tell me what is missing." A maximum exposure of 20 sec is allowed for each card. Some typical cards: a dog with a missing ear, a suit jacket with buttons but no corresponding button holes, profile of a man

Figure 8.10
The Picture Completion Subtest of the WISC-R.

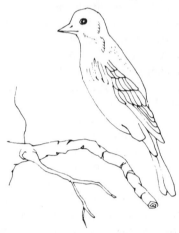

with a missing eyebrow. The maximum raw score is 26. The raw score is converted to a scaled score by reference to the conversion table for the child's age bracket. The mean scaled score is 10. The WISC-R does have a table (not frequently utilized) that directly provides age-equivalents for each subtest. A 10-year-10-month-old boy obtains a raw score of 20. Referring to the conversion table for children his age (10-8 to 10-11), we note that a raw score of 20 corresponds to a scaled score of 12, which is above average. By referring to conversion tables for age-equivalents we note that a raw score of 20 is average for a child of 12-6.

I consider the Picture Completion subtest to assess long-term visual memory because if the child is to be successful, he must have stored information about the complete figure. Also, he must be able to retrieve such data and form an internal visual engram of the object. The test is not simply one of visual memory. Successful performance requires sustained attention. The child must carefully view the picture, and attend to many details if he is to detect the omission. This is especially true of the more difficult pictures near the end of the test. For example, a cow is shown and all major parts seem to be present. Only on careful observation may one note that one of the hoofs is not cleft. The distractable child will also not attend well to the picture. Such distractability may be a manifestation of organicity, but it may also be secondary to anxiety that is psychogenic.

The Object Assembly Subtest of the WISC-R

The Object Assembly subtest of the WISC-R also assesses long-term visual memory. This is a jigsaw-puzzle type test in which the child is asked to assemble the parts into a completely recognizable entity. (Figure 8.11 depicts a facsimile of a typical test item.) As a demonstration, the child is presented an assortment of four wooden pieces and told, "If these pieces are put together the right way, they will make an apple. Watch how I do it." The examiner then demonstrates how the object is formed from the pieces. There are four more objects and these the child is asked to form himself. For the first two, the girl and the horse, the child is told the name of the object that is to be made. For the last two, the car and the face, the child is given no other instructions than "Put this one together as quickly as you can." The child is timed with maximum time allowances ranging from 120 to 180 seconds. Each item is scored on the basis of the number of cuts (pieces) that have been correctly joined by the end of the time limit. Bonus points can be obtained for perfect assemblies completed before the time limit, the shorter the time taken to execute the task the greater the number of bonus points. The maximum possible raw score is 33 points. Conversion to scaled scores and age-equivalents is identical to the procedure described for the Picture Completion subtest. For example, a 7-year-2-month-old girl

Figure 8.11
The Object Assembly Subtest of the WISC-R.

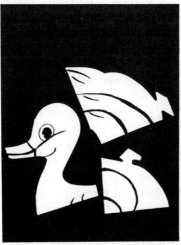

Items similar to those found in the Wechsler Intelligence Scale for Children-Revised. Copyright © 1974 by The Psychological Corporation, New York, N.Y. All rights reserved.

gets a raw score of 14 points. Referring to the conversion table for ages 7-0 to 7-3, we note that this score corresponds to a scaled score of 10. Therefore, we can conclude that this child's performance on this test is in the normal range. A 9½-year-old boy gets a raw score of 15. Referring to the table for ages 9-4 to 9-7, we see that this score corresponds to a scaled score of 8. This boy's performance then is below average. By referring to the age-equivalent table we note that a raw score of 15 corresponds to age 7-6. In short, this boy's score is approximately that of a child 2 years his junior.

The Object Assembly subtest assesses long-term visual memory because the child has to have stored information regarding the object to be formed with the pieces. When the examiner instructs the child to make a horse, the child must have information that will enable him to form an internal image of a horse. He must be able to retrieve from storage that information that will enable him to form such an engram. In the last two items, the child must utilize another function, namely, visualizing a whole from a part. Visual conceptualization capacity is also being evaluated here. When the child is told to make a horse, he must have the concept of what a horse is. When the child recognizes that a piece depicts a nose, he must also appreciate that a nose is part of a face. He must have developed the concept of a face in order to correctly place together its various parts. Visual organizational capacity is also being evaluated as well as planning capacity. Lastly, the test is a measure of persistence. This is especially true of the last two items where the child is asked to experiment with the various pieces, and to try to put them together in different arrangements until there is recognition of the object to be made.

Letter Reversals Frequency Tests

Most, if not all children will reverse letters when they first learn to write. Typically children will confuse letters that are mirror images of one another, hence the proverbial "Mind your p's and q's." Most examiners subscribe to the general rule of thumb that by the third grade children should no longer exhibit reversals. Children with neurologically based reading disabilities, especially those referred to as dyslexic, are said to exhibit greater reversals frequency than normals and to persist in such confusion beyond the age when normal children hardly ever do so (Critchley, 1970; Owen et al. 1971). The fact that written English utilizes symbols that are mirror images of one another contributes to the burden of the child who is learning to write. Reading problems are said to be less common in Japanese (Makita, 1968) where both the Kana phonetic symbols and the Kanji ideographs (word and concept characters derived from the Chinese) have no mirror-image representations that are of linguistic significance. A greater understanding of the causes of the reversals tendency in dyslexic children can perhaps provide us with clues about the more basic etiology(ies) and pathogenesis of dyslexia.

Before one can reasonably discuss and understand reversals errors, it is important to appreciate that the term is really a rubric under which is subsumed a variety of phenomena. Confining ourselves first simply to letters written in isolation, one can divide reversals into four categories (Kinsbourne, 1973):

1. mirror image: b for d
2. inversions: p for b
3. inverted reversals: p for d, u for n, 6 for 9
4. rotations: ႕ for b

Clearly, different operations are involved in making each of these reversals errors. In addition, reversing the *sequence* of letters within a word is different from reversing letters in isolation: strok for stork, cluod for cloud. And reversing whole words entirely: *was* for *saw*, *tac* for *cat*, may represent yet another phenomenon. Generally children tend to reverse palindromic words (those that spell other bona fide words when reversed) more frequently than words that do not have palindromes. The aforementioned examples are all visual. When an auditory component is introduced, that is, when the child is asked to write letters and words from dictation, auditory processing problems may contribute to what may appear to be a defect in written expression. One does well then when comparing studies of reversals to be sure that one is comparing the same thing; it is rare that two different studies do so.

Studies of Reversals Manifestation and Frequency

Before one can meaningfully speculate on *why* children reverse, it is useful to know something about reversals frequency in both normal children and children with learning disabilities. Davidson (1935) found that first-grade boys made more reversals errors than first-grade girls. Her findings were among the first in which boys were found to be more likely to have learning difficulties than girls. She found that "upside-down" errors (n-u, q-b, q-d, b-p, b-q) tended to drop out by age 6. Mirror image errors (d-b, p-q) tended to persist later (until 7 to 7½). Unfortunately, Davidson's groups above 7½ were so small that no meaningful conclusions can be made with regard to these older children's reversals tendency.

Gilkey and Parr (1944) studied reversals frequency in 324 elementary school pupils in four tests: (1) copying geometric forms, (2) writing the numbers 1–18 and the letters a–z in sequence, (3) connecting the two words in a series that are identical (e.g., nut, not, cut, ton, nut ...), (4) underlining the correct one of a visualized word pair that corresponds to the word verbalized by the examiner (for example, the child was presented with the written words *owl* and *low* and instructed to underline the word "owl," or he or she was presented with *froth* and *forth* and told to underline "forth"). The total number of reversals on all four tests was used to determine reversals frequency.

This study had many of the methodological problems that can confuse the reader trying to learn about the reversals phenomenon. The first test uses geometric forms, the assumption being that linguistic and nonlinguistic reversals will correlate. It is probable that letter processing of geometric forms, as spatial entities, take place mainly in the right hemisphere. The second test requires the child to write numbers and letters in the correct sequence. In my opinion, executing the figures in this way is less likely to bring out reversals errors than if the child were asked to write the numbers and letters in a specific random sequence. Such rote execution carries the child along in a fixed patterns with less thinking necessary about correct orientation. Test three appears much too easy to me; one doesn't even have to know language (English or other) to get the correct answer. Although test four comes closest to a true test of reversals frequency, it is not without its deficiencies. It is easier to detect reversals in a word than when letters are presented in isolation. The letters surrounding the reversed letter(s) provide clues about correct orientation. For example, u not n follows a q. There is no word *breab*, but there is a word *bread* (The first four letters clearly provide some hint as to what should be the orientation of the fifth. In addition, test four utilizes an auditory element (the examiner verbalizes the words), so that additional processes are introduced that might contribute to the errors observed.

Another problem that made this study suspect was the authors' claim that all children in the study were "normal" because they were in regular classes. Yet one seventh-grader made 8.5 reversals in test 1 and had an IQ of 88. This child would probably be diagnosed as neurologically learning-disabled (MBD) were this study done today. Accordingly, it is reasonable to assume that some of the other children in the study were dyslexic. In spite of these drawbacks, the authors' findings tend to confirm general clinical impressions. Forty-six percent of the first-grade children exhibited reversals and 88% of all the reversals were exhibited by children in the first three grades. The fact that 12% of the reversals were seen in children in grades 4-7 could be explained in two ways. Either they were exhibited by the undetected dyslexic children or normal children still manifest reversals in these grade levels.

Shankweiler (1964) found that there was no consistency regarding reversals errors: a child might just as well call a b a b as he would call it a d. He also pointed out that some children try to hide their reversals problem when writing lower case letters by using upper case letters instead. For example, it is less likely to confuse B and D than b and d.

Lyle and Goyen (1968) presented letters and words tachistoscopically to both normal and retarded readers. After each presentation the subjects were shown cards on which were printed the flashed words, both accurately and with reversals. The subjects had to point to what they had seen under speed conditions. Two types of errors were recorded: (1) letter reversals (bog for dog) and (2) sequence reversals (cloud for could). The total number of errors were also recorded. The ratio of letter and sequence reversals to the total number of errors was determined. The authors found that the normal group did not differ from the reading-disability group regarding the *fraction* of reversals errors over total errors. Although the reading-disability group made more reversals errors, they also made more total errors. The authors concluded that reversals per se are not a particular problem for children with reading disabilities. Rather, reversals are just one manifestation of their general problem in reading correctly under speed conditions.

Liberman et al. (1971) asked 15 boys and 3 girls, known to have reading problems, to read a list of words (samples: tar, was, saw, rat...). Errors were divided into four categories and the percentage of errors in each category determined. The results:

Reversals of sequence	10% of total reading errors
Reversals of orientation	15% of total reading errors
Other consonant errors	32% of total reading errors
Other vowel errors	43% of total reading errors
	100%

These results tend to confirm what many teachers know well: reversals problems are less common than errors of letter recognition in general, with vowel problems more frequent than consonant problems. These findings tend to confirm those of Lyle and Goyen (see above) that the reversals problem is just one manifestation (possibly minor) of the broader reading problem that dyslexic children have.

In another part of the Liberman study, the subjects were presented with isolated letters in a tachistoscope and asked to match the observed letter with the correctly oriented one of five written letters, some of which were mirror images of the one that was tachistoscopically presented. Only 7.4% of the errors were made in this manner. From this the authors concluded that reading letters alone produced a lower reversals frequency than when the letters were presented in the context of a word. I personally am dubious of this finding. As mentioned, I suspect that other letters of a word provide cues about the orientation of letters that may easily be confused. I believe that if more than 18 children had been studied, the results might have been different. Elsewhere in the study the authors describe more reversals errors when nonsense words were read than when real recognizable words were presented. This finding supports my view that the surrounding letters provide information that can lessen reversals frequency.

The 18 children that Liberman et al. studied were the worst readers among 54 children with reading problems. The authors considered the reversals problem to manifest itself primarily in children with significant reading problems. Ginsberg and Hartwick (1971) found significant reversals errors in the worst 10 of 43 children considered by their teachers to have reading problems. They considered reversals to be a sensitive test of reading disability.

If the above selections from the literature have impressed upon the reader the complexity of the reversals phenomenon, they will have served their purpose. Further reference to the significance of these studies will be made in my discussion of reversals etiology.

The Reversals Frequency Test

In the attempt to gather data on reversals frequency in normal and MBD children, I devised a reversals frequency test (Gardner, 1978; Gardner and Broman, 1979b). Five hundred normal children and 343 with MBD were tested with the instrument. The normal group consisted of 251 boys and 249 girls who were in regular classes. When IQs were available, only children in the 90 to 110 range were included. When not available, national achievement test scores were utilized and only students in the average range (twentieth to eightieth percentile) were selected. Any child with a history of reading or other academic difficulty was excluded from the study. The MBD group consisted of 245 boys and 98 girls, all of whom were either in special education classes or schools for children with MBD. All had been placed in these classes because of neurologically based learning disabilities. However, they all exhibited other mild neurological signs, justifying, therefore, the broader MBD categorization. Children who had been so labeled and were in regular classes, i.e., "mainstreamed," were excluded from the study. In this way children of questionable diagnosis were not included. Children on psychostimulant medication were also not utilized.

Each child was administered a two-section test (Gardner, 1978). The first measures the frequency of reversals on *execution*, and the second measures reversals *recognition*. In column I of section I (Figure 8.12) the child is simply asked to write the following numbers, one

Figure 8.12
The Execution Section (I) of the Reversals Frequency Test.

under the other: 5, 2, 6, 3, 9, 4, and 7 (excluded are 0, 1, and 8, which cannot be written in reversed form, as generally executed by the child). The numbers are always given in this exact random sequence. In column II the child is asked to write the following lower-case letters (using whatever term the child uses to define lower case, e.g., "small" or "little letters"): h,c,q,f,j,b,k,s,r,d,y,p,t,z,g,a, and e (the letters i,l,m,n, o,u,v,w, and x were omitted because they are either identical to or very similar to their mirror image form). Again this exact random sequence is used. The examiner then totals the number of errors in columns I and II and places this figure at the lower left corner of the page. In formulating the Reversals Execution Test the problem arose as to how to deal with children who were just learning how to write, who had mastered some of the letters and numbers but not all of them. To use only children who had mastered the numbers and letters completely would have deprived us of reversals-frequency data from the group most likely to reveal such errors. However, to include all children, even those who could only write a few letters or numbers, would have introduced data that could not be very convincing because the concept of reversals error only has meaning for children who have previously demonstrated reasonable competence with basic letter and number writing. To solve this problem, it was decided to record two types of errors in this section: execution reversals and unknowns. In order to remove from the study those who were insufficiently knowledgeable about writing letters and numbers, it was decided to exclude all children who did not know how to write more than 16 of the total of 24 numbers and letters contained in section I. In addition, if a child knew how to write a letter in upper-case form (which often does not reveal a reversals error) but could not write it in the lower-case form (the more likely form to reveal a reversals error) the letter was scored as an unknown. Therefore, when scoring section I the examiner records separately the total number of execution reversals and the total number of unknowns.

In section II,[1] the Reversals Recognition Test (Figure 8.13), the child is told, "In this first row" (examiner runs his or her finger along the first row) "are pairs of numbers, that is, two numbers together. In each pair, one of the numbers is pointing in the *right* direction and the other is pointing in the *wrong* direction. Draw a cross or an X over the number that is pointing in the *wrong* direction." Similar instructions

---

[1] Section II is a modification of a reversals test designed by Dr. Samuel T. Orton and given to me by Mrs. Katrina de Hirsch. To the best of my knowledge, no normative data were ever collected on the Orton test.

Figure 8.13

The Recognition Section (II) of the Reversals Frequency Test.

II

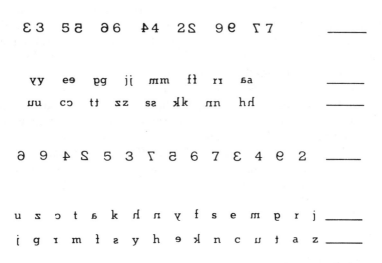

are then given for the next two rows of letters. For row four the child is told, "In this row some of the numbers are pointing in the *right* direction and some in the *wrong* direction. Put a cross or an X over the number pointing in the *wrong* direction." And similar instructions are given for the letters in rows five and six. The examiner then counts all recognition reversals errors in section II. When designing the scoring system for section II, a similar problem arose about what to do with children who were in the transition stage of learning to recognize letters. The maximum number of errors that a child can make in section II is 69 (assuming that only one of a pair can be crossed out). If a child knew nothing about letter orientation and guessed on every item, he would most likely make about 35 errors. Because some children seemed to be knowledgeable about some letters, made bona fide reversals errors with others, and guessed with others, it was decided to exclude all children who made more than 42 errors. In addition, when it was apparent that the child was guessing on most, if not all, of the items, he or she was also excluded from the study.

Execution-errors frequencies (means, ranges, and standard deviations) in section I for normals and MBDs is presented in Table 8.4. The same data are provided graphically in Figures 8.14–8.16. The frequencies (means, ranges, and standard deviations) of unknown errors in section I is presented in Table 8.5. (Because there was no significant difference between boys and girls with regard to the frequencies of unknown errors, the data from the two groups were combined.) The same data are provided graphically in Figures 8.17 and 8.18. Recognition-errors frequencies (ranges, means, and standard deviations) in section II is presented in Table 8.6. The same data are provided graphically in Figures 8.19–8.21. Whereas errors in section I for both execution and unknowns tended to reach very low levels after ages 7 and 8, errors in section II were seen with significant frequency at older age levels for MBD children. Accordingly, meaningful percentile rank data could be formulated for such recognition errors and these are presented in Tables 8.7 and 8.8.

Table 8.4

The Execution Section (I) of The Reversals Frequency Test: Error Ranges, Means and Standard Deviations.

	Normal Boys					Normal Girls				
Age	N	Low	High	Mean	S.D.	N	Low	High	Mean	S.D.
5-0 to 5-11	25	0	7	3.16	2.29	28	0	13	4.46	3.1
6-0 to 6-11	28	0	8	2.68	2.19	31	0	11	2.16	2.3
7-0 to 7-11	25	0	4	0.40	0.96	25	0	3	0.44	0.9
8-0 to 8-11	26	0	0	0.00	0.00	27	0	1	0.07	0.2
9-0 to 9-11	27	0	1	0.07	0.27	25	0	0	0.00	0.0
10-0 to 10-11	30	0	2	0.10	0.40	27	0	0	0.00	0.0
11-0 to 11-11	26	0	2	0.12	0.43	25	0	2	0.12	0.4
12-0 to 12-11	25	0	0	0.00	0.00	25	0	0	0.00	0.0
13-0 to 13-11	27	0	1	0.04	0.19	25	0	0	0.00	0.0
14-0 to 14-11	12	0	0	0.00	0.00	11	0	0	0.00	0.0
	251					249				
	MBD Boys					MBD Girls				
5-0 to 5-11	6	0	9	4.17	3.19	0	—	—	—	—
6-0 to 6-11	18	0	7	2.28	2.49	6	0	7	2.83	2.9
7-0 to 7-11	25	0	9	1.85	2.28	16	0	7	0.88	1.7
8-0 to 8-11	28	0	8	1.21	2.01	8	0	2	0.25	0.7
9-0 to 9-11	31	0	7	0.68	1.45	15	0	6	0.66	1.5
10-0 to 10-11	28	0	8	1.11	2.03	9	0	1	0.11	0.3
11-0 to 11-11	25	0	2	0.16	0.46	15	0	2	0.40	0.6
12-0 to 12-11	30	0	4	0.47	0.98	10	0	2	0.20	0.6
13-0 to 13-11	28	0	5	0.43	1.20	12	0	2	0.33	0.6
14-0 to 15-7 (Boys)	26	0	1	0.08	0.27	7	0	0	0.00	0.0
15-9 (Girls)	245					98				

Figure 8.14

Error Ranges and Means for Boys from the Execution Section [I] of the Reversals Frequency Test.

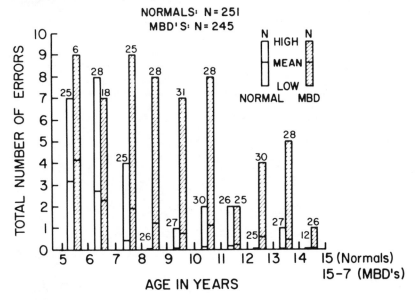

Figure 8.15

Error Ranges and Means for Girls from the Execution Section [I] of the Reversals Frequency Test.

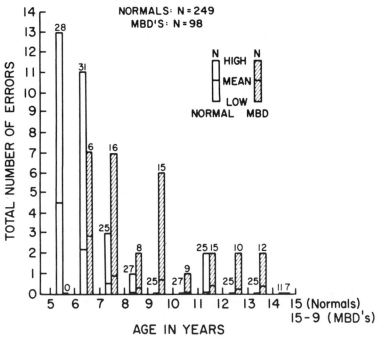

Figure 8.16

Mean Number of Errors from the Execution Section [I] of the Reversals Frequency Test.

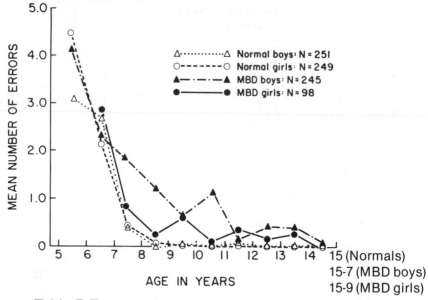

Table 8.5

Execution Section [I] of the Reversals Frequency Test: Error Ranges, Means, and Standard Deviations for Unknown Errors.

Age	N	Low	High	Mean	S.D.
Normals—Boys and Girls Combined					
5-0 to 5-11	53	0	11	4.26	2.74
6-0 to 6-11	59	0	7	1.54	1.87
7-0 to 7-11	50	0	2	0.08	0.34
8-0 to 8-11	53	0	1	0.02	0.12
9-0 to 9-11	52	0	1	0.02	0.14
10-0 to 10-11	57	0	1	0.05	0.23
11-0 to 11-11	51	0	1	0.02	0.14
12-0 to 12-11	50	0	2	0.08	0.34
13-0 to 13-11	52	0	0	0.00	0.00
14-0 to 14-11	23	0	1	0.09	0.23
	500				
MBDs—Boys and Girls Combined					
5-0 to 5-11	6	2	9	4.83	2.79
6-0 to 6-11	24	0	16	5.00	4.16
7-0 to 7-11	41	0	11	2.98	3.25
8-0 to 8-11	36	0	9	1.78	2.23
9-0 to 9-11	46	0	8	0.74	1.64
10-0 to 10-11	37	0	3	0.76	1.09
11-0 to 11-11	40	0	6	0.95	1.57
12-0 to 12-11	40	0	7	0.40	1.17
13-0 to 13-11	40	0	5	0.45	1.08
14-0 to 15-9	33	0	3	0.33	0.74
	343				

Figure 8.17
Ranges and Means for Unknown Errors from the Execution Section
[I] of the Reversals Frequency Test.

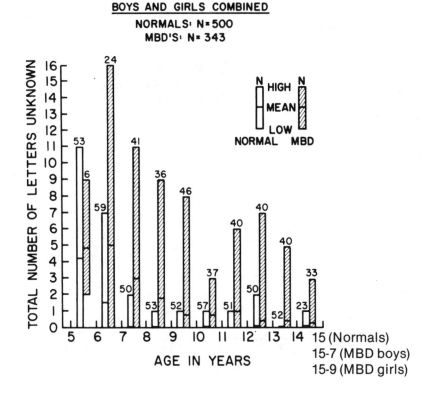

Figure 8.18
Mean Number of Unknown Errors from the Execution Section (I) of the Reversals Frequency Test.

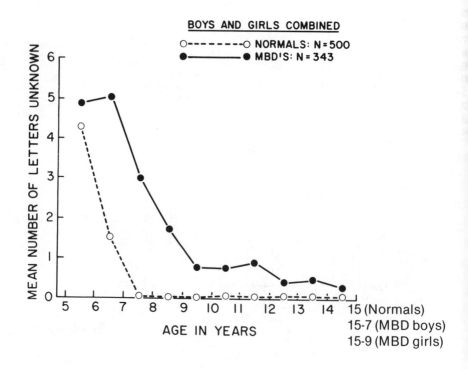

Table 8.6

The Recognition Section [II] of the Reversals Frequency Test: Error Ranges, Means, and Standard Deviations.

Age		Normal Boys					Normal Girls			
	N	Low	High	Mean	S.D.	N	Low	High	Mean	S.D.
5-0 to 5-11	25	4	42	23.76	11.11	28	3	39	21.20	10.25
6-0 to 6-11	28	2	36	18.54	11.52	31	0	34	13.00	9.49
7-0 to 7-11	25	1	22	8.16	5.31	25	0	29	5.64	6.48
8-0 to 8-11	26	0	19	3.73	4.07	27	0	9	2.63	2.80
9-0 to 9-11	27	0	13	3.15	3.03	25	0	9	2.24	2.22
10-0 to 10-11	30	0	14	2.07	2.73	27	0	7	1.74	1.68
11-0 to 11-11	26	0	11	2.81	3.12	25	0	10	2.36	2.78
12-0 to 12-11	25	0	7	1.56	1.66	25	0	6	1.36	1.68
13-0 to 13-11	27	0	8	1.96	2.24	25	0	5	1.08	1.35
14-0 to 14-11	12	0	7	2.42	2.06	11	0	5	1.20	1.60
	251					249				

Age		MBD Boys					MBD Girls			
	N	Low	High	Mean	S.D.	N	Low	High	Mean	S.D.
5-0 to 5-11	6	0	32	22.70	12.19	0	—	—	—	—
6-0 to 6-11	18	2	34	19.33	11.20	6	1	38	17.00	14.20
7-0 to 7-11	25	0	39	16.36	12.12	16	1	38	15.13	12.68
8-0 to 8-11	28	0	33	13.10	11.01	8	2	39	11.60	12.35
9-0 to 9-11	31	1	37	10.70	9.86	15	0	30	8.53	7.95
10-0 to 10-11	28	0	35	9.96	10.28	9	1	22	9.44	6.54
11-0 to 11-11	25	0	26	6.60	8.63	15	0	38	9.33	9.70
12-0 to 12-11	30	0	31	7.70	7.96	10	1	10	5.30	2.79
13-0 to 13-11	28	0	29	5.54	6.35	12	0	11	3.75	3.72
14-0 to 15-7 (Boys)	26	0	15	3.77	3.52	7	1	7	3.00	2.00
15-9 (Girls)	245					98				

Figure 8.19

Error Ranges and Means for Boys from the Recognition Section [II] of the Reversals Frequency Test.

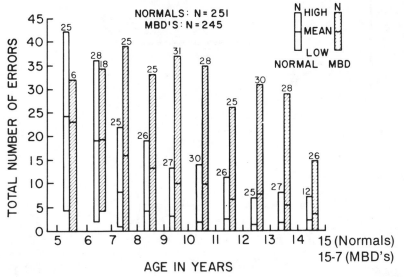

Figure 8.20
Error Ranges and Means for Girls from the Recognition Section [II] of the Reversals Frequency Test.

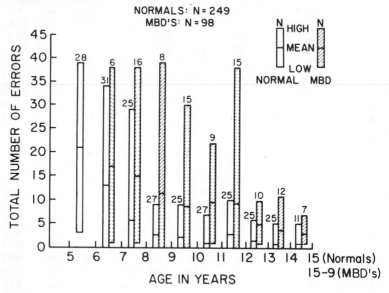

Figure 8.21
Mean Number of Errors from the Recognition Section [II] of the Reversals Frequency Test.

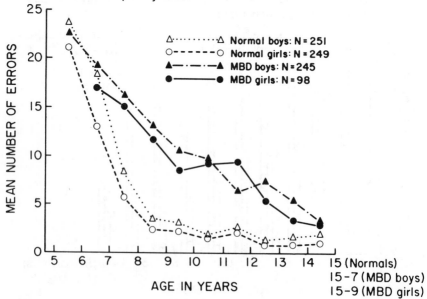

Table 8.7
The Recognition Section [II] of The Reversals Frequency Test: Percentiles for Number of Errors.

Age	N	Normal Boys								
		10	20	30	40	50	60	70	80	90
5-0 to 5-11	25	37.70	34.60	30.20	28.00	26.00	20.00	14.80	12.00	7.90
6-0 to 6-11	28	34.10	30.00	28.00	25.00	20.00	14.00	8.70	5.60	3.00
7-0 to 7-11	25	15.40	12.00	10.20	9.60	8.00	6.20	4.80	3.00	1.00
8-0 to 8-11	26	10.00	5.60	4.00	3.00	3.00	2.00	2.00	1.00	0.00
9-0 to 9-11	27	8.20	4.40	3.60	3.00	2.00	2.00	1.00	1.00	0.00
10-0 to 10-11	30	5.00	3.80	2.00	1.60	1.00	1.00	1.00	0.20	0.00
11-0 to 11-11	26	7.90	5.60	3.00	3.00	2.00	1.00	1.00	0.00	0.00
12-0 to 12-11	25	4.00	3.00	2.00	1.00	1.00	1.00	1.00	0.00	0.00
13-0 to 13-11	27	6.20	3.40	3.00	1.00	1.00	1.00	0.40	0.00	0.00
14-0 to 14-11	12	6.40	3.80	3.00	3.00	2.50	1.20	1.00	0.60	0.00
	251									

Age	N	Normal Girls								
		10	20	30	40	50	60	70	80	90
5-0 to 5-11	28	34.20	31.00	28.30	25.20	23.50	19.00	15.70	12.80	3.90
6-0 to 6-11	31	27.80	22.20	18.00	15.40	11.00	8.80	7.20	4.00	1.00
7-0 to 7-11	25	15.00	9.40	6.00	4.60	4.00	3.00	2.00	1.20	0.00
8-0 to 8-11	27	7.20	6.00	4.00	2.00	1.00	1.00	1.00	0.00	0.00
9-0 to 9-11	25	5.60	3.80	2.00	2.00	2.00	1.40	1.00	1.00	0.00
10-0 to 10-11	27	4.00	3.00	2.00	2.00	2.00	1.00	1.00	0.00	0.00
11-0 to 11-11	25	8.00	4.60	3.00	2.00	1.00	1.00	1.00	0.00	0.00
12-0 to 12-11	25	4.20	2.00	2.00	1.60	1.00	0.40	0.00	0.00	0.00
13-0 to 13-11	25	3.40	1.80	1.00	1.00	1.00	0.40	0.00	0.00	0.00
14-0 to 14-11	11	4.60	2.60	1.40	1.00	1.00	0.00	0.00	0.00	0.00
	249									

Table 8.8

The Recognition Section [II] of The Reversals Frequency Test: Percentiles for Number of Errors.

MBD Boys

Age	N	10	20	30	40	50	60	70	80	90
5-0 to 5-11	6	—	31.60	—	29.40	—	24.40	—	7.20	—
6-0 to 6-11	18	33.20	32.00	29.40	25.60	22.00	15.80	11.80	6.20	3.60
7-0 to 7-11	25	32.30	29.60	23.90	19.60	16.50	12.80	6.20	3.00	1.70
8-0 to 8-11	28	32.10	27.40	18.00	13.20	9.00	6.00	5.00	3.80	1.90
9-0 to 9-11	31	28.00	17.40	13.00	10.20	7.00	6.00	3.00	2.00	1.00
10-0 to 10-11	28	32.00	14.40	9.60	8.00	7.00	5.60	3.70	2.00	0.90
11-0 to 11-11	25	25.30	15.60	4.00	4.00	3.00	2.00	2.00	1.00	0.00
12-0 to 12-11	30	20.00	14.60	8.70	6.00	5.50	3.00	2.00	1.20	1.00
13-0 to 13-11	28	16.30	7.00	5.30	5.00	4.00	3.60	2.00	1.00	0.00
14-0 to 15-7	26	9.30	6.00	4.90	4.00	2.50	2.00	2.00	1.00	0.00
	245									

MBD Girls

Age	N	10	20	30	40	50	60	70	80	90
5-0 to 5-11	2	—	—	—	—	—	—	—	—	—
6-0 to 6-11	6	—	34.00	—	21.60	—	7.80	—	3.40	—
7-0 to 7-11	16	37.00	29.20	23.30	16.20	11.50	8.60	5.20	3.00	1.00
8-0 to 8-11	8	—	23.80	—	7.80	—	6.60	—	2.80	—
9-0 to 9-11	15	24.60	12.60	10.20	8.00	6.00	4.80	3.00	3.00	1.20
10-0 to 10-11	9	—	17.00	—	9.00	—	6.00	—	5.00	—
11-0 to 11-11	15	26.60	15.40	10.60	10.00	9.00	7.40	2.80	1.20	0.00
12-0 to 12-11	10	9.90	8.40	6.00	6.00	5.50	4.40	4.00	2.40	1.10
13-0 to 13-11	12	10.40	7.80	5.20	4.60	3.00	1.40	0.90	0.00	0.00
14-0 to 15-9	7	—	5.20	—	2.80	—	2.00	—	1.60	—
	98									

Statistical Analysis of Data.   Frequencies of execution reversals errors, recognition reversals errors, and unknowns for normal and MBD boys and girls at 10 age levels (5 through 15½ years), were entered into separate three-way analyses of variance, age by sex by group. The following findings emerged:

Age effects.   For all three types of errors, age was a highly significant main effect ($p < .001$ in each case), reflecting a linear decline in the frequency of errors with increasing age in each case. For recognition errors and unknowns, the age effect interacted significantly with group ($p < .01$ and $p < .001$, respectively); indicating that age trends differed between the normal and MBD groups. Means for individual age levels were compared separately for the two groups according to the Duncan Multiple Range procedure (1955). For normal children, both in the case of recognition errors and unknowns, age differences were significant only at the youngest age levels: In the case of recognition errors, 6- and 7-year olds made significantly more errors than every succeeding age group; and in the case of unknowns, 6-year olds made significantly more errors than every succeeding age level (all p's < .05). Beyond age 6 (unknowns) or 7 (recognition errors) there were no significant age differences. Regarding the recognition errors for MBD children, age differences were significant between (all p's < .05) but not within the age groupings 6–7 years, 8–10 years, 11–12 years, and 13–14 years. In the case of execution errors, age and group did not interact significantly. For the sample as a whole, 6- and 7-year olds differed significantly from succeeding age levels (all p's < .05), but age differences were not significant after age 7.

Group effects.   For execution and recognition reversals errors and unknowns, the main effect of group was highly significant (all p's < .001), reflecting an overall superiority of normal children in each case. The significant age by group interaction, previously mentioned, for recognition reversals errors and unknowns, indicated that the magnitude of group differences were not consistent across ages in the case of these two variables. Individual comparisons revealed a significant superiority for normal children at every age level except the youngest (ages 5 and 6) and the oldest (13 through 15 years) in the case of recognition reversals (all p's < .05). Stated otherwise, normals were signficantly superior to MBDs over the age range 7 through 12. MBD children obtained higher frequencies of unknown errors than normals at age levels 6 through 9 and 11 years (all p's < .05), but differences between the two groups were nonsignificant at older age levels 5, 10, and 12 through 15–9. The age-by-group interaction was nonsignificant for execution reversals errors. However, inspection of the graph in Figure 8.16 indicates that group differences were not consistent across age for this variable. Individual comparisons of normal and MBD groups at each age level reached a significant superiority for normal children, i.e., a smaller frequency of execution reversals errors, at age levels 7, 8, and 9 only (all p's $< .05$). Normal and MBD subjects did not obtain differing frequencies of execution reversals at any other age level. As the graph suggests (and as the statistical data confirm), the significant differences between MBDs and normals at ages 7 and 8 appear to be due mostly to more errors on the part of MBD boys, but not of MBD girls.

Sex effects.   Sex was a significant main effect in the case of recognition reversals ($p < .025$) and this effect approached significance ($p < .10$) in the case of execution reversals. Overall, girls made fewer errors of both types than boys. For neither type of error did the sex difference vary significantly as a function of age or group, as indicated by nonsignificant sex by age, sex by group, and sex by age by group interactions. The sex effect was not significant for unknowns. Girls and boys did not obtain differing scores, overall, for this variable.

Clinical Applications.   The study confirms the general clinical impression that MBD children exhibit letter and number reversals errors more frequently than normal children. Regarding the generally held view that normal children do not reveal reversals beyond the second grade (age 7), the study indicates that this is true for execution reversals errors and unknowns, but not for recognition reversals. Although there is a sharp drop in the frequency of recognition errors between ages 6 and 8 (Figure 8.21), the average youngster still exhibits 1–3 such errors through the mid-teens. Of the three types of errors evaluated (execution, unknowns, and recognition), the Recognition Reversals Test appears to be the most useful in differentiating MBD from normals in that differences between the two groups were significant over age ranges 7–12. For execution reversals the two groups differed significantly only in the age ranges 7–9 and for unknown errors the groups differed significantly over the age ranges 6–9.

In addition to its theoretical value, the data has practical clinical use as part of the MBD diagnostic battery. For example, a 7-year-1-month-old boy is found to have the following scores on the test: section I (Figure 8.22), 10 execution reversals and 1 unknown; section II (Figure 8.23), 21 recognition reversals. Referring to Table 8.4, one sees that this child's execution error frequency is 10 standard deviations (0.96) above the mean (0.40) for normal boys. For MBD boys his execution error frequency is over 3.5 standard deviations (2.28) above the mean (1.85). His 1 unknown error is above average for normal boys, but within the normal range for MBD boys (Table 8.5). His 21 recognition

Figure 8.22

Sample Paper from the Execution Section [I] of the Reversals Frequency Test.

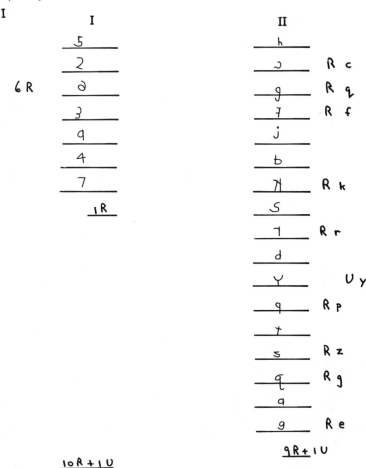

errors place him 2.4 standard deviations (5.31) above the mean (8.16) of normals his age (Table 8.6) but within 1 standard deviation (12.12) of the mean (16.36) of MBD boys his age. Referring to Table 8.7, we note that his 21 recognition errors places him significantly below the tenth percentile of normal boys and from Table 8.8 we find that he is at about the thirty-fifth percentile of MBD boys his age. The findings then, in this boy's case, are strongly suggestive of a neurologically based learning disability. However, one would not want to make the diagnosis on the basis of this examination alone. One would want to utilize other diagnostic criteria as well.

Figure 8.23
Sample Paper from the Recognition Section [II] of the Reversals Frequency Test.

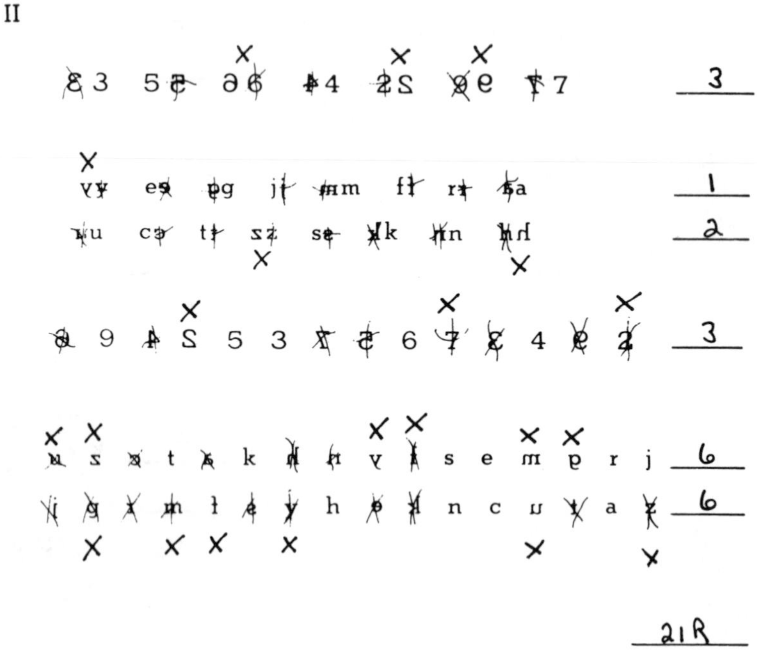

II

&3 5ɘ ɘ6 #4 2S ɘe ʇ7   3

vɣ eʂ ɘg jʇ mm fʇ rʇ ɕa   1

ʮu cɘ tʇ sʑ sɘ ʞk ʞn ʮrl   2

ɕ9 #2 5 3 ʒ ɕ6 ʇ ʒ 4 ɒ ʒ   3

ʮ s ɒ t ʀ k ɖ ʜ v ʇ s e m ɒ r j   6

ʮ ʂ ʮ ʍ ɫ ɕ ʮ h ɒ ʮ n c ʊ ʮ a ʮ   6

                                            21 R

Theories of the Etiology of Reversals.   Many theories have been put forward to explain the reversals phenomenon and its increased frequency in those with neurological learning disabilities. All of these must still be considered speculative. Some seem more reasonable than others. Those that are ultimately confirmed will be welcomed as definite contributions to our understanding of dyslexia.

Orton's Theory.   Samuel Orton (1925, 1929, 1931, 1937) proposed that reversals were the result of the failure of the dominant hemisphere to properly suppress the nondominant. His explanation is based on the premise that the images transmitted from the retinas to the occipital lobes are mirror images of one another. When the dominant hemisphere is impaired in its function of suppressing the nondominant, the reversed image projected on the nondominant is the one that is perceived and may even be the one that is executed when the patient is asked to write or draw that image. Actually, Orton was not the first to conceive of this explanation for reversals. As far back as 1881, Ireland described the same theory. However, it was Orton who collected extensive data in the attempt to confirm it, and his numerous publications on the subject have contributed to the widespread idea that this was "Orton's Theory." The failure of the dominant hemisphere to express its dominance was also viewed by Orton to explain weak laterality. Thus a unified theory was presented, one that explained the correlation between mixed laterality and increased reversals frequency by attributing both phenomena to the failure of the establishment of strong cerebral dominance. Harris (1958) found a definite correlation between the incomplete establishment of strong laterality and reversals frequency, thus tending to confirm Orton's theory.

Davidson (1935), Money (1962), and Critchley (1970) point out that Orton's theory might explain b-d and even p-q reversals, but it does not provide an adequate explanation for b-p and d-p reversals, so commonly seen in both young normal and MBD children. Other clinical observations as well tend to raise questions about the validity of Orton's theory. Most children, without any specific practice, can read sideways and even upside-down. If the mirror-image projections Orton describes occur for letters and numbers, why not for all other objects? Why don't patients with left hemispherectomies exhibit reversals problems immediately after the operation? The nondominant hemisphere in such patients would then, according to Orton, be the only source of information about how letters should be oriented and, according to Orton's theory, should cause a significant reversals problem. But it doesn't occur, suggesting that the orientation knowledge is stored bilaterally.

The most convincing refutation of Orton's theory comes, in my opinion, from neuroanatomical and neurophysiological research on the transmission of retinal impulses to the brain. Orton's theory is based on the notion that there is a one-to-one relationship between the image that is projected on the retina and that which is transmitted back to the occipital cortex. As mentioned, there is every evidence that this is not the case. The retinal rod and cone cells are connected to a complex network of interconnecting cells, which in turn interconnect with many ganglion cells that carry the retinal impulses to the occipital cortex. Light falling on a specific point on the retina is therefore spread throughout certain areas in both occipital lobes. This evidence against the Orton theory of reversals is so compelling that the theory should best be discarded.

Handedness, Scanning, and Writing Direction Tendency. Right-handed children will generally find it easier to write from left to right with arcs in the counterclockwise direction and lines going from NE to SW. Left-handed children seem to be more comfortable writing from right to left with arcs in the clockwise direction and lines going from

NW to SE. Along with this tendency, the left-handed children's letters would seem to be more naturally written as mirror images of the standard. Many left-handed children can mirror write without too much difficulty. And Leonardo da Vinci could do it routinely as many of his extant written documents will testify. Da Vinci was left-handed and it is well known that most of his writings after age 20 were mirror written (Burt, 1957). The theory that he did this in order to conceal his heretical writings from the Church does not seem reasonable in that it is hard to imagine a person as inventive as he resorting to so obvious a subterfuge (Corballis and Beale, 1976). The "correct" orientation of our letters is that of the right-handed person, not the left-handed. Reversals then can be considered to be a manifestation of the mirror-writing tendency. It is no surprise then that letter-reversals errors are described by some to be more common in the left-handed (Harris, 1957; Benson and Geshwind, 1968). Wolfe (1939) found that boys who were poor readers did better than normals in reading mirror-reversed printing.

Because it is the left-handed person's tendency to mirror write, he or she has to learn to suppress it in order to comply with social convention. Hildreth (1950a), a strong supporter of this theory, found reversals frequency greater in low-IQ, left-handed children than those with high IQs. She believes this is due to the fact that low-IQ children, having less capacity to comprehend, do not learn as readily the suppression of their natural tendency to reverse letters. She states, "The strongest tendency to mirror write occurs when left-handedness and mental defect coincide." Hildreth (1950b) and Burt (1957) describe how the right-handed person writing from left to right can easily see what has been written because the right hand "follows" the writing which is to the left of the hand. When the left-handed person writes left to right, the hand tends to cover what has just been written, and so one cannot easily monitor one's writing. By mirror writing, right to left, the left-handed person does not cover with the hand what has just been written. Furthermore, when the right-handed person writes from left to right the individual *pulls* the pen along the line. When the left-handed person writes in the traditional left to right direction the pen must be *pushed*, a maneuver that requires greater effort and is less likely to produce accurate letters. By mirror writing from right to left, the left-handed person can enjoy the advantages of pulling the pen. In order to overcome these drawbacks many left-handed persons "hook" the writing hand above the line of writing and so flex their wrist that they can pull rather than push the writing instrument (Barsley, 1970).

Proponents of this theory hold that the left-handed reader, when required to read in the conventional left-to-right direction, is likely to exhibit frequent "regressions" to his or her natural right-to-left reading direction. Or such readers will not proceed smoothly in the left-to-right direction but stop and "fixate" frequently. Such fixations represent an abortion of the tendency to revert to their more natural right-to-left scanning. Confirmation that children with reading problems do indeed exhibit more regressions and fixations come from studies conducted by Taylor (1966), Blakemore (1969), Zangwill and Blakemore (1972), and Rubino and Minden (1973). The main problem with this theory is that of ascertaining cause and effect. It may be that left-handed poor readers are exhibiting more fixations and regressions than normals because of a tendency to scan from right to left. But it is also possible that their increased frequency of such phenomena is merely the *result* of poor reading ability, that is, poor readers are more likely to have to go over what has been read (regress) or stop and think longer (fixate) about its meaning. Vernon (1960) is a proponent of the latter explanation. A further consideration is that of whether an increased frequency of fixations and regressions does indeed contribute to poor reading. Certainly they reduce reading speed; but they may also increase, rather than decrease, reading comprehension. It is reasonable to suspect that fixating longer on words and going back more frequently to words that have already been read is likely to improve the reader's retention.

In the aforementioned study of reversals frequency (Gardner and Broman, 1979b), the examiners recorded the hand preference for writing of 326 of the normal group and 330 of the MBD group. Ninety-one-and-nine-tenths percent of the normal boys and 90.8% of the normal girls were right-handed as compared to 81.2% of the MBD boys and 78.1% of the MBD girls. The differences between the two groups were significant at the $p < .001$ level. There was no significant difference between the boys and girls in the frequencies of left- and right-handedness in the normal group ($p < .8765$), nor was the difference between boys and girls in the MBD groups of significance ($p < .6278$). In short, with regard to handedness the study bears out common impressions that about 5–10% of normal children are left-handed, and that the frequency of left-handedness in MBD children is significantly greater.

The relationship between hand preference and reversals frequency for execution, unknowns, and recognition was assessed by means of the Wilcoxen rank-sum procedure. Scores on each of the dependent variables were converted to ranks, and right-handed and left-handed children were compared in terms of the sum of the ranks obtained in the case of each of the dependent variables. These comparisons were made separately for normal and MBD boys and girls at each of the 10 age levels from 5–14 years. Of all these comparisons only one was significant (and that barely so). Specifically, there was some correlation between the frequency of recognition reversals made by 12-year-old MBD girls and left-handedness. Essentially, this study did not find any significant correlation between reversals frequency and left-handedness in general.

In the course of the same study, 309 normal children and 317 with MBD were asked to draw a circle. The examiner recorded whether the circle was drawn in a counterclockwise or clockwise direction. (Henceforth the term *torque* will be used to refer to circle directionality, either clockwise or counterclockwise.) In both groups there was a significant increase with age in the tendency to draw circles to the left (counterclockwise), the direction used by most right-handed people. (Normal group, $p < .001$; MBD group, $p < .001$). There was no significant relationship between torque and sex in either the normal group ($p < .7609$) or the MBD group ($p < .4519$). Nor was there any correlation found between torque and membership in either the normal or MBD group ($p < .566$). In short, it appears that there is no significant difference between normal and MBD children with regard to torque, even though an increasing percentage of children in both groups do assume counterclockwise directionality with increasing age.

When all 626 subjects were combined, the majority of both right- and left-handeds were found to draw in a counterclockwise direction. However, a significantly greater proportion of left-handed children drew in a clockwise direction ($p < .0001$). This is true both of the normal group ($p < .0001$) and the MBD group ($p < .0084$). These findings tend to confirm the previously made observation that left-handed children tend to draw circles in the clockwise direction and right-handed children tend to draw them in the counterclockwise direction.

The relationship between torque and scores on the execution, unknown, and recognition reversals frequency tests was assessed by means of the Wilcoxen rank-sum tests. Each of the variables was converted to ranks, and clockwise and counterclockwise children were compared in terms of the sum of the ranks obtained in the case of each of the dependent variables. Of all the comparisons, the only one that was significant (and that, barely so) was between clockwise torque and recognition reversal frequency in 7-year-old normal boys. In essence, the study did not demonstrate a general relationship between torque and reversals frequency.

These studies, then, do not confirm a relationship between handedness and reversals frequency or torque and reversals frequency. They do, however, confirm the general notion that left-handedness is more common among MBD children and that left-handed children are more likely to draw circles in a clockwise direction.

Right-Left Discrimination. The preference for the right or left hand regarding use must be differentiated from the ability to discriminate right from left in general. Shankweiler (1964) studied 12 children with developmental dyslexia. Eight exhibited reversals on reading and 8 (not all the same children) demonstrated writing reversals. Six of the 12 had difficulty differentiating right from left in accordance with the Benton (1968) criteria. Benton points out that right-left discrimination tasks can be quite complex and that many factors may operate in producing errors in such discrimination. Dysphasic patients may have a primary linguistic problem in that they may not understand the meaning of the word symbols "right" and "left." Dyspraxic patients may understand but may not be able to execute correctly the request to point to the right or left. Clearly patients with such problems may only appear to have difficulties in right-left discrimination. For those who actually do, one must differentiate between right-left differentiations made unilaterally on oneself, crossed laterally on oneself, unilaterally on another person, and crossed laterally on another person. Shankweiler did not conclude, however, that the reversals were necessarily caused by the impairment in right-left discrimination. He considered the possibility that both could be manifestations of a more basic underlying disorder and that more complex factors are probably operative.

Belmont and Birch (1965) studied 150 9- and 10-year-old boys from the lowest 10% in reading ability in Aberdeen, Scotland. This group was compared to 50 boys from the upper 90%, matched for age and class placement. Twenty-nine of the poorest readers failed a test of right-left discrimination of parts of their own body, whereas only one of the superior readers failed the test. Again, the question as to whether the right-left discrimination problem causes the reversals or whether both problems are manifestations of a more basic difficulty is not answered by this study.

Orientation Focus.   When a child learns the name of the object we call chair, the name remains the same regardless of the direction in which the chair is facing. Whether pointing north, south, east, or west; whether upright or upside-down, the object is still called a chair. When the child learns to read, however, he or she finds that the orientation of an object is vital to the name one assigns to it and the meaning it has. The letters b, d, and p are all identical regarding their form. Yet they have entirely different names and meanings. The confusion regarding the fact that the child must now concern him- or herself with orientation is viewed by some as the cause of reversals error (Davidson, 1935; Money, 1962; Gibson, Gibson, and Pick, 1962; Kinsbourne, 1973). Even adults are less concerned with orientation than they are with more significant aspects of a visual stimulus. Corballis and Beale (1976) point out that most will readily conjure up a visual image of *Whistler's Mother*, but few are certain in which direction she is facing.

Some confirmation of this theory comes from the work of Teuber and Weinstein (1956) who found that damage to the frontal lobes results in distraction by irrelevant stimuli and attraction to the most prominent element in the stimulus field. Chalfant and Scheffelin (1969) refer to the frontal lobes as controlling active searching and scanning. Those with frontal lobe lesions only sluggishly examine for identifying signs, and conclusions are reached utilizing inappropriate criteria. Proponents of this theory gain support from those who claim that dyslexia is less common in children whose language does not have letters that are reversals of one another. In Chinese and Japanese, for example no character is the mirror image of another. The reversal tendency to these theorists is an artifact, a problem created by those who gave us letters that are mirror images of one another. If the language does not have letters or characters that are mirror images of one another, the problem is obviated.

Stein and Mandler (1974), who are also proponents of this theory, claim that children who exhibit this problem can easily be taught to overcome it by being instructed to attend more to the orientation element. In their study, however, they used geometric forms, not letters. Since linguistic symbols may very well be in a different class than non-linguistic, findings relevant to one class may not be applicable to the other. Johnson and Myklebust (1967) provide children with exercises in correctly orienting geometric figures in the attempt to correct this defect. My own experience has been that many dyslexic children continue to exhibit reversals difficulty in spite of assiduous attempts of teachers, parents, and the children themselves to correct this problem.

Newland (1972) presented a small asymmetric stimulus on a screen and had her subjects state whether the picture faced left, right, up, or down. Children with reading problems made more left-right errors than normals, but the two groups did not differ regarding error frequency for up-down responses. Sidman and Kirk (1974) studied 15 children with reading problems who were known to reverse letters and words. The children were presented with a sample letter and asked to match it to a sample that could be right-left reversed, up-down reversed, or correctly oriented. Left-right errors were more common than up-down errors. If the letter reversals problem were simply one of orientation, then one would expect left-right errors to be as frequent as up-down. These studies, like most, reveal that right-left errors are usually significantly more common than up-down, suggesting that simple unfamiliarity with the orientation element is not likely to be the sole, or even significant factor, in letter reversals problems.

Kinsbourne (1976a) believes that a related factor in the dyslexic child's reversals problem is the tendency to focus on the more salient features of a stimulus. The form is far more important than orientation to the child. The child simplifies a challenge by avoiding distractions by what is considered nonessential. Recognizing that the letter is a b, d, or p is far more important than differentiating one from the other by virtue of its orientation. The principle was described earlier by Piaget who found that at early levels of cognitive development the child uses the most apparent stimulus to derive conclusions. Elsewhere, Kinsbourne (1976b) describes three recognition steps in the child's learning to read: (1) form discrimination, (2) orientation, and (3) sequence. In short, the child must first learn to identify letters by form and differentiate one from the other. When this is accomplished, the child then concerns him- or herself with the more sophisticated task of differentiating orientation. And only after this is accomplished is the child concerned with the correct sequence of letters.

Attentional Deficit and Impulsivity.   In recent years many investigators (Douglas, 1972, 1974a, 1974b; Dykman et al. 1974; Conners, 1974, 1976; Cantwell, 1975a, 1977; Ross and Ross, 1976) have emphasized the importance of the attentional deficit in many children with neurological learning disabilities. And the improvement of many of these children's symptoms by psychostimulant medication has lent support to this theory (Conners, 1974; Peters et al., 1974; Fish, 1975; Cantwell, 1975b). Pertinent to this discussion is the question of whether reversals errors are also a manifestation of the attentional deficit. Does the child who writes a b when asked to write a d, do so because he or she is not properly paying attention. Kinsbourne (1976b) postulates that the child's focusing on the most salient features of a stimulus (form rather than orientation) may be a manifestation of a more fundamental attentional problem. Were the child to concentrate better, there would be more efficient scanning of the stimulus letter and the orientational elements would be better appreciated.

Kinsbourne (1976b) also considers such children's impulsivity problem to contribute to reversals errors. The child does not approach the problem in a systematic way. There is little, if any pause for forethought as to whether the letter is correctly or incorrectly oriented. Kinsbourne presents, as confirmation of his theory that the attentional deficit and impulsivity are important contributing factors in producing reversals errors, the observation that these children are accurate about half the time in identifying correctly oriented letters. This suggests that they leave this matter to chance and that this is what is done by impulsive children and those with attentional deficits.

In my own studies, most of the children did not impulsively go through the test. The few that were starting to do so were slowed down and encouraged to proceed with greater forethought and deliberation.

Most appeared to be concentrating to the limit of their capacity. (This does not mean, however, that they were necessarily concentrating as well as normals.) Accordingly, at the clinical level, impulsivity and impaired concentration did not seem to be a prominent factor. More important, those few children who were tested twice usually attained similar scores (within a few points) and many made the same mistakes, thereby suggesting that chance guesses were not the cause of their deficient performances.

Visual Discrimination. It might appear reasonable that reversals problems are simply a manifestation of a problem in visual discrimination, i.e., differentiating one visual stimulus from another. Just as the child who does poorly on the Wepman Test of Auditory Discrimination (1973) has trouble differentiating between words that sound similar but are not identical, so the child with a visual discrimination problem would have trouble differentiating between visual stimuli that are similar but not identical, like b and d. I will discuss below my own studies in which I attempted to determine whether children with high reversals frequencies also exhibit difficulty in differentiating letters that are mirror images of one another. The study was structured to remove the memory and retrieval elements and focus primarily on the ability to visually discriminate between mirror image letters and numbers.

Psychoanalytic Theory. I know of no article in which a psychoanalytic theory of reversals errors is presented. However, Fliess (1956) attributes to Abraham (1927) the theory that right-left confusion (a possible cause of reversals error) is a manifestation of a more basic confusion between anal and genital impulses. Corballis and Beale (1976) have my full agreement regarding the plausibility of this theory when they state that it is "more predictive of a back-front than of a left-right confusion!"

The Theory of Reversals Frequency That Appears Most Reasonable to Me. I believe that a presentation of the reversals theory that seems most reasonable to me is best accomplished by considering again the various phases of visual processing described at the beginning of this chapter, that is, specifically by considering the probability that the reversals problem is likely to result from impairments at each particular level.

Although the lens inverts the usual image that is projected on the retina, this image is not projected as an engram to the visual cortex; rather it is spread throughout the visual field by coded information. Accordingly, the visual reception-transduction system is not likely to be playing a role in producing reversals errors. There is also little reason to believe that the processes that correct potential distortions resulting from literal interpretation of the retinal projection (seeing a door as trapezoidal, for example) are involved. There is no reason to believe that the processes that enable us to appreciate depth and distance are involved either, because such functions are not required for letter recognition.

The previously discussed studies by Lyle and Goyen (1968) and Liberman et al. (1971) would seem to suggest that a problem in visual discrimination might be operative in producing reversals errors. Their dyslexic patients made more reversals errors than normals when asked to match an image presented tachistoscopically with the correct item in a series of possibilities, some of which were mirror-image reversals. However, in both of these studies the child was asked to make the match *after* visualization had been terminated. Accordingly, visual memory and retrieval were also being tested here, and impairments in these functions could account for the errors.

I know of no studies in which normal and dyslexic children were compared on their ability to match a letter with the one of a series of letters that is identical with it, the other letters in the series being reversed in various ways. Gibson et al. (1962) did collect data on the ability of normal children ages 4–8 to perform such a task. As expected, they found that there is a gradual improvement in children's ability to do this and that by age 8 such errors drop out almost entirely. However, these examiners did not administer their test to dyslexic children. Such a study might shed light on the question of whether the letter-reversals problem is related to impaired visual discrimination. In order to investigate this problem further, a study was conducted by me and my colleagues in which a group of MBD children was divided into two groups: (1) those whose reading level was not below two years the expected reading level for their age and (2) those whose reading level was two or more years below the expected reading level for their age. The children were all students in special classes and schools for MBD children with learning disabilities. None of the subjects was in a regular class. All had been well diagnosed as having neurologically based learning disabilities. Expected grade level was calculated according to age. Specifically, a 6-year-old was assumed to be able to read at first-grade level, a 7-year-old at second-grade level, an 8-year-old at fourth grade level, etc. However, children under 7 were excluded from the study because one cannot meaningfully consider children below that age to be two years behind in reading. Children between 10-0 and 10-11, for example, were expected to be reading at mid-fifth-grade level at the time of the study because it was conducted in the middle of the school year. All children in this age bracket who were reading at the 3-6 level and above were classified as "good" readers, i.e., reading within two years of their expected reading level for age. All those in this age bracket, reading at the 3-5 level and below, were considered to be "poor" readers, i.e., they were more than two years behind their expected reading level for age.

One hundred MBD children were included in the study. Each child was administered all three sections of the Reversals Frequency Test (Execution, Recognition, and Matching). It is my belief that the Execution (I) and Recognition (II) sections require adequate visual memory (storage and retrieval) functioning, whereas the Matching (III) section does not. In order to perform successfully in sections I and II, the child must have stored information about what the correctly oriented letter looks like. He must be able to convert that information into an internal display of the letter or number. He must then be able to write a duplicate of the engram he is internally visualizing (Execution section) or compare it with the one he is viewing on the test paper (Recognition section). The Matching section (III) requires no such storage and retrieval. In fact, as mentioned, I believe that a child with no previous familiarity with English letters and Arabic numerals could successfully accomplish the task. What is required to perform this test adequately is competence in visual discrimination, in the ability to see the difference between correctly oriented letters and numbers and their mirror images. It follows then, that if the problems that dyslexics have is primarily one of discrimination, then the poorer readers would do worse than the good ones on the matching test and they would not differ significantly on the execution and recognition tests. If the dyslexia problem is primarily one of memory, then the poor readers would do worse than the good readers on the execution and recognition tests, and not differ significantly from one another on the matching test.

The 100 MBD children were divided into good and poor readers as defined above. The data for the 7-10-year-old children were analyzed separately from that of the 11-14-year-olds because, as previously discussed, the 7-10 bracket is the age at which there is the greatest disparity between normals and MBDs. The results of the study are tabulated in Table 8.9. As can be seen, there was no significant difference between the good and poor readers on the Matching section in both age brackets. (Fisher's Exact Test was used and probabilities below the .05 level were taken to indicate significance.) On the Recognition section, the poorer readers did significantly worse than the good readers in both age brackets. This was also true of the older children with regard to the Execution section, but the differences between the good and poor readers in the younger (7-10) group was not significant. Were there a significant difference between the 7-10-year-olds on the Execution section, then the theory that memory, more than discrimina-

Table 8.9
Comparisons of "Good" MBD and "Poor" MBD Readers on Three Tests of Reversals Frequency.

	N	Execution Reversals Errors [I]				Recognition Reversals Errors [II]						Matching Reversals Errors [III]			
		0		1+		0-4		5-9		10+		0		1+	
		N	[%]	N	[%]	N	[%]	N	[%]	N	[%]	N	[%]	N	[%]
MBD Ages 7-10															
Poor readers	19	14	(74)	5	(26)	6	(32)	6	(32)	7	(36)	9	(47)	10	(53)
Good readers	9	6	(67)	3	(33)	6	(67)	0	(0)	3	(33)	7	(78)	2	(22)
p [Fisher's Exact Test, 1 tailed]		N.S.[a]				p < .05						N.S.			
MBD Ages 11-14															
Poor readers	46	38	(83)	8	(17)	32	(70)	7	(15)	7	(15)	31	(67)	15	(33)
Good readers	26	25	(96)	1	(4)	20	(77)	6	(23)	0	(0)	21	(81)	5	(19)
p [Fisher's Exact Test, 1 tailed]		p < .05				p < .05						N.S.			
	100														

[a] Not significant.

tion, is a primary problem for poor MBD readers would have been strongly supported. All we can conclude with regard to this study is that the results support the memory theory much more than they do the discrimination theory. A discrimination theory would have been supported if the poorer readers did significantly worse on the Matching section at both age levels, and if there was no significant difference between the good and poor readers on the Execution and Recognition sections in both age brackets. The aforementioned drawback notwithstanding, I consider the study to be much more supportive of the theory that a memory impairment is responsible for reversals deficit than one that postulates a "perceptual" (discrimination) deficit as an important contributing factor.

In an attempt to shed further light on the question of whether reversals errors are more likely to be discriminatory or related to memory impairments, a second study was conducted. Ninety-nine normal children, ages 7-0 to 8-11, were administered the Matching section of the Reversals Frequency Test. These children were all in normal classes with no history of learning impairment. They were all of average intelligence, either on the basis of IQ scores or average standing on national tests of academic performance. Their scores were compared to the 9 MBD good readers and the 19 MBD poor readers in the 7-10 age bracket from the study described above. The results of the study are shown in Table 8.10. Again, Fisher's Exact Test was used in the data analysis, and probabilities below the .05 level were taken to indicate significance. Strong support for the memory theory would come from findings that indicated no significant difference at all among the three groups, that the worst readers do as well as normal children with regard to their ability to visually differentiate correctly oriented letters from various types of reversals. If, however, the normals did significantly better than the good MBD readers, and the good MBD readers did significantly better than the poor MBD readers, then one would have to conclude that a discrimination problem was very likely to be contributing to these children's reading disability.

Again, the findings (Table 8.10) are equivocal, but more supportive of the memory than the discrimination theory. There was no significant difference between the normals and the good MBD readers. This would support the memory theory. There was no significant difference between the good MBD and the poor MBD readers. This finding also supports the memory theory. There was, however, a significant difference between the normals and the poor MBD readers, lending support to the discrimination theory. It is not unreasonable, however, to attribute the poor performance of the poor MBD readers to such factors as impaired concentration and impulsivity. If one accepts this explana-

Table 8.10

Comparisons of Normals, "Good" MBD, and "Poor" MBD Readers on the Matching Section [III] of the Reversals Frequency Test.

| | Number of Errors | | | | |
| | 0 | | 1 + | | |
	N	[%]	N	[%]	Total
Normals (ages 7–10)	75	(76)	24	(24)	99
Good MBD readers (ages 7–10)	7	(78)	2	(22)	9
Poor MBD readers (ages 7–10)	9	(47)	10	(53)	19

Normals vs. good MBD readers, not significant
Normals vs. poor MBD readers, p < .026.
Good MBD readers vs. poor MBD readers, not significant

tion, then the memory theory is strongly supported. If one does not, then the results, in my opinion, are still more supportive of the memory than the discrimination theory. Another explanation for the significant difference between the normals and the MBD poor readers is that the errors of the MBD group were increased by a small percentage who do indeed have a visual-discrimination problem. If this is the case, then one can say that most MBD children's reversals problems are related to memory impairment, but that a small percentage do have a discriminatory deficit.

I have attempted to apply my findings from the Reversals Frequency Test as well as from handedness frequency and circle drawing direction data, collected on normal and MBD children, to shed further light on the more common theories of reversals-errors etiology. My findings, combined with those of other studies, do not lend support to Orton's theory of impaired cerebral dominance. Nor do my findings support the theory that suppressed mirror writing in left-handed children induces directional difficulties in writing that contribute to reversals errors. My observations do not support the notion that lack of experience with orientation as a consideration in naming an entity is an important contributing factor in persistent reversals errors. I do not consider attentional deficits and impulsivity to be of fundamental etiological significance in reversals errors, although it cannot be denied that such manifestations can compound the problem. The notion that a simple problem in visual discrimination is important is also not supported by my findings.

In my opinion, the most convincing theories are those that consider an impairment in visual memory to be central to the problem. De Hirsch's (1965) notion of plasticity seems to be the most tenable. Symbols, especially linguistic, do not get firmly embedded in the psychic structure. There is a looseness to their accurate and precise storage and possibly an impairment in their retrieval as well. Corballis and Beale (1976), as well, in an excellent study of the subject of right-left discrimination, consider the reversals problem to be at the level of memory, rather than of perception. However, one does well to appreciate that the reversals problem is only one small part of the MBD child's difficulties with letter usage, and that problems with consonants and vowels (especially the latter) are more common than reversals errors. In addition, one does well to view MBD children's problems with letters to be one aspect of a more general problem of language decoding (understanding the entity that a linguistic symbol denotes) and encoding (forming the linguistic symbol that denotes an entity). Increased reversals frequency is a dramatic clue to such difficulties, and with my test reversals frequency can easily be measured and the degree of deviation from the normal readily ascertained.

The reader may have wondered why I have devoted such a lengthy discussion to the subject of reversals. My principal reason relates to my belief that there is a high correlation between reversals errors and the neurologically based learning disabilities. Many children whose reading is impaired are often automatically considered to be suffering with a neurophysiological impairment. Accordingly, there are many children with purely psychogenic reading disturbances who are being misdiagnosed. Reversals errors are, in my opinion, specifically "organic" in etiology. Therefore they are useful diagnostically, and the normative data on reversals frequency that my colleagues and I have collected will, hopefully, serve to objectify the diagnosis of the neurologically based learning disabilities. I do not believe that high reversals frequency is automatically diagnostic of a neurologically based reading disorder. I am only saying that it is highly correlated with such an impairment. In addition, from the theoretical point, an understanding of this typically organic sign can help us gain further insight into the causes and manifestations of MBD. The study described on reversals etiology is the kind of inquiry that can provide such information.

VISUAL SEQUENTIAL MEMORY

Visual sequential memory appears to be a special category of visual memory. A child, for example, may be able to recall all the letters of a word, but not in the correct order. Therefore, he will do poorly in spelling even though he has recalled correctly all the letters in a word and not included letters that do not belong. On the Digit Span subtest of the WISC-R, no credit is given if numbers, even though correctly recalled, are not in the proper order. As will be discussed in chapter 9, there are some who believe that a central problem for children who do poorly on the Bender Gestalt Test is not one of "visual perception" but of visual sequencing and construction dyspraxia. The tests described here enable the examiner to assess objectively this aspect of visual memory.

The Digits Backward Section of the Digit
Span Subtest of the WISC-R

As discussed in chapter 7, the Digit Span subtest of the WISC-R is actually two separate tests. In chapter 7, I described the Digits Forward section as a test of short-term auditory memory. Here I will discuss in greater detail the rationale for considering Digit Span to be two separate tests and then describe the use of Digits Backward as a test for short-term visual memory, especially visual sequential memory.

Designers of the most commonly used tests of intelligence have generally appreciated that what we refer to as *intelligence* is really a composite of capabilities, and that any test, no matter how comprehensive, can only assess a fraction of capacities in the human repertoire. They have generally recognized, as well, that a subtest rarely, if ever, evaluates a single function. Accordingly, the final IQ score is best viewed as a statistical average of a wide range of functions, numbering far more than the number of subtests in the particular instrument. Although averages provide some information, one clearly learns more from the particular data utilized in determining the average. Meaningful data get lost in averages. Abnormal highs counterbalance abnormal lows and both get buried in the resultant average. But even the subtest should be viewed as an average, that is, a composite of the various functions that have contributed to its resultant score. The more we can isolate and quantify the particular entities within the subtests, the better will be our understanding, not only of intelligence, but of the wide variety of functions that we have selected to include in the test being utilized.

An analogy from medicine is applicable here. Most patients would not particularly appreciate being told that the average value of 10 of their blood tests was in the normal range, that is, that the sum of their hemoglobin, free blood sugar, blood urea nitrogen, white count, etc., when divided by 10 resulted in a figure that was in the average range. But even when the specific figures are given, one wants to know the reasons why a particular value is abnormal. There are literally thousands of causes of an elevated white-blood-cell count. To say that it is elevated is only a *clue* that something is wrong. It puts us on the track to pathology. Further inquiry is made, further testing or examinations conducted, in order to ascertain the specific cause of the abnormality.

My study, described below, attempts to isolate and quantify factors that contribute to the score that one obtains on the Digit Span subtest of the WISC-R (Wechsler, 1974). In the first half of the test, Digits Forward, the examiner presents the child with a three-digit number, given at the rate of one digit per second. If the child repeats the sequence correctly he is given a score of 1; if not, he is scored 0. Then a second three-digit number is presented. Next, two four-digit numbers are given and similarly scored. Each pair of sequences is one digit longer than its predecessor. The increasingly longer number sequences are presented until the child misses both series of the same length. The longest trial pair are two nine-digit numbers. The child's score on this part of the subtest is the total number of sequences recalled correctly.

In the Digits Backward section, the child is instructed to repeat the presented sequence in reverse order. Trial pairs range from 2- to 8-digit numbers. Scoring is identical to the Digits Forward section, with the child receiving one point for each sequence correctly repeated backwards. The scores on the two sections are then *combined* to obtain the raw score. This is converted to the *scaled score* by reference to the proper table. For the purposes of subsequent discussion I wish to emphasize here that the two scores are combined; there is no way of obtaining a scaled score (thereby comparing the child to others) for Digits Forward or Digits Backward as separate entities.

What the Test Measures

Wechsler (1958) emphasized the Digit Span's value in assessing immediate auditory memory, sustained auditory attention (especially Digits Backward), anxiety level (the anxious child will not attend well to the examiner's recitation of the numbers and will not concentrate well on recalling them), and the suspension of irrelevant thought processes (if one is preoccupied with other material, one is not going to concentrate well on the immediate task of number recall). Wechsler considered the capacity to recall rote material to be of less value than most other functions in his battery in ascertaining intelligence. Accordingly, he combined Digits Forward and Digits Backward into one subtest (Wechsler, 1958) in order to reduce its influence on the total IQ. By combining the two, Digit Span contributes only 1/12 of the score; if used as two tests, they would contribute 2/13. Furthermore, he designated Digit Span (along with the Mazes subtest) as optional, i.e., it should be one of the first to be omitted if one chose (as most do) not to administer the total battery of 12 subtests. Accordingly, it is one of the least frequently utilized of the WISC and WISC-R subtests. When utilizing the WISC (Wechsler, 1949) one can include Digit Span (and Mazes) in the Full Scale IQ by prorating from 5 to 6 subtests. This is not possible in the WISC-R (Wechsler, 1974). One can, however, use Digit Span or Mazes as a substitute for another test in computing the Full Scale IQ.

Glasser and Zimmerman (1967) emphasize that Digit Span is not correlated with general intelligence for *all* levels, but is sensitive to intellectual deficit and organic defect because of the concentration and memory impairments that such patients so frequently exhibit. Because such functions become impaired when there is psychogenic disorganization, the subtest may detect anxiety and varying degrees of disorganization. They consider the primary value of Digit Span to be that of measuring immediate auditory recall, capacity for grouping operations, attention, ability to suspend irrelevant thought, and the self-control of mental operations. They point out that performing Digits Forward is a relatively passive procedure (listening); whereas Digits Backward is a more active operation (requiring greater concentration and cogitation). They (like Wechsler) do not consider it to be well correlated with high intelligence in that there are people with good rote memories who are not particularly bright.

Of particular pertinence to this discussion are Glasser and Zimmerman's comments on significant discrepancies between the two sections of the subtest. They hold that it is probably impossible to genuinely obtain a higher score on Digits Backward than on Digits Forward because the digits backward operation requires one to review the forward series before conversion to reverse order. Yet most examiners agree that one occasionally sees a child who does better on Digits Backward than on Digits Forward. Such superiority may be specious and might be explained by the child's not "catching on" until the Digits Backward section is reached. Or the child may be one who rejects "easy" tasks and only applies himself diligently (from the desire to excel) when more difficult tasks are presented. Independent types, who only strive in areas of their own choosing, may selectively reject the Digits Forward section. And negativistic children may get some morbid gratification from rejecting certain aspects of the tests. There are probably some children whose visual learning is significantly superior to their auditory and so they do better on the Digits Backward section because visual functions (as I will elaborate below) are called into play when one verbalizes the presented sequence in reverse order.

I believe that there is another factor that one must consider when a child appears to have Digits Backward superiority. The Digits Forward section begins with three-digit numbers; whereas the Digits Backward begins with two-digit numbers. Let us take, for example, a child who on the Digits Forward section correctly recalls both three-digit and four-digit numbers, but misses both five-digit numbers. Such a child's raw score would be 4. Now if this child were to repeat correctly in reverse order both two-digit, three-digit, and four-digit numbers, and then miss both five-digit numbers, his raw score would be 6. It would appear that his Digits Backward capacity was superior to his Digits Forward. Actually only his *score* here is superior, his *capacity* is identical. The superiority, then, is specious, an artifact of the test. The child who is truly superior on the Digits Backward would have to be able to recall longer digit series on the Digit Backward section, not merely obtain a higher score.

When the Digits Backward scores are significantly lower (generally considered to be 3 or more points) than Digits Forward, pathological factors are possibly operative. Costa (1975) and Lezak (1976) consider such discrepancy to be strongly suggestive of brain damage. Such children may be very anxious and have a tendency to "fragmentize" under pressure. They may have trouble shifting their frame of reference (from the forward to the backward task), or even of comprehending the reversed-function operation. Combining the forward and backward scores will cause such discrepancies (higher Digits Backward or significantly lower Digits Backward) to be lost to the reader of the psychological test report, unless this has been specifically pointed out by the initial examiner.

Sattler (1974) points out that Digits Backward not only requires memory but also the capacity for remanipulation and reorganization. He also refers to the more active participation required for Digits Backward as compared to Digits Forward. He considers Digit Span, along with Arithmetic, to be an excellent test of concentration, especially at younger ages. Sattler makes reference to the visualization of the digits (an issue that I will discuss subsequently) but does not differentiate between the two sections of the test with regard to this element.

Weinberg et al. (1972) and Lezak (1976) make specific reference to the internal visual-scanning operation in the Digits Backward section of the subtest. Lezak describes, as well, the "feat of mental double-tracking" involved in the Digit Backward section, i.e., the subject must scan the sequence both forward and backward in order to perform the task. Rudel and Denckla (1974) also consider the Digit Span to be two separate tests that reflect the differential functioning of the two hemispheres. Digits Forward requires primarily verbal repetition of numbers and is primarily a left-hemisphere function. Digits Backward, requiring "visualization" and conversion into spatial coordinates, is primarily a right-hemisphere function. Their studies of 297 school children with learning disabilities confirmed this hypothesis. They found that those children whose neurological signs were primarily right-sided (indicative of left-hemisphere dysfunction) did most poorly on Digits Forward. Those with predominantly left-sided neurological signs (indicative of right-hemisphere dysfunction) characteristically did worse on Digits Backward. Weinberg et al. (1972) came to similar conclusions after administering the two Digit Span sections to right- and left-sided adult hemiplegics. Thirty percent of Rudel and Denckla's subjects exhibited a difference of 3 or more points between Digits Forward and Backward, giving support to the commonly held view that a differential of this magnitude is strongly suggestive of organic disease of the brain.

It is my view that both sections of the subtest test *auditory* memory. The Digits Backward section, much more than the Digits Forward, is likely to assess *visual* memory as well. In repeating the presented digits forward, most subjects do not need to form an internal visual image (engram) of the numerical sequence. Repeating the digits backward requires most, if not all, subjects to form an internal display that is then scanned, at least for the backward operation and probably, for most subjects, for both forward and backward operations. It is, thus, *formation of an engrammatic display* and subsequent *scanning* that distinguishes the two sections of the subtest. Digits Backward, then, is a test (among other things) of the capacity to form an internal *visual* display from an auditory stimulus, that is, to transform an auditory presentation into a visual engram. Furthermore, internal scanning processes are *necessary* for successful performances of the task. In Digits Forward, scanning is probably an optional feature (probably not used at all by most for the shorter sequences and probably used only to a limited degree for the longer ones).

Digits Forward and Digits Backward as Separate Tests

Considering the aforementioned limitations of the Digit Span subtest as an indicator of intelligence, Wechsler was probably justified in combining Digits Forward and Digits Backward in order to reduce their importance in the total IQ determination. As a result of combining them, however, the examiner may be deprived of important information. A child, for example, who has good auditory memory, but poor visual memory (a common problem among children with neurologically based learning disabilities), may do better than average on Digits Forward and below average on Digits Backward. When the two scores are combined he may end up with a raw score (and, therefore, a scaled score) that is in the normal range. Because the examiner generally only records the combined score, the defect gets buried in the average score that results. The short-term visual-memory problem and/or internal-scanning defect is therefore not detected.

Because of my interest in objectifying the diagnosis of neurologically based learning disabilities, and because of my appreciation of the valuable role that the WISC-R battery can play in this regard, I have collected separate Digits Forward and Digits Backward scores on 1,567 school children (782 boys and 785 girls) ages 5-0 through 15-11.

(There were 2,200 children used for standardization of the WISC-R.) The children were from schools in Bergen County, New Jersey (a suburb of New York City). They came primarily from working-class (blue-collar and lower-to-middle-income white-collar) families and were generally in the average range of intelligence. Their scores on standardized national achievement tests were primarily in the average range. Boys and girls in special classes, those with a history of grade repeat, or children who required special tutoring were excluded from the study.

The subjects' scores were divided into 1/2-year age brackets. The average number of children for each of the 22 1/2-year age levels from 5-0 through 15-11 was approximately 35 (number range for boys 16–53, for girls 27–52). The data for Digits Forward has been presented in chapter 7. For Digits Backward, means, standard deviations, and percentile ranks for boys are presented in Table 8.11. The same data for girls are to be found in Table 8.12. With such data, the examiner is in a position to gain the same information provided by the Wechsler Digit Span subtest (as to be described below, the data are comparable), but can, in addition, detect those children with the aforementioned kinds of visual-processing problems, namely, impaired formation of an internal visual

Table 8.11
Digit Span—Digits Backward for Boys

Age	N	Mean	S.D.	Percentiles								
				10	20	30	40	50	60	70	80	90
5-0 to 5-5	26	1.69	1.12	0.0	1.0	1.0	1.0	2.0	2.0	2.0	2.6	3.0
5-6 to 5-11	29	1.66	1.47	0.0	0.0	0.0	1.0	1.0	2.0	2.0	3.0	4.0
6-0 to 6-5	33	2.48	1.44	0.4	1.0	2.0	2.0	2.0	2.0	3.0	4.0	4.0
6-6 to 6-11	43	3.23	1.17	2.0	2.0	3.0	3.0	3.0	3.0	4.0	4.0	4.6
7-0 to 7-5	45	3.62	1.39	2.0	3.0	3.0	3.0	4.0	4.0	4.0	4.0	6.0
7-6 to 7-11	53	3.87	1.00	3.0	3.0	3.0	4.0	4.0	4.0	4.0	5.0	5.0
8-0 to 8-5	36	3.69	1.43	2.0	2.4	3.0	3.0	4.0	4.0	4.0	5.0	6.0
8-6 to 8-11	47	3.85	1.22	2.0	3.0	3.0	4.0	4.0	4.0	4.0	5.0	5.0
9-0 to 9-5	38	4.26	1.27	2.0	3.0	4.0	4.0	4.0	4.0	5.0	5.0	6.0
9-6 to 9-11	34	4.82	2.05	2.5	3.0	4.0	4.0	4.0	5.0	5.0	7.0	8.5
10-0 to 10-5	29	4.31	1.37	2.0	3.0	4.0	4.0	4.0	4.0	4.0	6.0	6.0
10-6 to 10-11	22	6.09	2.07	3.3	4.0	5.0	5.0	6.0	6.0	7.1	8.0	9.7
11-0 to 11-5	34	5.09	1.75	3.0	4.0	4.0	4.0	5.0	5.0	6.0	7.0	7.0
11-6 to 11-11	35	4.89	1.37	3.0	4.0	4.0	5.0	5.0	5.0	5.2	6.0	7.0
12-0 to 12-5	35	5.14	1.88	3.0	4.0	4.0	4.0	5.0	5.0	5.2	6.8	8.4
12-6 to 12-11	40	5.43	1.75	3.1	4.0	4.0	5.0	5.0	6.0	6.0	7.0	7.9
13-0 to 13-5	51	5.22	1.85	3.0	4.0	4.0	5.0	5.0	5.0	6.0	7.0	7.0
13-6 to 13-11	38	5.82	2.14	3.0	4.0	4.0	5.0	6.0	6.0	7.0	7.2	9.0
14-0 to 14-5	35	4.68	1.54	3.0	4.0	4.0	4.0	4.0	5.0	6.0	7.0	8.4
14-6 to 14-11	36	5.17	1.59	3.0	4.0	4.0	5.0	5.0	6.0	6.0	6.6	7.0
15-0 to 15-5	27	4.52	1.58	2.8	3.0	4.0	4.0	4.0	5.0	5.0	5.4	6.2
15-6 to 15-11	16	5.13	1.36	3.7	4.0	4.0	4.8	5.0	5.0	5.9	6.6	7.3
	782											

Table 8.12

Digit Span—Digits Backward for Girls

Age	N	Mean	S.D.	10	20	30	40	50	60	70	80	90
								Percentiles				
5-0 to 5-5	27	1.22	1.36	0.0	0.0	0.0	0.0	1.0	2.0	2.0	2.4	3.2
5-6 to 5-11	22	1.36	1.09	0.0	0.0	0.0	1.0	2.0	2.0	2.0	2.0	3.0
6-0 to 6-5	30	2.67	1.42	0.0	2.0	2.0	2.4	3.0	3.0	3.7	4.0	5.0
6-6 to 6-11	36	3.47	1.13	2.0	2.0	3.0	3.0	4.0	4.0	4.0	4.0	5.0
7-0 to 7-5	43	3.72	1.47	2.0	3.0	3.0	3.0	3.0	4.0	4.0	5.0	5.0
7-6 to 7-11	42	3.76	1.25	2.0	3.0	3.0	4.0	4.0	4.0	4.0	5.0	5.0
8-0 to 8-5	37	3.97	1.17	2.0	3.0	3.0	4.0	4.0	4.0	4.0	5.0	6.0
8-6 to 8-11	51	4.02	1.39	2.0	3.0	4.0	4.0	4.0	4.0	5.0	5.0	6.0
9-0 to 9-5	38	4.05	1.63	2.0	3.0	3.0	3.6	4.0	4.0	5.0	5.0	6.0
9-6 to 9-11	28	4.79	1.50	3.0	4.0	4.0	4.0	4.0	5.0	5.3	6.0	7.1
10-0 to 10-5	30	4.53	1.50	3.0	3.0	4.0	4.0	4.0	5.0	5.0	5.0	6.9
10-6 to 10-11	29	5.00	1.67	3.0	3.0	4.0	5.0	5.0	5.0	6.0	6.0	7.0
11-0 to 11-5	52	5.35	1.82	3.0	4.0	4.0	5.0	5.0	6.0	6.0	7.0	7.7
11-6 to 11-11	36	5.72	2.16	3.0	4.0	5.0	5.0	5.5	6.0	6.9	7.0	9.0
12-0 to 12-5	37	5.30	1.68	4.0	4.0	4.0	5.0	5.0	5.0	6.0	6.0	8.0
12-6 to 12-11	47	5.68	1.75	3.8	4.0	5.0	5.0	5.0	6.0	6.0	7.4	8.0
13-0 to 13-5	42	5.74	1.68	4.0	4.0	5.0	5.0	6.0	6.0	6.1	7.0	7.7
13-6 to 13-11	36	5.31	1.85	3.0	4.0	4.1	5.0	5.0	5.0	6.0	6.0	8.3
14-0 to 14-5	36	5.08	1.90	3.0	3.4	4.0	4.0	4.5	5.0	5.9	7.0	8.0
14-6 to 14-11	34	6.12	2.52	4.0	4.0	4.0	5.0	5.5	6.0	7.0	9.0	10.5
15-0 to 15-5	25	5.72	1.37	4.0	4.0	5.0	5.0	6.0	6.0	6.2	7.0	7.4
15-6 to 15-11	27	6.26	2.16	3.8	4.0	5.0	5.2	6.0	7.0	7.0	8.0	9.2
	785											

engram from an auditory stimulus and/or defective internal visual scanning. In addition, discrepancies between the two figures (Digits Backward higher than or three or more points lower than Digits Forward) are automatically reported.

Comparison of the Gardner Data with Wechsler's

In order to ascertain whether my data were comparable to Wechsler's, the *raw score* totals (Digits Forward *plus* Digits Backward) of the two instruments were compared. My subjects ranged in age from 5-0 through 15-11; Wechsler's 6-0 through 16-11. Accordingly, only the 6-0 through 15-11 group of the two instruments could be compared. [My lowest year (5-0 through 5-11) and Wechsler's highest year (16-0 through 16-11) were omitted from comparison.] Wechsler's data is divided into 1/3-year groupings, mine into 1/2-year groupings. To facilitate comparison, full-year groups were compared. This was done by first calculating the average raw score totals for each full-year age level in my study. For example, for 7-year-old boys, the average total raw score is 9.06. With the Wechsler data the raw score corresponding to a scaled score of 10 was recorded for each of the 1/3-year age brackets. The average of the three raw scores for each one-year level was calculated. For example, at the 7-0 to 7-3 age level, the Digit Span (total) raw score corresponding to a scaled score of 10 is 8. At the 7-4 to 7-7 age level the raw score is 9. And at the 7-8 to 7-11 year level it is 9. The average, therefore, for these three figures is 8.67. The difference between my figures and Wechsler's is $+0.39$ (when my figure was higher, it was assigned a plus sign, when lower a minus). The differences between the two sets of data for each of the one-year age levels are shown in Table 8.13. The average difference for all age levels between my boys' scores and Wechsler's subjects (boys and girls combined) was -0.28. For my girls, the difference was $+0.21$. Because scores can only exist at full integer levels (6.00, 7.00, etc.) it is reasonable to consider a deviation of less than 0.5 to make the data comparable. These deviations are far below this level. If one combines my boys' and girls' deviations (to make my data even more comparable to Wechsler's) the average deviation is only -0.035. It is reasonable to conclude, then, that my data are comparable to Wechsler's. Furthermore, they confirm Wechsler's conclusion that there are no significant differences between the performance of boys and girls on this instrument and that the data from the two groups can justifiably be combined.

The data can be used clinically in the following way. A 7½-year-old girl gets a raw score of 5 on Digits Forward and 4 on Digits Backward. We see from Table 8.12 that the mean Digits Backward score for girls her age is 3.76 ± 1.25. Her score, therefore, is in the normal range, within 1 standard deviation of the average. From the table of percentile ranks, we see that her score is at the fortieth to seventieth percentile level. A 9-year-7-month-old boy gets a raw score of 8 on Digits Forward and 3 on Digits Backward. From Table 7.1 (chapter 7), we note that the mean score for boys this age is 6.85 ± 2.22. The patient's Digits Forward score is above average but within the normal range. From the table of percentile ranks, we note that this score is at about the seventy-fifth percentile level. From Table 8.11, we note that the mean Digits Backward score for boys this age is 4.82 ± 2.15. The patient's score is less than 1 standard deviation below average. Referring to the percentile rank data, we note that a score of 3 is at the twentieth percentile level. If we add the two scores in accordance with Wechsler's instructions, we obtain a raw score of 11, which corresponds to a scaled score of 10 for children this patient's age. Using the Wechsler scoring system, we would conclude that his child's Digit Span performance is average. Using the breakdown data provided here, we see that this boy's Digits Forward performance is above average and Digits Backward is below average. Scores of this kind suggest that auditory memory is intact

Table 8.13

Comparison of Gardner and Wechsler Digit Span Data. Raw Scores: Digits Forward Plus Digits Backward.
Gardner: N = 1,567; Wechsler: N = 2,200.

Age	Gardner [Boys]	Wechsler [Boys and Girls Combined]	Deviation	Gardner [Girls]	Wechsler [Boys and Girls Combined]	Deviation
6-0 to 6-11	7.52	7.00	+ 0.52	7.80	7.00	+ 0.80
7-0 to 7-11	9.06	8.67	+ 0.39	9.26	8.67	+ 0.59
8-0 to 8-11	9.54	9.83	− 0.29	10.40	9.83	+ 0.57
9-0 to 9-11	10.94	11.00	− 0.06	11.31	11.00	+ 0.31
10-0 to 10-11	11.70	11.00	+ 0.70	11.90	11.00	+ 0.90
11-0 to 11-11	12.13	12.00	+ 0.13	12.42	12.00	+ 0.42
12-0 to 12-11	13.02	13.00	+ 0.02	13.14	13.00	+ 0.14
13-0 to 13-11	13.47	14.00	− 0.53	14.00	14.00	0.00
14-0 to 14-11	12.93	14.00	− 1.07	13.13	14.00	− 0.87
15-0 to 15-11	11.92	14.50	− 2.58	13.72	14.50	− 0.78
		Boys, average deviation	− 0.28		Girls, average deviation	+ 0.21

The average deviation of Gardner's total group (boys and girls combined) from Wechsler's group (boys and girls combined) = − 0.035

(Digits Forward is above average) and that the primary impairment is in visual memory. In addition, the 5 point discrepancy supports the conclusion that a neurological impairment is present. Such discrepancies, both for above and below average scores, get buried in the Wechsler scoring system, as was the case in this example.

The Numbers Subtest of Cancellation of Rapidly Recurring Target Figures

In chapter 3, I discussed Cancellation of Rapidly Recurring Target Figures (Rudel et al., 1978) as a test of attention-sustaining capacity. Earlier in this chapter, I described the Geometric Forms section of this instrument as a test of visual discrimination. Here I discuss the Numbers section as a test of short-term visual sequential memory. As mentioned, the child is presented with the model number sequence 592, below which is an array of three-digit numbers, each of which begins with 5, has as its second digit a 6 or a 9, and as its third digit 1, 2, 3, 4, 5, 8, or 9 (Figure 3.2). The child is asked to go through the array and place a line through each 592 sequence and none other, as rapidly as he can. Means and standard deviations for the time to complete the test and for numbers of errors are provided (Table 3.2), enabling the examiner to compare the child's score with children known to be free from neurological impairment. An 8¼-year-old boy, for example, takes 205 sec to complete the test and he makes 7 errors. From Table 3.2 we see that the mean time for children his age is 116.00 ± 33.71 sec and that the mean number of errors is 2 ± 2. We see, then, that this boy's time to perform the task is about 2.7 standard deviations above the average and that his number of errors is about 2½ standard deviations more than normal. If the child has no problems in visual acuity (of the kind described at the beginning of this chapter), then we must consider the following possibilities: attention-sustaining impairment, visual discrimination deficit, short-term visual sequential memory impairment, and impulsivity. Other tests for concentration (chapter 3) might help the examiner determine whether this factor was operating. The tests of visual discrimination described earlier in this chapter could help one ascertain whether this function was impaired. Considering the significantly long time it took this child to complete the task, it is not likely that impulsivity is a factor in this child's case. (Typically, the impulsive child takes a short time and gets a large number of errors.) If this boy showed no significant concentration and visual discrimination deficits, then we would be highly suspicious of a visual sequential memory problem. One would want, however, to do the other tests of visual sequential memory described in this section to either confirm or refute this supposition.

The Visual Sequential Memory Subtest of the ITPA

The Visual Sequential Memory subtest of the ITPA (Kirk, et al., 1968) is a useful test of short-term visual sequential memory. The examiner shows the child 17 tiles, each of which has an imprinted geometric design (Figure 8.24). Next to these is an empty tray on which the child is to place specific design sequences. Lastly, there is the examiner's booklet that contains the various sequences that the child is asked to reproduce. The child is first provided with demonstration sequences to ensure that he understands that he is to reproduce with the chips the sequences depicted on the examiner's cards. The examiner takes from the pile of 17 chips only those required for the particular task. These are placed randomly in front of the tray, and the remaining ones are placed at the side. The examiner must be sure not to place the chips in the order that the child is being asked to reproduce. The model patterns are exposed for 5 sec (examiner times with a stopwatch), and the child may be given a second 5-sec exposure to each pattern that is to be copied. Tile sequences range in length from three to eight chips. The scoring system is somewhat complex, but the basic principle is that the

Figure 8.24
The Visual Sequential Memory Subtest of the ITPA.

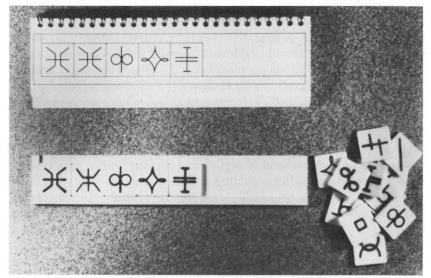

child receives 2 points if he reproduces the sequence accurately on the first trial, 1 point if he does so on the second trial, and no points for failure on both trials. The child's raw score can be converted to an age-equivalent or scaled score by referring to the proper table. As mentioned, the mean scaled score on the ITPA is 36 with a standard deviation of 6.

A 6½-year-old girl obtains a raw score of 10. Referring to the age-equivalent table, we note that this corresponds to age 4-4. Referring to the conversion table for scaled scores, we note that a raw score of 10 corresponds to a scaled score of 22. Accordingly, this girl's performance is more than 2 standard deviations below the mean. Turning back the tables, we note that a scaled score of 36 corresponds to a raw score of 10 at the 4-4 to 4-7 age level, confirming the data from the age-equivalent table. We can conclude then that this child may have a problem in short-term visual sequential memory. If there are no problems found on administration of the general tests of visual memory described in the previous section, then it is likely that there is a specific sequencing problem present. Again, one would want to administer other tests of visual sequential memory before coming to any definite conclusion.

The Spelling Subtest of the Wide Range Achievement Test

The spelling subtest of the Wide Range Achievement Test (WRAT) (Jastak and Jastak, 1976) is a good test of long-term visual sequential memory. There are two tests, level I and level II. Level I is for children ages 5-0 to 11-11 and level II is for people 12-0 and above. The level I spelling test consists of three sections. In section 1 the child is presented with a series of 18 simple geometric forms and asked to copy each one in an empty box below it within a 60-sec time limit. The maximum score for this section is 18 points. This section of the test is obviously not one of spelling. It serves to help the examiner determine whether the child has attained a minimal level of writing and copying ability, which needs to be present if one is to accomplish the more complex task of writing. Actually, section 1 is primarily a test for the presence of dysgraphia and fine-motor-coordination deficit and could be considered a contaminant of the test. In order to obviate this possibility, the child can automatically be given full credit for this section and for section 2 if he spells 6 words correctly in section 3. In section 2, the child is asked to write his name within a 60-sec time limit. The child gets 1 point for one letter and 2 points for two letters, with a maximum score of 2 points as long as at least two letters are written correctly. In section 3 (Figure 8.25), the examiner dictates a series of words which the child is asked

Figure 8.25
Level I—Spelling from The Wide Range Achievement Test.

15. reach	He couldn't *reach* the ball	rēch
16. order	The captain's *order* was obeyed	ôr' dĕr
17. watch	My *watch* is fast	wôch
18. enter	*Enter* this way	ĕn' tĕr
19. grown	Potatoes are *grown* in the field	grōn
20. nature	The study of *nature* is interesting	nā' chĕr
21. explain	*Explain* how it happened	eks plān'
22. edge	He sat on the *edge* of the chair	ĕj
23. kitchen	Our *kitchen* is small	kĭch' ĕn
24. surprise	He may *surprise* you	sĕr prīz'
25. result	The *result* of your work is good	rē zŭlt'
26. advice	My *advice* was forgotten	ăd vīs'
27. purchase	We did not *purchase* the car	pĕr' chĭs
28. brief	I received a *brief* note	brēf
29. success	*Success* makes people happy	sŭk sĕs'
30. reasonable	His request was *reasonable* and just	rē z'n ă b'l

Reproduced with the permission of Jastak Associates, Inc., Wilmington, Delaware.

to write. The total list consists of 45 words from the simplest (go, cat, in ...) to the most difficult (... prejudice, belligerent, occurrence). Each word is presented with a sentence that includes the word ("cat ... The cat has fur"). The test is discontinued when the child makes 10 consecutive errors. A pronunciation guide is provided so that there will be some degree of uniformity for all testees. The examiner is allowed to repeat a word if necessary or requested. The time limit for each word is 15 sec, but this may be extended for children with known motor-coordination handicaps. In fact, if there is a severe writing impairment, oral responses are acceptable.

The maximum possible score is 65 (18 + 2 + 45). The raw score is directly converted into grade norms, ranging from the prekindergarten to the 16-7 grade level. Scaled scores, standard scores, and percentile ranks are also provided for raw scores at each 1/2-year age level from 5 through 11½. For example, a 9-year-2-month-old boy obtains a raw score of 39 points. From the table on the examination sheet, we note that this corresponds to the 4.2 grade level. By referring to the table in the manual for children 9-0 to 9½ years of age, we note a raw score of 39 places a child at the fifty-eighth percentile level and is equivalent to a scaled score of 11 (10 is the mean scaled score for the WRAT). This child's standard score is 103, with 100–108 being the + 1 standard deviation level. We can conclude then that this child's spelling level is in the normal range.

A 10¼-year-old girl gets a raw score of 35. She is reading at the 3.2 grade level, and is at the eighteenth percentile. Her score corresponds to a scaled score of 7 and a standard score of 86 (85–91 represents the – 2 standard deviation range). This child is significantly behind in spelling. Although a problem in visual sequential memory may be present, other causes must be considered. Educational deprivation is possible. Psychological problems that may have interfered with learning may be operative. Other organic impairments, unrelated to visual-sequential-memory deficit, may be present. Hyperactivity and/or a concentration problem may have interferred with her learning how to spell. A problem in auditory processing may not only have compromised her learning how to spell in the classroom (teachers traditionally verbalize and write simultaneously when teaching spelling), but may have interfered with her hearing accurately the examiner's verbal presentation of the words. Dyspraxic difficulties may have interfered with her executing correctly the letters she wishes to write. And, then there are the linguistic impairments that may interfere with the child's capacity for linking the auditory stimulus (the word that has been verbalized by the examiner) with the written symbols that have been designated by social convention to denote these particular sounds. The linkage is by no means obvious. The two entities have absolutely no intrinsic relationship with one another and are only linked by what might appear to be rather arbitrary associations. There is really no good reason why the sound of the word *cat* should be associated with the written symbols c - a - t. One could designate an infinite number of other symbols if one wished to, e.g., d - o - g, p - i - g, g - j - t, 6 - k - %, etc. All that is required for communication is to get general agreement regarding which written symbols should be utilized to denote which particular sounds. Considering the many factors that can cause a spelling deficit (and the aforementioned are only some of them), the examiner must carefully consider the child's scores on other tests described in this book if he or she is to be in a position to decide whether a child's spelling problem is related to a visual sequential memory defect or whether other functions are impaired.

Level II of the WRAT covers ages 12-0 to adult (65). Forty-six words ranging from the simplest (cat, run, arm...) to the most difficult (...charlatan, pusillanimous, iridescence) are presented by the examiner. A sample sentence follows the presentation of each word. A pronunciation key is also provided. If a patient gets a raw score that is lower than 4, then sections 1 and 2 of the level I test are administered. Scores on these two sections, under the level II scoring system, can range from 0 to 5. All patients who correctly spell four or more words are automatically credited with 5 points. Accordingly, the maximum score is 51 (46 + 5).

The raw score is readily converted to the grade level by referring to the chart on the score sheet. The manual provides percentile ranks, scaled scores, and standard scores.

VISUAL ORGANIZATION AND GESTALT

I use the term visual organizational capacity to refer to the ability to place visual stimuli into a specific arrangement. It is a different task from differentiating and identifying visual stimuli. It involves taking such stimuli and arranging them in a specific way warranted by the situation. It is the same process that is sometimes referred to as visual *integration*. In fact, for the purposes of this discussion, I use interchangeably the terms *organization* and *integration*. Visual organizational capacity is closely allied to the phenomenon of visual Gestalt. To form Gestalten, one must be able to arrange the separate entities into a unified *whole* or composite *form*. The term Gestalt refers to the final product, the desired consultation; the term organization refers to the *process* by which one arrives at the Gestalt.

The Block Design Subtest of the WISC-R

The Block Design subtest of the WISC-R is a good test for visual organizational capacity. The test materials consist of 9 blocks and 11 cards of designs. Each block is colored red on two sides, white on two sides, and red/white on two sides. Each of the 11 cards depicts a design that can be reproduced by proper alignment of the blocks.

The test begins with the child being shown the blocks and told, "See these blocks? They are all alike. On some sides they are all red; on some all white; and on some half red and half white." (The examiner turns the blocks to show the different sides.) "I am going to put them together to make something with them. Watch me." The examiner then creates a simple 4-block design (copied from demonstration card A) and asks the child to reproduce the same design with 4 other blocks. The child is given 45 sec to reproduce the design. Two points credit is given if the child accomplishes this. If he fails, a second 45-sec trial is given for which 1 point credit can be obtained for success. The second demonstration design is also made from blocks by the examiner. For the third demonstration, the child is asked to copy a printed design from card C. Again, two trials of 45 sec each are given, with either 2 or 1 point credit for successful performance. Eight more patterns are then presented for reproduction. The first five utilize 4 blocks and the remaining three require 9 blocks. There is a time limit on each task, ranging from 45 sec–120 sec. Four points credit is given for successful completion within the time limit, and as much as 3 points bonus can be won for perfect reproductions completed before the time limit. The maximum score is 62 points.

A 7½-year-old boy, for example, obtains a score of 19 points. This corresponds to a scaled score of 12. (As mentioned, 10 is the average scaled score for all WISC-R subtests.) By referring to the conversion tables for age-equivalents, we note that his score corresponds to age 8-10, about 1⅓ years above that expected for his age. An 8½-year-old boy obtains a raw score of 8. This corresponds to a scaled score of 7. The age-equivalent table informs us that this score corresponds to age 6-6. We can conclude, therefore, that this child is functioning 2 years below age level on this test. It is likely that he is suffering with a problem in visual organization. He does not seem to be able to organize the separate visual elements (red, white, and red/white) into an integrated pattern (Gestalt).

The test may also detect persistence problems in that some children give up easily and do not try to construct the various combinations that might give them the desired results. Others work tenaciously at the task, even though they might not be successful. The Block Design test also measures the child's capacity to use trial and error materials for solving problems, as well as his tolerance for making errors. As mentioned, I do not like the terms analysis and synthesis because they are so loosely used in psychology, but the Block Design test does measure visual analysis and synthesis, when narrowly defined. The child must break down (analyze) the observed model pattern into its component parts and then build up (synthesize) the total pattern with specific block designs. Bortner and Birch (1960) hold that most children who do poorly on this test do so not because of a perceptual (visual organizational) problem, but because of difficulties in organizing sequential action (dyspraxia). In their study, patients who made errors on this test were shown three pictures: one depicted the correct pattern; the second, the patient's incorrect pattern; and the third, another incorrect pattern designed by the examiner. Ninety-three percent of nonhemiplegic patients correctly identified all three patterns as did 93% of patients with right hemiplegia (left cerebral damage). Only 68% of those with left hemiplegia (right cerebral damage) correctly identified the three pictures. They concluded that with right cerebral damage, perceptual problems can interfere with Block Design performance; but with left cerebral damage, apraxic difficulties are a more likely explanation for low performance on this test. Lastly, we must never forget the anxious and distractible child who may not have any problems at all in visual processing, but who does poorly on the test because he isn't concentrating well on the task.

The Spatial Relations Subtest [V] of the Developmental Test of Visual Perception

The Spatial Relations subtest (V) of the Developmental Test of Visual Perception (Frostig, 1961) is a good test of visual differentiation, organization, and Gestalt. It assesses the child's capacity to execute increasingly complex graphomotor tasks. Hence, the child with a coordination problem and/or one who is dyspraxic may do poorly on this test. The child who does well on the tests of coordination disorders, discussed in chapter 5, as well as the tests for dyspraxia, to be discussed in chapter 9, may do poorly on the Frostig V because of deficits in visual processing.

A typical test item is shown in Figure 8.26. The left side of each page depicts a pattern that the child is requested to reproduce on the right. Specifically, the child is told, "Do you see the picture on this side?" (Examiner points to pattern on the left.) "It has dots and sticks. Now look at this side." (Examiner points to right side of page.) "It has dots but it doesn't have any sticks. Take your pencil and draw sticks or

Figure 8.26
The Spatial Relations Subtest [V] of the Developmental Test of Visual Perception.

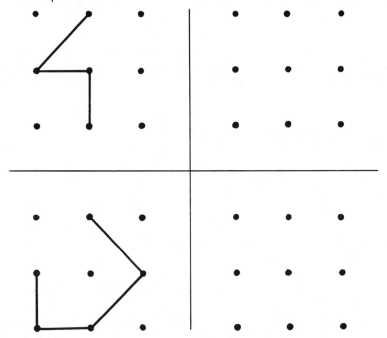

lines so that this side looks just like the other side." Nursery-school children are asked to do six items of increasing complexity. First graders and older children are given two more tasks, the last of which is quite complicated.

In the Eye-Motor Coordination subtest (I) of the Frostig test the child loses credit if lines are not drawn straight (within certain limitations), but in the Spatial Relations subtest no credit is lost for "crooked" lines. As long as the correct dots are connected by the lines, credit is given. Each item in the test is scored either 0 or 1. Scoring is stringent. The reproduction must be completely accurate and erasures are not permitted, i.e., even if the child recognizes an error after a line has been drawn, he still gets a 0 score on the item. Raw scores can be converted to age-equivalent and scaled scores by reference to the proper table. Normative data is provided only for a relatively narrow range, ages 4-0 through 8-3. As mentioned in chapter 5, this is one of the drawbacks of the Frostig test, even though one can "expand" the data a little by making a statement regarding how the older child's score compares to the group on which normative data is provided. For example, an 9½-year-old boy gets a raw score of 6. By referring to the 7-9 through 7-11 table of normative data, we note that this corresponds to a scaled score of 10 (the average). Or by referring to the age-equivalent table we note that a raw score of 6 corresponds to age 7-6. Therefore, one can conclude that this child's score is below average because at 9 he is performing at the level of the 7½–7¾-year-old child.

Frostig recommends summing the scaled scores on the five subtests in order to ascertain the child's "Perceptual Quotient." I do not consider this figure as meaningful as the individual scores on each of the subtests, and generally view them as separate assessment instruments. And each one of them is far from "pure." The Spatial Relations subtest is a good example of such complexity. First, the child must concentrate well in order to successfully complete the task. He must be able to *organize* visual stimuli. The confusion that some children exhibit when doing the task (especially the more difficult items) may relate to a problem in organizing visual stimuli. There must be an appreciation of the total form and pattern *(Gestalt)*, not merely the individual segments, if the child is to reproduce the pattern accurately. The child has to be able to *compare* the designs on the two sides and differentiate between them with regard to whether they are the same or different. In addition, all these functions may be operating normally but the child does poorly because of a coordination or dyspraxic problems. The child who does well is not likely to have a visual problem of the aforementioned types. (The test is less sensitive for ruling out the motor problems because irregular lines that connect the correct dots receive full credit.) If the child does poorly, and the examiner considers the poor performance to be related to a visual processing problem, he may be hard put to ascertain which of the impairments described above is responsible. To say that the deficit is in the area of spatial relations may be all that one can do. But it behooves the examiner to appreciate that such a conclusion is broad and that far more specificity is desirable.

Organizational and Gestalt impairments can interfere significantly with a child's functioning, especially in the linguistic area. A child must be able to organize letters into a whole word if he is to spell and write. He must learn to go from phonetic breakdown and slow fusion of phonemes to word recognition if he is to read with a reasonable degree of speed. He must be able to organize the words of a sentence into a Gestalt if he is to understand more than the particular meaning of each word. De Hirsch (1975) describes this impairment well in the 6-year-old boy who said, "It's just a jumble. It looks like ants crawling around the page."

VISUAL LANGUAGE

As the reader by now probably knows well, I use the term language to refer to the phenomenon in which the individual associates an entity with a symbol (usually auditory or visual) that specifically denotes the entity. Accordingly, *meaning* is given to stimuli that do not intrinsically mean anything. Visual linguistic symbols can be divided into two categories: nonalphabetical and alphabetical. Nonalphabetical visual linguistic symbols would include such entities as a red light (meaning stop), green light (meaning go), skull and crossbones (meaning poison or danger), and a red cross (meaning medical or emergency aid). Alphabetical visual symbols are letters, combined into words, that convey specific communications, each word having its own meaning. The alphabetical symbolization process is the more difficult to master and the one that generally causes MBD children more difficulty. Accordingly, I will focus here only on this one of the two categories of visual linguistic problems.

The Comprehension Section of the Gilmore Oral Reading Test

The Gilmore Oral Reading Test (Gilmore and Gilmore, 1968) assesses objectively three aspects of oral reading: accuracy, comprehension, and speed. The test was standardized on a total of 4,455 pupils in six parts of the U.S.: Belmont, Massachusetts; Hammond, Louisiana; Milwaukee, Wisconsin; New York, New York; Santa Rosa, California; and St. Petersburg, Florida. The standard population, then, represents a reasonably good cross section of the U.S.

The manual contains 10 paragraphs of progressively increasing complexity. (Figure 8.27 shows a sample paragraph.) A basal level is obtained by starting with the paragraph that corresponds to the child's actual class placement. The examiner records the number of errors the child makes while reading the paragraph. There are eight categories of errors: substitutions, mispronunciations, words pronounced by the examiner, disregard of pronunciation, insertions, hesitations, repetitions, and omissions. The manual of instructions describes the

Figure 8.27

The Gilmore Oral Reading Test.

Mary is just twelve years old.

Her brother Dick is fourteen.

They both go to the same school.

Mary is in Grade Seven.

She likes her class in cooking.

Dick is now in Grade Nine.

Although he enjoys all his school work,

Dick likes the work in art class best.

TIME_____Seconds

1. Who is the older child?
2. How old is Mary?
3. What grade is Dick in?
4. What is Mary's favorite class at school?
____ 5. What school subject does Dick prefer?

ERROR RECORD	Number
Substitutions	
Mispronunciations	
Words pronounced by examiner	
Disregard of punctuation	
Insertions	
Hesitations	
Repetitions	
Omissions	
Total Errors	

Reproduced from the Gilmore Oral Reading Test. Copyright © 1968 by Harcourt Brace Jovanovich, Inc. Reproduced by special permission of the publisher.

specific criteria that the examiner should utilize to score each of these types of error. The basal level paragraph is the one in which the child makes no more than two errors. The ceiling level is the paragraph in which the child makes 10 or more errors. The time to read the paragraph is also recorded by the examiner.

For the purposes of this discussion of visual language, I will focus only on the comprehension section of the test, the other sections being irrelevant, or hardly relevant, to the issue of *meaning*. (One could read the paragraph with totally correct pronunciation of all words, and do so at an above average rate, without understanding one word of what one was reading.) After each paragraph has been read, it is removed from the child's view, and he is asked five questions that determine whether he has understood what he has been reading. One point is given for every correct answer for questions following paragraphs between the basal and ceiling levels. The method of assigning scores for paragraphs below the basal level and above the ceiling is described in the manual. There are two forms of the test, C and D, enabling the examiner to repeat the test without the child's benefiting from "practice effect."

The data are used in the following way. A sixth-grade boy gets a total comprehension raw score of 29 on form C of the test. Referring to the table that converts raw scores to grade levels, we note that a score of 29 corresponds to grade level 6-7. Referring to the table of ranges, percentile ranks, and stanines, we note that the score of 29 is in the mid-average range, the fifth stanine, and at the fortieth to fifty-ninth percentile. We can conclude that this boy's reading comprehension is at grade level and in the normal range. A fourth-grade girl gets a raw score of 15 on form C. This corresponds to a grade level of 2.1. The score is found to be in the low part of the below average range, in the second stanine, and at the fourth to tenth percentile level. This child clearly has a problem in reading comprehension. One must consider it probable that she has a problem in decoding visual linguistic symbols, i.e., in understanding the meaning of the written word. One must consider the possibility, however, that other processes might be operative. Perhaps this child's poor score is related to faulty educational exposure, psychological learning disorder, visual attentional deficits, impulsivity, or another visual processing defect that could interfere with reading (for example, an impairment in letter discrimination or visual memory defect). Only by carefully evaluating other factors as well is one in a position to make a definite statement about the probable cause of this child's reading deficit.

The Oral and Silent Reading Sections of the
Standard Reading Inventory

The Silent Reading Inventory (McCracken, 1966) contains oral and silent reading sections that enable the examiner to assess objectively a child's comprehension of written language. Like the Gilmore Oral Reading Test, there is a series of paragraphs of increasing complexity from the preprimer to the seventh-grade level. The child's errors and reading time are scored for the oral reading paragraphs. Seven kinds of errors are evaluated: pronunciation, mispronunciation, omission, substitution, addition, repetition, and punctuation. Two forms, A and B, of the test are provided, enabling the examiner to repeat the test without contamination by practice effect. For the purposes of this discussion of visual linguistic capacity, I will only discuss the comprehension aspect of the subtest.

Each paragraph story is followed by 10 questions that relate to it. After the child has read the paragraph, either orally or silently, he is asked the general question, "Tell me about _____" (Story title). While the child is relating the story, the examiner checks off those of the 10 questions that the child is answering in his telling about the story. After the child has told as much about the story as he can, the examiner then asks him those questions that have not yet been answered. A sample paragraph and questions are shown in Figure 8.28. The child's total score is then computed, the maximum score being 10. There is a complex system for determining basal- and ceiling-level stories, and this is based on the number of word errors. I find it equally useful to start at the level of the child's grade and then go down and then up so that one can make comments about functioning at two or even three grade levels. The child's score at each level is described in the following terminology: 9–10 correct—*independent*; 7–8 correct—*definite instructional*; 6 correct—*questionable instructional*; and 0–5 correct—*frustration*. I consider these terms injudicious and somewhat misleading. One does better to substitute: 9–10 correct—excellent; 7–8 correct—good; 6 correct—borderline; and 0–5—poor (and these are the terms I will use here).

A boy in the fifth grade gets a score of 9 on the fourth-grade level silent-reading paragraph, a score of 8 on the fifth-grade level, and a score of 5 on the sixth-grade level. Accordingly, he is excellent at the fourth-grade level, good at the fifth-grade level and poor on the sixth-grade level paragraph. One can conclude from these findings that this boy is an average silent reader for a fifth-grade student and is essentially reading at grade level. A girl in the sixth grade obtains the following scores on the silent reading paragraphs: third-grade level, 10

Figure 8.28

The Silent Reading Comprehension Section of the Standard Reading Inventory.

Circus Time (130 words)

SECOND SILENT

Bob and Jack were working in the pumpkin field. They were pulling weeds. It was summer and was very warm. It was hard to work and not cut the vines. Bob and Jack wanted to get enough money to go to the circus. The circus was coming next Saturday. The train would pull into the station early in the morning. There would be a parade to the circus grounds with lions and elephants and clowns and every-thing. Bob and Jack worked very hard. By night time they had pulled all the weeds. Mr. Green was very glad all the work was done. He gave the boys some money. Bob and Jack were very hungry. As they hurried home they counted their money. They had enough to go to the circus.

__1. Where were they working?
__2. What were they doing?

__3. Why was it hard work?
__4. Why were they working?.
__5. When was the circus coming?
__6. How would the circus come?

__7. How long did they work?

__8. What did Mr. Green do?

__9. What did the do as they hurried home?
__10. Did they have enough money?

Time__ seconds

Comprehension unaided __: total _____

__a. How much money did the boys earn? (Why?)
__b. What time did they start working? (Why?)
__c. EVERYTHING

Reproduced with the permission of the publisher: Klamath Printing Co., 320 Loewell St., Klamath Falls, Oregon 97601.

points; fourth-grade level, 8 points; fifth-grade level, 5 points; sixth-grade level, 2 points. One can reasonably conclude that this girl's silent reading comprehension is at the fourth-grade level. She may have a visual linguistic impairment. However, she may be suffering with other problems that may have interfered with her reading functioning, such as the kind described in my discussion of the Gilmore Oral Reading Test.

As I am sure the reader has come to appreciate, breaking down visual-processing problems into component parts may be a difficult task. However, separate functions are operative and the careful examiner, by administering a series of tests should be able to isolate some clusters or trends that provide a greater understanding of the child's deficits.

Dyslexia

It may have occurred to the reader that I have not yet devoted a section to the evaluation of dyslexia. This was by no means an oversight. Such omission relates to my belief that the word dyslexia, like the words perception and agnosia, has come to mean so many different things that they have become almost useless for purposes of communication. Strictly defined, dyslexia means difficulty in reading. Twenty-five years ago it was considered to be a neuropathological manifestation categorized under the aphasias and agnosias. Many today use the term more broadly to include any kind of reading deficit that is related to a neurologic problem. And there are some who would use the term to describe any type of reading deficit, regardless of its etiology. In order to avoid the problems that one now encounters with the term, I generally try to avoid using it and prefer to discuss the specific kind of deficit that may be contributing to a child's reading difficulties. Accordingly, I have been talking about dyslexia in many ways throughout this book. Some children have trouble reading because of hyperactivity; others because of an attentional deficit; others because of impulsivity. Many of the auditory processing problems discussed in the last chapter can contribute to reading disabilities and every one of the visual processing problems described in this chapter is likely to cause difficulty in reading. And the aphasic impairments that I will discuss in the next chapter can also interfere with reading capacity.

When one says that a child has difficulty reading, little information is actually being provided. It's almost like saying that a person has fever. There was a time when fever was viewed as a disease per se; we now recognize it to be a symptom of a wide variety of diseases. Similarly, we do well to view difficulty in reading as the final result of any number of deficits. The person who states that a child does not read well may not differentiate among the various kinds of reading disorders that a child may manifest. Reading single words is different from reading sentences. There is phonetic reading of words and "look-say" (total word at once). There is silent reading, reading aloud, comprehension of what one is reading (either silently or aloud), and there is comprehension of what is being read to the child. Information about which specific kind of problem the child exhibits clinically can provide clues about the kind of impairment that is contributing to the reading deficit.

One does well to appreciate that reading capacity is a distinctly human trait (although with great labor one can train some of the higher apes to "read" a few simple words). It is one of the latest developments in the evolution of living forms. It is reasonable to conclude that some individuals will be more advanced than others with regard to this facility, that some may be a few million years ahead of others in the acquisition of this capacity. Whether one wants to call such poor readers dyslexic is not important, in my opinion. What is important is that we recognize this possible cause of some people's reading impairment. Then there is the individual developmental factor. Some children start to walk at 9 months, and others not until 18 months of age. By 30 months their gaits may be equally good and no one would be able to tell who the late walker was. To provide the late walker with a special pathological label (derived from the Greek or Latin, perhaps) would not be particularly useful and to say that he or she has a disease might even be detrimental. Similarly, there are children who can be taught to read at age 2 and there are others who do not get the "hang of it" until 11 or 12. By age 14 children from each group might be reading equally well and no one could differentiate between the two. Some call the late readers dyslexics, but many of them outgrow the pathological designation and end up with "a history of dyslexia." It is of interest that in Sweden, where children do not begin to be required to learn how to read until age 8, there is reported a very low prevalence of reading disabilities. It is reasonable to assume that were reading required of younger children, many more would be so diagnosed, but they have escaped the label by not having been required to read before they had developed the basic capacity or "readiness." When teachers say that a child has developed "reading readiness," they mean (whether or not they realize it) that he has come to appreciate the decoding process, the process by which he can link the visual linguistic symbol with the entity that it denotes.

Another factor that must be considered in reading difficulties is the child's language. It is much easier to learn to read a phonetic language like Spanish than a nonphonetic language like English. Languages that use ideographs or characters are probably easier to read than phonetic languages. This may relate to the fact that the ideograph may give some hint of its meaning, because many were originally designed to resemble the object they symbolize. Letters rarely provide such cues. In Japanese, children must learn both ideographic words derived from the Chinese (Kanji) and phonetic symbols (Kana) which are generally used for words of more recent origin (often derived from the West). Tatara (1974) claims that most teachers in Japan agree that children have more difficulty reading the Kana than the Kanji script.

We must appreciate, as well, that our Western culture places a great premium on reading capacity. It has selected this function from the multiplicity of skills in the human repertoire and given it an importance that is immense. Poor readers, regardless of the cause of their deficit, are severely stigmatized in such a society. Lumping all such individuals into the category of dyslexics is like telling a patient with a headache that he has cephalgia; nothing really has been learned or gained. Only by understanding the various causes of reading disorder can we help these unfortunate individuals.

9

Aphasias, Agnosias, and Apraxias

I have previously discussed how all the signs and symptoms of MBD could be considered to be *soft neurological signs,* i.e., mild forms of the "harder" more obvious signs generally described in classical neurology (especially for the adult). The soft neurological signs discussed in chapter 6 are best viewed as having been somewhat artificially selected to warrant the rubric. Considering the wide variety of neurological signs and symptoms that may be found in children with MBD, it is to be expected that some of them might exhibit milder forms of aphasia, agnosia, and apraxia, the "Three A's" of classical neurology. Yet we do not hear these terms used frequently when discussing MBD (with the exception of the word *dyslexia* which was once viewed narrowly as one form of aphasia and/or agnosia). But a careful consideration of some of the traditional signs and symptoms of MBD leads us to the conclusion that we are indeed dealing at times with one or more of the three A's. However, we may not have recognized the presence of such a sign(s) because a different name was being utilized, or it (they) was mixed in with or buried by other neurological entities. In this chapter I will delineate the kinds of aphasias, agnosias, and apraxias one may see in MBD children and present tests that specifically focus upon these impairments. It is important for the reader to appreciate that one rarely sees any of the three A's in pure form. The more clearly we are able to define the various elements that contribute to a clinical manifestation, the greater are our chances of determining its etiology and the more efficaciously we can devise treatment.

APHASIAS

The study of aphasias can be a mind-boggling experience. This is often the case when we venture into a field in which relatively little is known. Theories abound and there are contradictions everywhere. When this is the situation, then we can be sure of one thing only: We are swimming around in a sea of ignorance and there is still much to be learned. Although this is the state of the *art* (the word *science* must be used cautiously here) as it pertains to aphasias, there are a few things that we do know that are more of theoretical interest than therapeutic value. As is true with many forms of neurological disorder, there is good reason to doubt the efficacy of many forms of therapy. It is more often a matter of waiting and hoping that the patient will outgrow the disorder (often the case for the child) or recover via the body's own reparative mechanisms (usually the situation for the adult).

I believe the best way to introduce the concept of what aphasias are is with a clinical vignette. An elderly man, previously fully conversant with an excellent command of the English language, suffers a stroke. He becomes hemiparetic on his right side, indicating that the site of his cerebrovascular disorder is in the left hemisphere. One manifestation of his disorder is that he finds himself having trouble speaking. But he has a very specific kind of speech disorder: he has great difficulty finding the right words to verbalize what he is thinking or would like to say. This is especially true when he attempts to identify objects. He has trouble retrieving from memory the proper words for the occasion. For example, when shown a fork, and asked to name it he may say, 'That's a ... a ... knife. No, no that's not it. That's ... a ... a ... scissors. No, no it's a thing you eat with. It's a ... a .... " The patient may become frustrated to the point of crying and yet the word just won't come to mind. The patient is ever aware of the impairment and knows well that he is not using the correct word. The examiner then says, "I'm going to say three words, one of which correctly identifies this object and the other two do not. Now, you tell me which is the correct word: *spoon, tongs, fork.*" Without hesitation the patient will exclaim: "Fork! That's it. It's a fork!" This type of aphasia is generally referred to as *anomia* when the loss in naming capacity is severe, and *dysnomia* when it is mild to moderate. When searching for the correct word, the patient may even bang his head with his hand (not a wise thing to do if one has a stroke), as if he were trying to knock some loose connection into place or release some kind of a block. He cannot seem to connect the fork that he sees with the stored word that denotes it. He cannot make the correct association. The terms *connection* and *association* are useful to use when discussing aphasias because, as will be discussed below, they touch upon a central problem in the disorder (or, more accurately, group of disorders).

Now to a more specific definition of aphasia. Blakiston's *New Gould Medical Dictionary* (1951) defines aphasia as "Loss or the impairment of the capacity to use words as symbols or ideas ... caused by a lesion or lesions in the cortex and association paths of the dominant hemisphere. It does not refer to a defect in the mechanics of hearing or speaking but to an impairment of the highest function of the use of language as translating thought." Goodglass and Kaplan (1972) use this definition: "Aphasia refers to the disturbance of any or all of the skills, association and habits of spoken or written language, produced by injury to certain brain areas which are specialized for these functions. Disturbances of language usage which are due to paralysis or incoordination of the musculature of speech or writing or to poor vision or hearing or to severe intellectual impairment are not, by themselves aphasic." They also emphasize that "Virtually all aphasics suffer some restriction in the repertory of words which they have available for speech and require increased time to produce these words." Brock (1945) emphasizes the impairment in forming linguistic symbols as central to the aphasias. These definitions do not provide much information about the manifestations of the defect *per se*; rather they restrict the use of the term to those disorders of written and spoken language that result from lesions in certain parts of the brain (to be discussed below) and preclude the use of the term from situations in which peripheral organs and organ systems or other than the above mentioned brain areas are responsible for the disorder.

Geschwind (1971) considers aphasias to be a "disturbance of language output." He emphasizes that "however distorted the patient's speech may be, if when it is transcribed he is producing correct English sentences, he is not suffering from aphasia, but rather from some form of articulatory disability." It is in Geschwind's (1965a, 1965b) discussion of the "disconnexion syndrome" that we are provided with a theory that shows promise of explaining what may be a fundamental impairment in the aphasias (and possibly the agnosias and apraxias as well). His theory is based on the observation that the major sensory areas are not directly linked with one another. There are no intersensory connections, except with immediate adjacent parasensory areas. These sensory areas are connected with one another, with motor areas, and other parts of the brain via association tracts. Lesions in the association pathways (and in the areas that they connect) are primarily responsible for aphasias. For example, the failure to be able to verbalize the word that denotes a visualized object may relate to lesions in pathways that connect the visual cortex (reception and/or memory) of the occipital lobe with the speech area in the left inferior frontal lobe. One could almost say that the stroke patient described above, while hitting his head in frustration, was unwittingly trying to link two brain areas that had been "disconnected" from one another.

A brief review of the cerebral areas and pathways generally considered to be involved in aphasic disorders can help the reader gain a clearer picture of the nature of the various kinds of aphasias. The concepts presented here are those of Geschwind (1972) and represent present thinking on the subject. The most convenient place to start such a discussion is with Broca's area, which is located in the posterior part of the left inferior (third) frontal lobe. (See Figure 9.1 for visualizing this and all other neuroanatomical areas and tracts to be discussed in this section.) This area, commonly referred to as the "speech center," is responsible for encoding, i.e., formulating speech information into a recognizable speech pattern, in all right-handed people and the majority of left-handed people. Penfield and Roberts (1959) found that surgery of the left hemisphere produced aphasia in 115 of 157 right-handed patients and in 13 of 15 of those who were left-handed. Geschwind (1972) states that "out of 100 people with permanent language disorder caused by brain lesions approximately 97 will have damage in the left side." One can view Broca's area as the place where engrams for speech are formulated. Such programs are then transmitted to the adjacent area of the precentral gyrus (motor strip) that is responsible for the movement and coordination of the articulatory apparatus. Auditory stimuli are received in the auditory reception area (Heschl's gyrus) on the superior surface of the superior temporal lobe, deep within the Sylvian fissure. These are transmitted to the nearby Wernicke's area where they are decoded and given meaning (comprehended). Visual stimuli are received on the medial surface of the occipital lobe. These stimuli are given meaning in the visual association area on the lateral aspect of the occipital lobe. In short, we have two reception areas (auditory and visual) each connected with a nearby area that serves to provide the incoming stimuli with meaning (decoding). We also have a verbal expressive area responsible for controlling the peripheral articulatory apparatus and this region is programmed by Broca's area that is adjacent to it.

These two-part units do not function in isolation from one another; they are interconnected. The *arcuate fasciculus* connects Wernicke's and Broca's areas. Accordingly, areas receiving auditory stimuli are

Figure 9.1
Left Cerebral Hemisphere Showing Regions Involved in Aphasic Disturbances.

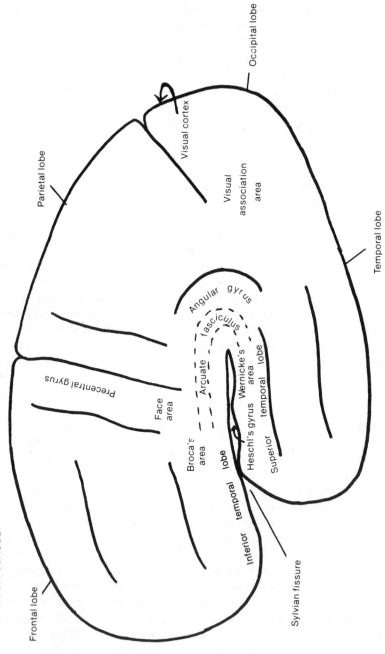

Parietal lobe

Occipital lobe

Visual cortex

Visual association area

Temporal lobe

Angular gyrus

Arcuate fasciculus

Precentral gyrus

Face area

Broca's area

Wernicke's area

Superior temporal lobe

Heschl's gyrus

lobe

temporal

Inferior

Frontal lobe

Sylvian fissure

linked with areas responsible for speech. In the repetition of a word that one hears, for example, sound is transmitted from the ear to Heschl's area in the temporal lobe by paths described in chapter 7. These impulses are then sent to the adjacent Wernicke's area where they are decoded. They are then transmitted via the *arcuate fasciculus* to Broca's area where the word is encoded. Impulses are then transmitted to the motor speech area that controls peripheral speech. With the information so provided, the individual now verbalizes the word that has been heard.

Similarly there are connections between the visual and the auditory regions. Such function is served primarily by the angular gyrus which lies between Wernicke's area and the visual association area. If one is asked to spell a word, for example, the sound of the spoken word is first transmitted from the auditory reception area (Heschl's gyrus) to Wernicke's area. It then gets translated in the angular gyrus from an auditory to a visual stimulus. This is then transmitted to the visual association area where visual information is formulated for transmission to the primary visual cortex in the occipital lobe. There the word engram is visualized. In order to verbalize the spelling of the word, the information must be relayed to Broca's area and then to the motor speech area in the precentral gyrus. This is probably done through Wernicke's area rather than via direct connections between the visual and speech areas. The pathway, then, is probably like this: visual cortex-visual association area-angular gyrus-Wernicke's area-arcuate fasciculus-Broca's area-motor speech center. A clinical verification that there are few, if any, direct connections between the visual and speech areas is the observation that most people, when they read, form an internal, nonverbalized auditory form of the word at the same time (or more accurately, a fraction of a second before) they read the word and give the visual symbols meaning. The process appears to be almost instantaneous, viewing the word, visualizing it in the brain, and "hearing" it internally, but it probably occurs in accordance with the sequence described above. Another confirmation of this comes from the observation that patient's with Wernicke's aphasia have trouble with written as well as spoken language. They cannot speak properly because they are not sending information to Broca's area via the arcuate fasciculus. They cannot write properly because they are not sending information to the visual cortex (via the angular gyrus and visual association area) for engrammatic display in the visual cortex, and because visual displays in the occipital cortex cannot be transmitted to the hand for writing. The pathway, whereby the word to be spelled is transmitted through the auditory areas on to Broca's area and then to the arm and hand motor areas in the precentral gyrus that control hand movement and writing, is interrupted by the lesion in Wernicke's area.

It is also probably the case that a visual stimulus cannot be comprehended until it is transmitted through auditory pathways. We apparently need to hear internally if we are to understand the meaning of a linguistic symbol—not simply auditory symbols, but visual as well. A patient with a lesion of the angular gyrus will not be able to transmit visual stimuli to Wernicke's area. Accordingly, such a person will not be able to understand what he reads because he cannot avail himself of the internal audition necessary for comprehension. The words appear as meaningless, visual symbols. Nor will the patient be able to spell a word that is auditorily transmitted because the auditory stimuli cannot travel from Wernicke's area to the visual cortex for engrammatic display. Without being able to spell the person cannot write dictated words either. But agraphia is present also because the patient cannot transmit impulses to the motor strip from the visual engrammatic display that might arise internally in the visual cortex. The damage to the angular gyrus interrupts such transmission quite early along its course.

Although the model presented above may appear somewhat simple (and future research may conclude that it is), it has been Geschwind's experience (1972) that it is a valid model. It has enabled clinicians to locate brain lesions with a high degree of accuracy on the basis of a patient's language disturbance.

Further insights into the nature of aphasic disorders can best be gleaned from a description of the most common types found in adults. The descriptions and theories described here are those of Geschwind (1965a, 1965b, 1971, and 1972) who, in my opinion, provides the most comprehensive and reasonable explanation for this complex phenomenon. It is important to appreciate that children do not generally exhibit these types of aphasia in as pure form as adults (not that adults frequently do so either). Not only do they exist in more primitive form in children, but it is harder to detect and define them because of the difficulty in accurately examining children for these disorders. In addition, the younger the child at the time of the cerebral insult that caused the disorder, the greater the likelihood that other parts of the brain will take over for the impaired functions. Such compensation is generally considered to be a manifestation of the plasticity (de Hirsch, 1965) that the brain exhibits. In addition, the other hemisphere may serve as a reserve for taking over impaired functioning; again, the younger the patient, the greater the likelihood of this occurring. This capacity is clearly adaptive but, unfortunately, the older the child the less likely he will be able to compensate for cerebral insults in this way.

Broca's Aphasia

Lesions in the posterior part of the left inferior (third) frontal gyrus (Broca's area) result in this type of aphasia. Broca's aphasia is often associated with a right hemiparesis as the lesion is rarely confined to the speech area alone.

Aphasias can be divided into the *fluent* and *nonfluent* types. In *fluent* aphasias, speech is well articulated and effortlessly produced. The sentences have a normal grammatical skeleton and rhythm. Often the speech is rapid. The primary abnormal characteristic of *fluent* aphasias is that the patient's speech is devoid of meaningful content (This will be elaborated upon in my discussions of the *fluent* types of aphasia). As the name implies, in the *nonfluent* type of aphasia, speech is not smooth flowing. Broca's aphasia is one of the *nonfluent* types. The speech is halting, slow, sharp, clipped, and monotonous. In short, the patient talks as if he were dictating a telegram ("Friend. Jim. Visit.") or like The Lone Ranger's friend Tonto ("Tonto hungry." "White man, no trust."). Impaired (but not totally incapacitated) in the capacity to retrieve or formulate all the desired words, the patient speaks slowly as he tries to form words and saves himself trouble by using as few as possible. Comprehension is intact in a pure Broca's aphasia, the patient generally understanding everything that is being said to him. Although the patient has trouble speaking, there is no basic articulatory deficit. The peripheral speech apparatus is intact and the motor centers that control speech (just posterior to Broca's area in the motor strip) are unaffected in a pure Broca's aphasia.

Wernicke's Aphasia

Lesions in the posterior superior temporal region, may result in Wernicke's aphasia. The person has difficulty understanding the spoken word (decoding). The patient recognizes that a language is being spoken, but it is as if it were foreign rather than his native tongue. (This impairment is different from the agnosias where spoken words are not recognized as language.) Isolated words are more difficult for such patients than those in a sentence because from those in a sentence the patient can often garner meaning from context. Sentences that are long and complex, however, also cause such patients great difficulty. Basically the patient has difficulty connecting the heard message with stored information related to it (information that enables the individual to recognize the meaning of the verbal message). The loss of understanding is primarily for language. The patient may still comprehend the meaning of nonverbal sounds (lunch whistle, bell that signals the end of the class period) and music.

In Wernicke's aphasia, verbalizations are fluent, well articulated, and sentences have a normal grammatical skeleton. Speech may be rapid. It may sound normal at first, but when listened to closely one notes that it is generally devoid of content. ("He was in over manager, before I left in there.") Sometimes the speech is pure jargon, in an attempt to feign verbal communication when there is little if any capacity to do so. Often the patient will use circumlocutions, i.e., he provides a *descriptive* rather than a *denotative* response when requested to name an object. For example, when asked what one uses to open a door, the patient may reply, "a thing that turns." When shown a shoe and asked what it is, the patient may state, "It's something you put on your foot." The circumlocution serves as a feeble attempt to provide a response when there is little capacity to do so.

Patients with Wernicke's aphasia may also exhibit one of a variety of *paraphasias*. In *verbal paraphasias*, one correct word is unintentionally substituted for another. When the substituted word is related to the originally intended word or in the same category (*knife* for fork, *mother* for wife, *screwdriver* for hammer), the term *semantic paraphasia* or *paraphasic substitution* is used. The term *paraphasic part-whole* error refers to the use of a part of an obect to name the whole (*wheel* for car, *nose* for face). *Half-right paraphasic errors* refer to the substitution of a word that is half correct (*kickball* for football, *burnman* for fireman). When the two words are unrelated (*rose* for pencil, *house* for book), the term *random paraphasia* is used. Also seen are *phonemic (or literal) paraphasias* in which the patient replaces one or more sounds in otherwise correct words (*pipe* for hike, *spoot* for spoon). Typically, patients with Wernicke's aphasia have trouble repeating what is being said to them. They also generally exhibit naming difficulties.

Conduction Aphasia

In conduction aphasia, the lesion is in the *arcuate fasciculus* that connects Wernicke's and Broca's areas. Usually the lesion lies deep in the portion of the parietal lobe just above the Sylvian fissure. Accordingly, the patient has trouble transmitting information from the healthy Wernicke's area to the healthy Broca's area. This is truly the kind of dysconnection syndrome described by Geschwind (1965a, 1965b). Speech is fluent (Broca's area is intact) and comprehension is also normal (Wernicke's area is functioning). Paraphasias, especially of the phonemic type, are characteristic of this disorder. Repetition of the examiner's words is also impaired in conduction aphasia. Typically, the repetition is more difficult for short than long words. Accordingly, phrases such as "She is there" is more difficult than words like "congregation." One of the most difficult phrases for such patients is, "No if's and's or but's."

Anomic Aphasia

The patient with anomic (or amnesic) aphasia with acute onset often has a vascular occlusion in the region of the left angular gyrus or the adjacent portion of the lower temporal lobe. Both comprehension and repetition are preserved. The problem is one of word finding or naming. The patient does not seem to be able to retrieve from storage the specific word he is looking for. Typically, nouns are more difficult for such patients to recall than other types of words, and the ability to name letters and numbers may be intact. Although speech is fluent, such patients' talk is relatively empty of content. Rather, one sees a flow of small talk and rambling, uninformative speech. Typically, such patients exhibit a circumlocutory type of paraphasia.

ASSESSING DYSPHASIAS IN CHILDREN

Children rarely exhibit clear-cut aphasias of the kind just described. The various factors that are considered to be of etiological significance in MBD usually affect the child in the pre-, para-, and early postnatal period. Accordingly, the brain's plasticity enables it to compensate to varying degrees for the damage that may occur during these early phases of the child's existence. The kinds of disorders one sees in such children are more properly called *dysphasias*, i.e., mild forms of aphasias. The tests for assessing such impairments rely on the quantification of some of the more subtle manifestations of aphasic and dysphasic disorders. The ones described here assess dysnomia, probably the most common form of dysphasia in children. Dysnomia is present in many children with "word finding" problems. Dyslexia, which I have discussed in chapter 8 is also related to dysphasic and dysgnomic problems.

   Naming something, i.e., providing a verbal symbol for an entity, is central to language acquisition. The question of whether one can think without language is ancient. Is thinking only covert speaking? If one cannot link an object or entity with its linguistic symbol, one cannot speak. But can such an individual still think? After language has been established, one can think of an object that one sees but whose name is unknown. It is more difficult, however, even for the person who has mastered a language, to think of a new abstraction that has not been given a specific name. It is difficult, if not impossible, to be able to know if these tasks could be accomplished without first learning a language. The earliest phases of language development involve naming objects ("ma-ma," "da-da," "cookie"). Naming something gives it stability and permanence. It helps differentiate the entity from others, it classifies, and it enhances concept formation. I am in agreement with Benton (1966) who holds that thinking is covert speaking as well as covert symbolization. If one doesn't learn words, then one cannot learn classes, and so conceptualization is not possible. De Hirsch (1974) quotes from a poem by O. Mandelstam who put this well: "I have forgotten the word I intended to say and my thought, unembodied, returns to the realm of shadows."

De Hirsch considers naming impairments to be a central problem for dyslexic children. Jansky (1972) found a high correlation between deficient picture-naming in preschool children and subsequent reading failure. She uses a picture-naming test in her screening battery for early detection of reading problems and considers it to be one of the most important contributing factors in reading disability. Denckla and Rudel (1976) found that dyslexic MBD children did poorly on picture-naming (on the Oldfield-Wingfield test, to be described below), whereas, nondyslexic MBD children did as well as normals. These findings confirm the relationship between dysnomia and dyslexia. The examiner should, therefore, give serious consideration to naming impairments and include tests for dysnomia in the MBD evaluation.

The Oldfield-Wingfield Picture-Naming Test

Oldfield and Wingfield (1965) used a series of pictures of common objects to test naming *speed* and *accuracy* in adult neurological patients. As mentioned, this impairment is referred to as dysnomia when mild to moderate and anomia when it is severe. Thirty-six pictures were selected of objects generally recognizable by the large majority of individuals. In addition, the objects selected were clearly and easily differentiated from one another. The authors point out that a thing must be recognized before it can be named. Accordingly, the test does not simply measure the ability to express correctly the name of an object; there is a receptive element that is being assessed as well in the test. They found also that the response latency for less common words is longer than for the more common. This is to be expected because we are not likely to recall as readily the name of an object that we only infrequently see. Subsequently, Newcombe et al. (1971) used the test on a group of adults known to be suffering with focal brain injuries. They found that patients with left hemisphere damage had longer latencies than normal controls on naming the objects on the cards. Regarding accuracy, they describe three kinds of errors: (1) Misnaming. The patient recognizes the object but can't verbalize the correct name. Accordingly a circumlocution may be used instead, e.g., a cigarette is called "a thing that you smoke." (2) Misidentification. The patient verbalizes the name of another object rather than providing the correct name of the object being viewed ("drill" for microscope or "violin" for stethoscope). (3) Unknown. The patient says that he doesn't know what the object is. The authors found that the patients with left hemisphere lesions also exhibited a higher frequency of misnaming and misidentification errors than normal controls.

Denckla and Rudel (1976) collected normative data on the Old-field-Wingfield Naming Test on 120 normal children at the four age levels from 8 to 11 (15 boys and 15 girls at each age). This was part of a larger study in which they compared normal children's scores with dyslexic MBD and nondyslexic MBD children. The 36 pictures used are shown in Figure 9.2. Each subject is told that he will be shown a series of pictures and that he should name the object he sees as quickly as possible. The 36 pictures are presented in random order. However, the first 10 serve as practice, so only 26 cards are effectively used and scored. Response latencies are timed with a stopwatch. If, after 30 sec, the subject fails to offer a name, the watch is stopped and he is told to give any description or associated thought regarding the picture. Only the first verbal response (exclusive of 'um," "er," or other similar vocalization) is recorded.

The number of items correctly identified from the 26 test cards by a group of 120 boys and girls is presented in Table 9.1. Denckla and Rudel (1976) found that MBD children with dyslexia made significantly fewer correct responses than normal children. However, the number of errors made by MBD children who were not dyslexic was not significantly different from normals. This study supports the view, discussed in chapter 8, that dyslexic children do not have a basic impairment in "perception," i.e., *recognizing* what they see. This study suggests that their problem relates instead to their impairment in *naming* what they see, i.e., they have a dysnomic type of dysphasia.

Denckla and Rudel divided incorrect responses into three categories: (1) *Circumlocutions.* The child uses a series of words to describe the object that is recognized but whose name cannot be verbalized. For example, when shown the picture of the stethoscope the child says "the thing that a doctor uses to listen to your heart." (2) *Wrong name.* The child verbalizes a word that is totally unrelated to the item shown on the card, e.g., tuning fork is responded to as "magnet." (3) *Not known.* The child can provide neither a word nor a description for the

Figure 9.2
The Oldfield-Wingfield Picture-Naming Test.

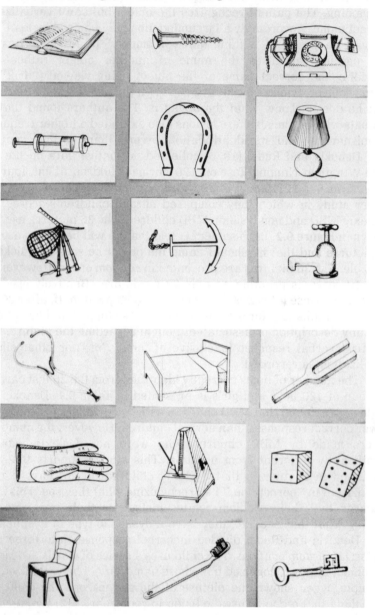

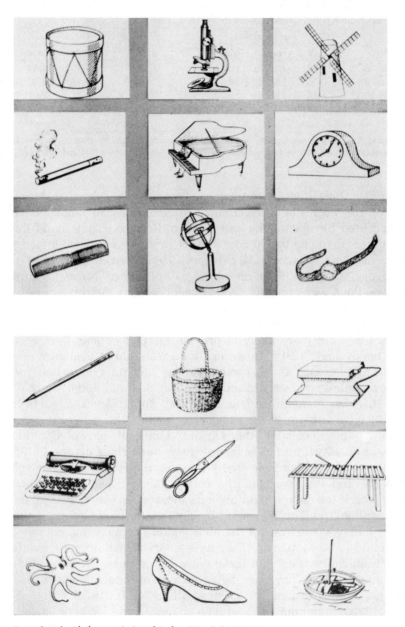

Reproduced with the permission of Arthur Wingfield, Ph.D.

Table 9.1

Total Number of Items Correctly Identified by Normal Children
on the Oldfield-Wingfield Picture-Naming Test.

Age	N	Boys Range	Mean	S.D.	N	Girls Range	Mean	S.D.
8-0 to 8-11	15	12–22	18.53	3.14	15	12–19	16.47	1.92
9-0 to 9-11	15	16–22	19.47	1.77	15	10–22	18.40	3.04
10-0 to 10-11	15	15–14	19.53	2.23	15	14–21	19.07	1.94
11-0 to 11-11	15	15–24	20.26	2.31	15	14–22	19.47	2.23
	60				60			

Reproduced with the permission of the authors and Academic Press Inc., from M. B. Denckla and R. G. Rudel, "Naming of Object-Drawings by Dyslexic and Other Learning Disabled Children." *Brain and Language*, 3:1–15, 1976.

item. (This classification is similar to that of Newcombe et al. described above. However, the terms *circumlocution* and *wrong name* have been substituted for misnaming and misidentification.) They found that of the errors made by the 90 normal 8-, 9-, and 10-year-olds studied 30% were in the *circumlocution* category, 33% were in the *wrong name* category, and 37% were classified as *not known*. Normal children's errors, then, were roughly divided evenly among the three categories. The authors found that nondyslexic MBD children were more likely to provide *wrong name* errors than normals and dyslexic MBDs, and that dyslexics were more likely to provide *circumlocutions* than normals and nondyslexic MBDs. However, there were only 10 subjects in each of the MBD groups and so one cannot use such data other than for the experimental purposes utilized in the Denckla and Rudel study.

In subsequent utilizations of the test, Rudel, Denckla, and Broman (1978) have attempted to categorize further the different types of errors. They consider the various kinds of paraphasic errors (substitutions within the same category, part-whole errors, half-right errors, and dysphonemic errors) to be related to left-hemisphere damage and they warrant the child's being considered dysphasic. However, if the child's error appears to be one of visual discrimination (perception), (calling the dice "blocks" or the stethoscope a "jump-rope"), they would suspect right-hemisphere damage and not consider the child to be dysphasic. They have no extensive normative data on the frequencies of each of these types of responses with the Oldfield-Wingfield cards. They have, however, obtained such frequencies on a related naming test on 202 children (Rudel, et al., 1978).

I have found the test useful as an instrument for assessing object recognition and naming ability. In the analysis of error type there are a number of intrinsic difficulties. One relates to the problem of placing the error in the correct category. Some children will readily say that they don't know the name for the object depicted in the picture. Generally, they are children with a high sense of self-worth and are not devastated by the admission of errors. In addition, there are children who say they don't know because of negativism or the fear that any response will be ridiculed. There are other children, however, who will try to conceal their ignorance of an item and make a "wild guess." This is a common practice among MBD children. Having failed in many areas they do not have the ego strength to admit easily their mistakes. Had they been psychologically strong enough to admit they did not know the word, their response would have been placed in the *not known* rather than the *wrong name* category. Psychological rather than neurological factors, then, have determined here the error classification. Some MBD children provide *wrong name* responses because of their impulsivity. Their self-control is so poor that they blurt out an answer without giving themselves time to contemplate the name. Others whose responses fall in the *wrong name* category might be truly dysnomic and have verbalized the incorrect word because they cannot link the visualized object with the word that denotes it. Typically such children might exhibit one of the types of paraphasias described earlier in this chapter.

It is also important for the examiner to appreciate that a child with an impaired educational experience (at home and/or at school), who may not have had the opportunity for the normal degree of exposure to words, may get a low score on this test. Although, as mentioned, the objects were chosen because the authors considered them to be widely recognized, a few (gyroscope, anvil, microscope, xylophone, tuning fork, and metronome) are not likely to be recognized by deprived children because of their curtailed experiences. Such a child may even utilize circumlocutions, not because he is dysnomic but because he has some vague recognition of the word's function but not its identity. A child's score on the Peabody Picture Vocabulary Test (described in chapter 7) can sometimes help the examiner determine whether a dysnomic problem is causing a child's poor performance on the Oldfield-Wingfield Test. In the PPVT the child is given a word and asked to point to the one of four pictures that best relates to it. No verbalization or even word finding is required by the child. If a child does well on the PPVT and poorly on the Oldfield-Wingfield Test then the probability of a dysnomic problem being present is increased.

In conclusion, then, at the present time I consider the Oldfield-Wingfield Test to be primarily useful as a way of determining the child's ability to *recognize* and to *name* correctly common objects. The child who scores normally on this test is probably not dysnomic. The child who does poorly may be dysnomic, but his low score may relate to other factors already described. The *nature* of the errors can provide a clue as to whether the child is dysphasic. Observations for circumlocutions and various kinds of paraphasic responses, are suggestive of a dysphasic disorder. Perceptual errors suggest another kind of neurological impairment (right-hemisphere dysfunction). However, until extensive normative data on the frequency of such responses in normal children are obtained, conclusions regarding the presence of true dysnomia have to be impressionistic and cautiously made. It is my hope that such studies will be forthcoming.

At the present time I use the Oldfield-Wingfield Test in the following way. A 10½-year-old boy, for example, correctly identifies 22 of the items. Referring to Table 9.1 we see that the mean number of correct responses for boys his age is 19.53 with a standard deviation of 2.23. His score lies between 1 and 2 standard deviations above the mean for boys his age. The likelihood of this child's being dysnomic is small. A 10½-year-old girl gives 15 correct responses. The mean score for girls her age is 19.07, with a standard deviation of 1.94. Her score is 2 standard deviations below the mean. Reviewing the 11 cards that were not correctly identified, we note that she called the metronome a "thing that ticks," the gyroscope a "spinner," the stethoscope a "tethacope," and the horseshoe "the thing on the bottom of a horse's foot." I would consider this child to be suffering with a dysnomic problem; however, I would not be certain. Her low accuracy score is established. Although the quality of her errors suggests the presence of a true dysnomia (circumlocutions and dysphonemic errors), we cannot be certain that the number of errors suggesting dysphasia is beyond the normal range. My own subjective clinical experience leads me to the *impression* that her dysphasic-type errors are abnormally high. Hopefully, frequency data will be forthcoming to enable examiners such as myself to be more definitive with regard to the conclusions we can come to on this aspect of the test.

Rapid "Automatized" Naming

Denckla and Rudel (1974) have introduced a battery of tests that are designed to detect mild dysnomias in children. The instruments are based on the observation that dysnomic children are not only *slower* than normals in naming objects, but make *more errors* as well. The tests do not attempt to formally assess the *nature* of the errors, e.g., whether circumlocutions or paraphasias were utilized. Rather, they merely measure the *number* of erroneous responses the child has made. The examiner may wish to consider the quality of the errors and surmise whether a true dysnomia is present. However, as mentioned, without normative data such conclusions must be tentative and cautiously made. Delayed response is more objectively measured in these tests and this is suggestive of the kinds of storage and retrieval problems one sees in dysnomia.

The authors describe nine tests, in each of which the child is to name as rapidly as he can the 50 items depicted. In each series there are 5 basic items each of which is represented 10 times, the total 50 items being presented in a random array. The nine sets are (1) Colors (red, green, black, blue, and yellow); (2) Numbers (2,6,9,4, and 7); (3) Capital Letters, High Frequency of Occurrence (A,D,S,L, and R); (4) Animals (dog, cow, cat, bird, and squirrel); (5) Lower-Case Letters, Low Frequency of Occurrence (b,q,e,c, and i); (6) Use Objects (comb, key, watch, scissors, and umbrella); (7) Capital Letters, Lower Frequency of Occurrence (V,U,H,J, and F); (8) Random Objects (flag, drum, book, moon, and wagon); and (9) Lower-Case Letters, High Frequency of Occurrence (p,o,d,a, and s). I have not found it necessary to utilize all nine of these tests. I have found five enough to establish whether or not a child exhibits an abnormal score. Accordingly, these five will be described in greater detail and are the ones I recommend for use by the examiner.

For each of the tests the child is given the following instructions. "You are going to name some things you see as fast as you can without making mistakes. First tell me, slowly, the names of each of these five things." (Examiner points to each of the five different items until the child responds with a name for it). "Good. Now go back to the first one and when I say 'Go,' name every single thing you see across this row" (examiner sweeps finger across first row) "and this" (examiner sweeps finger across second row, and then each subsequent row) "until you come to the very last one on the card. O.K. Get ready, get set, Go!" The trial period during which the examiner ascertains whether the child recognizes the 5 items is untimed. If at this time the child offers two alternative names for an object ("Is this a wagon or a cart?"), the child is advised to use the shorter name. If, however, the child does not know the name of the item, he is not given it, because to do so would defeat the whole purpose of the test.

Use Objects

Pictures of a comb, a key, a watch, a scissors, and an umbrella were selected from the Stanford-Binet Intelligence Test (Terman and Merrill, 1937). However, I believe that the same normative data, if obtained elsewhere, would be applicable for similar pictures of these common objects because these objects are generally recognizable to the large majority of children age 5 and over. Ten pictures of each of these 5 objects are randomly placed in an array of 5 rows (Figure 9.3).

Figure 9.3
Rapid "Automatized" Naming of Use Objects.

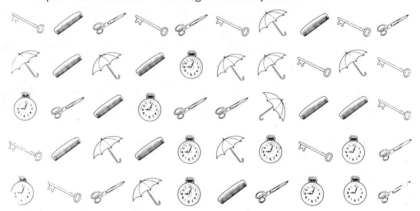

Reproduced from the Stanford-Binet Intelligence Scale (L. M. Terman and M. A. Merrill, 1937) by permission of the publisher, Houghton Mifflin Co., Boston, Mass.

After the untimed trial period in which the examiner asks the child to identify each of the 5 objects by pointing to it on the card, the child is requested to name the objects as quickly as he can while the examiner times him. Mean times for normal children are shown in Table 9.2 and the percentage of normal children in the Denckla and Rudel study who exhibited errors are shown in Table 9.3. In the latter table, two figures are shown. The first indicates the percentage of children in the study who made any number of errors at all, i.e., 1 or more. The second figure indicates the percentage of children at that age level who made 3 or more errors.

The test can be used in the following way. An 8-year-old boy, for example, names the 50 items in 86 sec. He makes 4 errors. Twice he called the watch a "tick tock," once he called the scissors a "cutter," and once he called the umbrella "a rain thing." Referring to Table 9.2, we note that normal children his age take 61.6 ± 12.6 sec. This child's score is about 2 standard deviations above the normal. Referring to Table 9.3, we note that only 3.3% of the normal children studied made 3 or more errors. It is reasonable to conclude that this child is likely to be dysnomic. In addition, the quality of errors (paraphasias and circumlocution) are also suggestive of the disorder.

Random Objects

The five objects depicted here (flag, drum, book, moon, and wagon) were also taken from the Stanford-Binet Intelligence Test (Figure 9.4). However, as is true for the Use Objects Test, I believe that

Table 9.2

Normative Data for Rapid "Automatized" Naming: Mean Times [in Seconds].

Age	N	Colors		Random Objects		Numbers[a]		Capitals [HF][a]		Use Objects[a]	
		Mean	S.D.	Mean	S.D.	Mean	S.D.	Mean	S.D.	Mean	S.D.
5-0 to 5-11											
Boys	15	109.5	37.7	112.9	36.9	85.3	34.9	90.8	38.9	105.2	43.9
Girls	15	92.9	47.7	96.5	27.0						
6-0 to 6-11											
Boys	15	68.5	14.8	90.2	16.6	57.2	26.7	56.1	21.9	89.8	26.7
Girls	15	66.7	21.5	76.0	32.1						
7-0 to 7-11											
Boys	15	56.3	10.9	63.5	13.1	34.4	6.8	34.4	7.9	69.9	24.2
Girls	15	52.4	8.8	56.9	10.3						
8-0 to 8-11											
Boys	15	54.7	6.9	61.0	8.0	30.8	5.8	30.3	5.3	61.6	12.6
Girls	15	49.0	11.7	56.6	11.9						
9-0 to 9-11											
Boys	15	46.5	11.4	53.4	15.4	25.8	8.6	25.2	5.8	48.7	10.7
Girls	15	40.4	6.9	44.5	8.6						
10-0 to 10-11											
Boys	15	42.3	8.2	48.3	13.6	24.2	3.5	24.4	3.9	50.6	10.8
Girls	15	41.1	5.9	47.3	3.8						
	180										

[a] Boys' and Girls' means combined because of no significant sex differences.

Reproduced with the permission of the authors and publisher from M. B. Denckla and R. R. Rudel, "Rapid 'Automatized' Naming of Pictured Objects, Colors, Letters, and Numbers by Normal Children," *Cortex*, X:186-202, 1974.

Table 9.3
Rapid "Automatized" Naming: Percentage of Children Making Errors [Boys and Girls Combined]

Age	N	Colors		Random Objects		Numbers		Capitals [HF]		Use Objects	
		Any Errors	3 or More Errors	Any Errors	3 or More Errors	Any Errors	3 or More Errors	Any Errors	3 or More Errors	Any Errors	3 or More Errors
5-0 to 5-11	30	40.0	16.7	56.7	6.7	40.0	13.3	20.0	10.0	50.0	16.7
6-0 to 6-11	30	13.3	3.3	13.0	0.0	13.3	6.7	0.0	0.0	16.0	3.3
7-0 to 7-11	30	13.3	0.0	26.6	0.0	6.7	0.0	10.0	3.3	23.3	6.7
8-0 to 8-11	30	23.3	0.0	16.6	3.3	13.3	0.0	13.3	0.0	13.3	3.3
9-0 to 9-11	30	13.3	0.0	10.0	0.0	10.0	0.0	3.3	0.0	6.7	0.0
10-0 to 10-11	30	13.3	0.0	16.6	0.0	13.3	0.0	3.3	0.0	16.0	0.0

Reproduced with the permission of the authors and publisher from M. B. Denckla and R. R. Rudel, "Rapid 'Automatized' Naming of Pictured Objects, Colors, Letters, and Numbers by Normal Children." Cortex, X:186-202, 1974.

Figure 9.4
Rapid "Automatized" Naming of Random Objects.

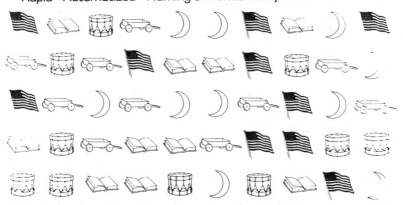

similar pictures taken from other sources would be equally useful for the purposes of this test. Mean response times for normal children are shown in Table 9.2, and the percentage of children who exhibited errors at each age level are shown in Table 9.3. A 10-year-old girl, for example, takes 43 sec to name the 50 items and makes no mistakes. Referring to Table 9.2, we note that normal girls her age average 47.3 sec with a standard deviation of 3.8 sec. We see that her score is over one standard deviation below the average. Referring to Table 9.3, we note that 16.6% of children her age make 1 or more errors. Considering that she made no errors at all and that her speed was significantly faster than the average, one can conclude that this girl does not have a dysnomic problem.

Numbers

The numerals 2, 6, 9, 4, and 7 were selected for random display (Figure 9.5). Normative data for speed and errors are again to be found in Tables 9.2 and 9.3. Whereas most children of age 5 will readily recognize the Use and Random Objects, some may not yet know how to read numbers and letters. Obviously, it would be inappropriate to consider a 5-year-old child dysnomic if he is not able to correctly identify numbers and letters. Accordingly, if a child of 5 does not correctly identify *all* letters and numbers in the untimed trial period, I do not administer the test. The child who correctly identifies all the numbers is, of course, tested. Such a child might still make errors in the testing period when, under the pressure of time, he gives a letter or number an incorrect name. Again, Tables 9.2 and 9.3 can be consulted for mean response times and percentage of children exhibiting errors.

Figure 9.5
Rapid "Automatized" Naming of Numbers.

7	4	7	9	6	6	2	6	4	6
6	9	2	2	2	9	4	4	6	4
4	6	2	9	9	2	2	9	2	4
7	4	9	2	9	7	7	9	9	7
6	6	6	4	7	4	7	2	7	7

Based on information described in M. B. Denckla and R. R. Rudel, "Rapid 'Automatized' Naming of Pictured Objects, Colors, Letters, and Numbers by Normal Children." *Cortex*, X:186–202, 1974.

Letters

Five capital letters of high frequency of occurrence (A,D,S,L, and R) were selected (Figure 9.6). As mentioned, there are some 5-year-olds who do not yet know how to read numbers, but who are not dysnomic (or dyslexic). Accordingly, I do not use this test if the child does not demonstrate full ability to correctly identify the numbers during the untimed trial period. Normative response data are to be found in Tables 9.2 and 9.3.

Figure 9.6
Rapid "Automatized" Naming of Capital Letters—Higher Frequency of Occurrence.

A	D	A	S	A	R	A	S	R	D
L	D	L	L	D	S	L	A	L	D
S	R	S	S	D	D	R	A	R	L
A	A	A	S	R	L	L	D	R	D
L	S	S	R	R	L	S	R	A	D

Based on information described in M. B. Denckla and R. R. Rudel, "Rapid 'Automatized' Naming of Pictured Objects, Colors, Letters, and Numbers by Normal Children." *Cortex*, X:186–202, 1974.

Colors

The five colors (red, green, black, blue, and yellow) that were selected for display are shown in Figure 9.7. (Unfortunately, the reader must use a little imagination to correctly identify these colors in the black-and-white rendition provided here). Normative data are to be found in Tables 9.2 and 9.3.

Figure 9.7
Rapid "Automatized" Naming of Colors.

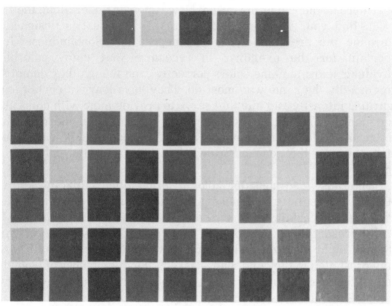

Based on information described in M. B. Denckla and R. R. Rudel, "Rapid 'Automatized' Naming of Pictured Objects, Colors, Letters, and Numbers by Normal Children." *Cortex,* X:186–202, 1974.

Testing the child's ability to recognize colors, as one test of naming capacity, may appear simple at first, but the more one looks into this phenomenon the more complex it becomes. I will discuss this issue in some detail in order to give the reader and examiners an appreciation of the complexity of these matters and how tentative one's conclusions must be regarding the kinds of assessments discussed in this book. Castner (1940) found that 61% of normal 5-year-olds successfully named the colors red, yellow, blue, and green when they were presented to them. This would appear to be a simple enough test. However, Denckla (1972) describes a number of considerations that indicate the complexity of this ostensibly simple evaluation.

The child should first be given a standard test for *colorblindness*. Obviously if the child is colorblind, one cannot properly evaluate his responses on any test involving color recognition. Denckla prefers the Dvorine Pseudo-Isochromatic Plates (Dvorine, 1953) to tests in which the child is asked to identify a dotted numeral embedded in an array of dots of similar colors and hues. The latter is not too reliable for pre-literate children and those who may, for psychological reasons, feign colorblindness. In the second section of the Dvorine plates, the child is asked to trace 8 trails with his finger. The child is instructed, "Put your finger here at the rim of the circle. Now run your finger along the trail so you find your way out of the forest." This test is designed to determine the presence, type, and degree of colorblindness. It is important for the examiner to recognize that many colorblind individuals learn to name colors correctly even though they do not see them exactly the same way most do. They have learned certain cues regarding intensity and hue that serve to provide them with clues as to what name to give a particular color. For example, the colorblind person may state that a fire engine is red, not because it is seen as such but because of the common knowledge that red is the color of fire engines.

One must also consider *color discrimination* capacity, i.e., the ability to differentiate between colors that differ from one another and to be able to ascertain when two colors are the same. Denckla tests for this by presenting the child with an array of 16 swatches of yarn. Although eight different colors are represented, they are all mixed when presented to the child who is asked, "Find the pieces of wool that are just the same color, like twins, and put them together, two-by-two, on the table." She does not use primary colors for this examination, but rather "burnt orange," "cinnamon," "fuchsia," "chartreuse," "beige," "moss green," "aquamarine," and "robin's-egg blue." The child who cannot easily differentiate colors from one another will make mismatched pairs.

One is also interested in whether the child has developed *color abstraction* capability, specifically the appreciation that the word *color*, per se, does not refer to any particular hue. Rather, the word is a rubric under which is subsumed all colors. The child who provides correct answers to questions involving color recognition, naming, memory, and association (all to be discussed below) can be presumed to have adequate color abstraction capability, i.e., he understands the meaning of the word *color*.

One must differentiate *color recognition*, i.e., the ability to point to a color that is named by the examiner ("Point to the red box") from *color naming*, which involves the child himself naming a color to which the examiner points ("What color is this box?"). Color recognition is an easier task than color naming and can generally be accomplished at a younger age. For recognition, the association between the color and its name need be less deeply entrenched than for color naming. In recognition testing, the examiner's question, by providing the name, gives information that helps the child remember. In color naming tests (such as the 50-item test described above) no such helpful data is provided. Also, naming involves verbalization capacity; recognition (with pointing) does not. Accordingly, naming tests can detect aphasias; simple recognition tests (with pointing) do not. As discussed above in detail, even the naming test can be further broken down into functional components. The child's speech and the nature of his errors provide information about the presence of dysnomia.

Color association refers to the child's ability to associate colors with known objects. Such capacity, like the functions discussed above, rely upon color storage and retrieval ability (memory). For instance, the child can be asked questions such as, "What color is a banana (grass, Santa Claus's suit, the sky, etc.)?" Answering such questions correctly involves the child's memory of both banana and yellow as well as the fact that the color of a banana is yellow. He must link (associate) the two.

It is beyond the scope of this discussion to present in detail Denckla's standardizations of the aforementioned tests. The reader who is interested in these should refer to her article (Denckla, 1972). Unless a more detailed inquiry is warranted, I generally use the above mentioned 50-item naming test. This not only tells me about how the child compares to others regarding color naming concepts, but also (via the speed and error quality) provides me with information about possible dysnomia as well.

AGNOSIAS

The word agnosia means absence of knowledge. Agnosias are traditionally defined as impairments in the ability to recognize the form and nature of objects. Blakiston's New Gould Medical Dictionary (1951) defines agnosia as "Total or partial loss of the perceptive faculty by which persons and things are recognized." Hinsie and Shatzky's Psychiatric Dictionary (1953) considers the central defect to be a "loss or disuse of the knowledge of objects." In attempting to determine whether a patient is agnosic, the examiner must rely on the patient's communications (usually verbal) that the object is recognized, and he must try to determine whether he and the patient are thinking about the same thing. Sometimes it may be difficult for the examiner to be certain that an object is truly recognized. For example, a patient who is impaired in seeing green like most people may say that grass is "green" because he has learned that that is the traditional color of grass. Demonstrating that a patient does not recognize an object, therefore, poses operational difficulties.

Impairments in perception are considered by many neurologists and neuropsychologists to be related, if not identical to, the agnosias. Perception is traditionally defined as the capacity to discriminate, organize, structure, and recognize stimuli, that is, provide a constellation of stimuli with *meaning*. Again, one must often surmise what is going on in the mind of the examinee in order to determine whether or not he is truly recognizing something or providing it with meaning. A more practical, objective, less philosophical, and less speculative concept of agnosia would consider it to be an impairment in which there is difficulty discriminating between two stimuli of a specific sensory modality when the ability to detect the sensation is intact. This definition has the advantage of avoiding the operational difficulties encountered when one attempts to ascertain what is going on in the patient's mind. But to say that agnosia is merely an impairment in the ability to differentiate between stimuli would be an oversimplification. The whole problem can probably best be solved by dispensing entirely with the word agnosia (just as I suggested in chapter 7 and 8 that we do well to dispense with the word *perception*) and utilize instead the various terms that are generally subsumed under the rubric. Many neurologists are doing just that. Here I will describe the traditional categories of agnosia and describe how they relate to some of the more well-defined phenomena that have been presented. I will not, however, describe any tests for agnosia in this section. Such tests have been presented in my discussions of the various kinds of visual and auditory processing phenomena that are generally referred to as perceptual.

Tactile Agnosia

In tactile agnosia (when defined simply as an impairment in tactile discrimination), the individual has difficulty feeling the difference between similar objects. (Such testing is usually done with the patient's eyes closed to prevent his gaining visual information.) This impairment is sometimes referred to as *astereognosis*. For example, when the person's eyes are closed and coins are placed in the palm of his hand, he cannot differentiate well between coins of different sizes and may even have trouble differentiating between objects as dissimilar as a pen and a pair of glasses. Using a broader definition, the person with a tactile agnosia has trouble identifying objects placed in his hand.

Auditory Agnosia

Defined narrowly as a discrimination problem, the patient with auditory agnosia cannot differentiate between various sounds. The auditory apparatus is intact; rather, cerebral processes are impaired. The person might not be able to differentiate bells from buzzers or he might not be able to recognize the sounds of speech, i.e., recognize speech as language. As the reader may recall, in Wernicke's aphasia the individual appreciates that a language is being spoken, but he cannot understand it. It is as if it were foreign. The agnosic patient cannot differentiate between language and nonlinguistic sounds. The child who does poorly on the Wepman test of auditory discrimination (described in chapter 7) could be considered to have agnosia. Defined more broadly, the patient has difficulty understanding the meaning of a sound, e.g., that the sound of a bell means that the class is over, or that the spoken word *water* refers to a particular kind of fluid.

Visual Agnosia

Colorblindness is one kind of visual agnosia. The person cannot differentiate between hues. On the standard tests of colorblindness, he does not differentiate the patterns from their backgrounds. Such people may learn what the social names are for a particular color but they do not see them as others do, nor do they differentiate them as clearly from other colors as the normal person. This may not be appreciated by the casual examiner but is readily picked up on tests for colorblindness.

The person who cannot differentiate between letters suffers with a visual agnosia, and this may contribute to alexia (a neurologically based inability to read). However, a person can be alexic on an aphasic basis in that he cannot verbalize the stored word that corresponds to what is being seen. Reading is silent verbalization. Externally uttered speech is secondary to internally thought speech, that is, the individual must mentally retrieve the word from his memory system before he can utter it. Even the silent reader can be aphasic, although one cannot prove it until he tries to speak, because aphasia by definition is a type of impairment in spoken language. The lesion can exist in Broca's area, in which case the individual cannot verbalize what he or she reads even though he or she recognizes what has been read. Or there can be a lesion in the association fibers to Broca's area which in effect produces the same kind of speech impairment. The impulses never get to Broca's area and so the person cannot verbalize what he has read. Lastly, in the aphasic who has a lesion in the memory areas in the parietal lobe, the reader again cannot properly retrieve the word that is associated with the one he is reading. In short, in alexia which is the result of visual agnosia (agnosic alexia), the patient doesn't perceive (recognize) the letters or differentiate them properly from one another. In alexia associated with aphasia (aphasic alexia), the patient cannot verbalize words that are recognized.

Denckla (1976) believes that only about 15% of alexic children suffer with visual agnosias and that the remainder (about 85%) are basically aphasic. The child who is alexic on an aphasic basis will generally exhibit other impairments in spoken language, either receptive or expressive. He often exhibits phonemic errors, substituting when speaking one phoneme for another (e.g., sheep for sheet). There are reversals in his speech, both letters and phonemes, and he may exhibit sequence errors in repeating digits. When asked to say the days of the week, he will often mix them up as he will the seasons. Many of these children exhibit dysnomic problems. In short, the child whose alexia is on an aphasic basis will exhibit other spoken language problems typical of aphasics in general.

The child whose alexic problem is on a visual-perceptual (agnosic) basis, will exhibit other difficulties in differentiating or recognizing what he sees. Accordingly, he will have trouble matching patterns, doing crossword puzzles, copying geometric forms, and performing adequately on such tests as Raven's Progressive Matrices. (Many of these functions were discussed in chapter 8.)

As the reader may appreciate at this point, there is little to be gained by retaining the term agnosia. Like the term perception, I try to avoid using it. Therefore, I do not have tests for agnosia per se in my battery. I do, however, test for the functions generally subsumed under the term. In the narrow sense these are the tests of auditory and visual discrimination; in the broader use of the term, these are the tests involving recognition and meaning of auditory and visual stimuli. These have been discussed in detail in chapters 7 and 8.

APRAXIAS

Apraxias are impairments in the skilled performance of purposeful movements without paralysis, paresis, or sensory loss. Benton (1973) defines apraxia as "an inability to perform purposive acts within the setting of intact motor capacity." In other words, the individual has no defect in the proper functioning of his extremities or any other parts of the body that may be involved in performing a purposeful movement. Rather, the central mechanisms that enable him to perform these accurately and in proper sequence are impaired. It appears that the body is not able to perform functions that the brain wills it to execute. I will first describe the various kinds of apraxias described in classical neurology and then discuss some tests useful in assessing for the presence of apraxias and dyspraxias in children.

Ideokinetic Apraxia

An impairment in the ability to perform a single act is referred to as ideokinetic apraxia. For example, if the patient is asked to throw a ball, he performs an act that may be totally unrelated. Or if asked to hammer a nail, he just doesn't seem to be able to know what to do to perform the act correctly. Hearing is intact as is probably the inner appreciation of what the request is.

Ideational Apraxia

The inability to perform a sequence of acts requiring several steps is called ideational apraxia. For example, if the person is asked to light a cigarette, he may put the match to his mouth before putting the cigarette in, or try to strike the cigarette against the matchbook, or otherwise involve himself in maladaptive and incorrect sequences.

Constructional Apraxia

An impairment in the ability to properly construct or put together a collection of objects is usually referred to as constructional apraxia. Such patients have great difficulty building models, doing jigsaw puzzles, or copying geometric designs and drawings. Here, the impairment is not a perceptual one in that the individual can properly differentiate and recognize accurately various perceptual forms. Rather, when the person is asked to *perform* he cannot put together correctly what he sees. Children who have difficulty building models may have motor coordination problems, but they also may be suffering with a constructional dyspraxia. I am in agreement with those who believe that children who have problems copying geometric designs more commonly suffer with a constructional apraxia than a visual-perceptual problem, that is, a visual agnosia. As will be discussed below, the Bender-Gestalt Test is *not* so much a test of visual-motor perception as it is a test for the presence of a constructional dyspraxia.

Dressing Apraxia

Occasionally one sees children who could justifiably be considered to be suffering with a dressing apraxia. Here, the child has trouble putting on his clothing in the correct way. Commonly, the problem exhibits itself for the left side of the body only, because lesions in the right hemisphere are the more common cause of this disorder. In constructional apraxias, as well, constructing the left side of a project may be impaired, again because of right-hemispherical deficit.

Agraphias

Agraphias can be apraxic in that the individual is unable to make his hands do what his brain wants them to. Accordingly, the person can think of a particular word but not be able to write it, even though there is no physical disorder of his hands or arms. However, agraphias can be agnosic (perceptual) when the individual cannot copy a particular word. This is related to an impairment in being able to differentiate letters from one another or recognize them. Agraphias may also be seen in Wernicke's aphasia. Because such patients cannot understand what they are being asked to write (although they recognize a language is being spoken), they are not able to successfully satisfy a request to write a particular word. The end result is that they cannot write, but the inability has nothing to do with an apraxia but with an aphasia.

Whatever its cause, objectively assessing dysgraphia in children (and even adults) may be very difficult. To merely look at a child's handwriting and say that it is poor, is not very convincing. One can ask, "poor, compared to what?" There are no norms for different ages and even if one were to attempt to collect them, he or she would be hard put to set up objective criteria for differentiating various levels of competence. What I do, therefore, is to ask the child to write his name. If he is second grade or beyond and if his handwriting is *almost illegible in spite of great effort*, I will consider it probable that dysgraphia is present. I then attempt to ascertain whether a fine-motor-coordination problem is present (by using tests described in chapter 5) or whether it is the result of a dysphasic, dysgnosic, or dyspraxic impairment (by utilizing tests described in this chapter).

As is true for the aphasias, children with MBD can be expected to exhibit apraxias. However, they are often less dramatic than those seen in adults with gross brain lesions. The term dyspraxia is therefore more appropriate. The tests I have found most useful in assessing for the presence of dyspraxia in children are here presented.

The Manual Expression Subtest of the ITPA

The Manual Expression subtest of the ITPA (Kirk et al., 1968), although not described as such by the authors, is an excellent objective test for the presence of ideokinetic and ideational dyspraxias. In the demonstration phase of the test the child is shown a toy hammer and told, "Show me what to do with a hammer." If the child does not understand, the examiner demonstrates its use. The child is then given the hammer and instructed to perform the same kind of hammering movements that the examiner has just demonstrated. If the child successfully accomplishes this, he is shown a *picture* of a hammer and told, "Good. Now, show me again. Pretend you have a real one." The same procedure is followed with a picture of a coffeepot and cup. If the child cannot spontaneously demonstrate what should be done with these utensils, the examiner demonstrates their use and encourages the child to perform the proper motions along with him or her. Other than the first demonstration hammer, all other objects are presented as pictures only. Whereas in the demonstration phase the examiner may help the child and show proper use of the device, in the test phase such assistance is not permitted. The examiner only shows the child the picture of the object and says, "Show me what we do with _____." If the patient only verbalizes the use of the object he is told, "Don't tell me about it. Show me what we do with it." If the patient still does not respond manually, he is told, "Do it so I can see. I want to see you do it."

There are a total of 15 pictures presented to the child: guitar, knife and fork, telephone, toothbrush and toothpaste, comb and mirror, cigarette and matches, pencil sharpener, doorknob, binoculars, eggs and egg beater, camera, stethoscope, suitcase, combination lock, and clarinet. The knife and fork card is shown in Figure 9.8. As the child demonstrates the use of the object, the examiner notes whether he is performing certain functions traditionally utilized when using the object. For example, when demonstrating the use of the knife and fork the child receives 1 point for pantomimes using the fork to cut or scoop, another point if he pretends that he is cutting with the knife, and a third if he brings his hand to his mouth. The child's total raw score for all 15 items is converted to a scaled score by referral to the table corresponding to the child's age. As is true for the other ITPA subtests, the mean scaled score is 36 with a standard deviation of 6. Accordingly, a 6½-year-old child who receives a raw score of 28 (out of a possible maximum of 41 points) would be found to have a scaled score of 43. This would be 1 standard deviation above the mean and the examiner can conclude that the child is not likely to be dyspraxic. A 10-year-1-month-old child gets a raw score of 18. This corresponds to a scaled score of 22, which is more than 2 standard deviations below the mean. Such a child may be dyspraxic. However, other factors must be considered. There may be an auditory processing defect which may be interfering with the child understanding the instructions. The child may be retarded or of borderline intelligence and not have been exposed

Figure 9.8
Illinois Test of Psycholinguistic Abilities, Manual Expression—Knife and Fork.

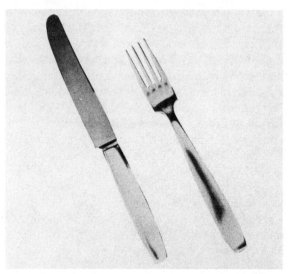

to or had the curiosity to learn about all the objects. A visual memory problem may interfere with the child recognizing the object or remembering the way it should be used. If these other factors can be ruled out, then one may be more certain that the child is indeed dyspraxic.

Visual Motor Gestalt Test

Bender (1938 and 1946) has devised a widely used instrument that is generally viewed as a test of "visual-motor perception." It was devised to detect organic disease of the brain and is based on the observation that many patients with known brain damage have difficulty copying geometric forms accurately. Bender considered a central problem of patients with such impairments to be integrating a constellation of stimuli into a well-organized, complete pattern, referred to as a Gestalt (German: form, shape, figure).

The test is relatively easy to administer. The child is given a blank sheet of paper, generally 8½ in. × 11 in.. One sheet usually suffices, but he can be given a second if he uses up significant space on the first. The examiner holds nine cards, each of which depicts a geometric pattern. Two of the patterns are shown in Figure 9.9. Each card in turn is

Figure 9.9
Visual Motor Gestalt Test.

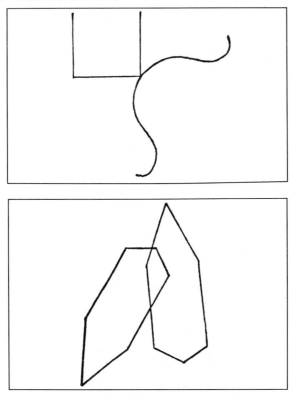

Cards 4 and 7 of the Visual Motor Gestalt Test, Lauretta Bender, M.D. Reproduced with the permission of the American Orthopsychiatric Association, publisher.

placed with its lower edge at the top of the child's paper so that the orientation of the design is correct. The child is told, "Here are some figures (or designs) for you to copy. Just copy them the way you see them." The child is not permitted to turn the card lest he draw a rotation and thereby compromise (possibly unnecessarily) his score. The child is permitted to erase and correct any errors he believes he has made. There is no time limit and each figure is removed only after the child has demonstrated maximum capacity to reproduce it.

Bender's original scoring system involved the examiner's referring to a chart that presented the most common types of rendition provided for each card by children ages 3 and over. Each rendition was accompanied by the percentage of children who drew the form in the manner depicted. By comparing all of the child's reproductions with the normal renderings, one could come to certain conclusions about the child's maturational level. In a typical report, one could make a comment about the age level at which each figure was reproduced and then make a general statement about the child's level of maturity. Children who performed at an immature level are considered to do so on the basis of some kind of neurophysiological pathology.

Koppitz (1964) introduced a scoring system that has generally been considered an improvement over Bender's. This was subsequently updated with further experience (Koppitz, 1975). This latter version is the one that I will discuss here.

Koppitz describes four kinds of errors that the child may make: distortion, rotation, integration, and perseveration. In errors of *distortion,* the reproduced figure is misshapen, lacks the correct number of sides or angles, exhibits minor errors of overlap, or is otherwise inadequately copied. *Rotation* errors involve 45° or more rotations around certain axes. In *integration* errors, the basic shape or pattern is lost or the various parts of the design are improperly aligned or positioned. Separate sections either overlap too much or do not have the proper amount of contact. In *perseveration* errors, the child adds significantly to the number of items depicted in a series. A score of 1 point is given for each error. The Koppitz scoring criteria are very specific and provide many examples of the kinds of errors one is likely to see in each category. Examples are given of the kinds of reproductions that justify being scored and those that do not. In this examiner's experience, it is rare to find a reproduction that is not similar to ones shown in the scoring criteria. Scoring criteria for Bender Figure 6 are shown in Figure 9.10. Bender Figure 6 depicts two wavy lines intersecting at almost a 90° angle. When the child's total number of errors are calculated (the process takes only a few minutes for the experienced examiner), one can compare the child's score to others his age by referring to the table of means and standard deviations for various ages. Age-equivalent data are also provided for each score. For example, an 8-year-3-month-old boy makes a total of 7 errors. Referring to the proper chart we note that the mean number of errors for children (boys and girls not differentiated) ages 8-0 to 8-5 is 4.2 ± 2.5. This patient's number of errors, then, is more than 1 standard deviation above the normal for his age. Referring to the same chart, we note that the average score for children ages 6-6 to 6-11 is 7.2 ± 3.5. It appears, then, that this child's score is more like that of children 1½ years his junior. Referring to the chart of age-equivalents, we note that a score of 7 corresponds to the age bracket 6-6 to 6-11, confirming the conclusions derived from the table of means and standard deviations. In recent years, it has become common practice for psychologists to describe "numerous" and "excessive" rotations, perseverations, etc.

Figure 9.10

Koppitz Scoring Criteria for Figure 6 of the Bender Visual Motor Gestalt Test.

Distortion

18a. Distortion of shape; three or more distinct angles or points instead of curves; in case of doubt do *not* score (see Plates 2, 6, 8, 9, 10, 11, 12, 13, 14, 16, 20, 22).

Examples:

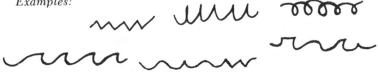

18b. Straight lines; less than two complete sinusoidal curves or no curves at all in one or both lines (see Plates 3, 25, 33).

Examples:

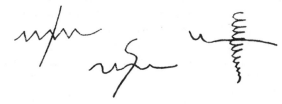

19. *Integration*

Two lines crossing not at all or at extreme end of one or both lines or less than one complete sinusoidal curve from end of line; two interwoven lines (see Plates 4, 19, 25, 31).

Examples:

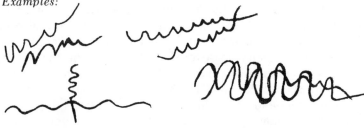

20. *Perseveration*

Six or more complete sinusoidal curves in either direction (see Plates 2, 8, 9, 10, 12, 13, 14, 20, 22, 23, 24, 27).

Example:

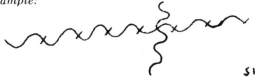

sinusoidal curve

Reproduced with the permission of the author and publisher from: Koppitz, E. M., *The Bender Gestalt Test for Young Children*, New York: Grune & Stratton, Inc., 1975.

without providing quantitative data. One should be very dubious about the validity of such impressionistic reports.

The reader may have wondered why I have chosen to discuss the Bender Gestalt Test in a section on dyspraxia rather than in chapter 8 in my discussion of visual processing. The answer is simple. I believe that most (but certainly not all) children who do poorly on this test have problems in reproducing what they see (dyspraxia) rather than in seeing accurately what is on the cards (impaired "perception"). When administering the test, I have often found that many children appreciate that they have not copied the forms accurately, but they just cannot reproduce them the way they know they should be done no matter how hard they try. Bortner and Birch (1960) and Diller and Birch (1964) describe the same observations and conclusions.

Owen et al. (1971) conducted an excellent study that confirms this examiner's observations. Seventy-six learning-disabled and 76 academically normal children were administered the Bender Gestalt Test. After the test was over, each child was again shown every card and asked whether his copy was the same or different from the original. If different, the child was encouraged to discuss the exact ways in which his renditions were different. When the number of items scored as errors by the children were compared with the number of errors that the psychologists found, there was an overlap of 76% for the LD children and 73% for the normals. There was no significant difference in accuracy of discrimination between the two groups. Not only were the LD children as good as the normals in identifying errors, but the agreement with the psychologists averaged about 75% for both groups.

The examiners then analyzed the four types of errors (distortion, rotation, integration, and perseveration) to determine the degree of agreement between the two groups of children as well as with the psychologists who scored the tests. Of the 158 reproductions considered by the LD children and psychologists to have errors, 110 (69%)were judged to be the same type of error. The normal children had 114 agreements of errors with the psychologists, of which 76 (64.9%) were judged to be the same type of error. The difference between the two groups was not significant. In short, LD children were as accurate as normal in identifying the type of error made and both groups were in agreement with the psychologists on about 66% of the errors.

The children, of course, did not use the same terminology utilized by Koppitz. They usually reported their errors in terms such as "Mine's too big," "That one's flatter," "It's pointing the wrong way," and "They don't touch." The LD children described 42.4% of their errors in exactly the same terms as the Koppitz criteria; the normal children did so for 47.4% of their errors. The difference between the two groups was not statistically significant.

The authors conclude that it is not because of an impairment in "visual perception" that the LD children do more poorly than normals on the Bender Gestalt Test. Rather, they consider these children's problems to lie in two areas. They noted that many of their errors were related to improper *sequencing* of the material. In addition, they observed that many of the children had trouble *"constructing"* what they were trying to copy.

Denckla (1976) believes that about 85% of children who do poorly on the Bender Gestalt Test have a constructional dyspraxia and only about 15% have a genuine problem in visual processing. If Denckla, Owen et al., and I are correct, then those who use the Bender Gestalt Test to assess "visual-motor perception" are likely to come to invalid conclusions regarding a child's deficits. The examiner should take these findings seriously and consider carefully whether the patient who does poorly has a genuine deficit in visual processing or whether the child is basically dyspraxic.

The Administration C Subtest of the
Revised Visual Retention Test

As the reader may recall from chapter 8, the Revised Visual Retention Test (Benton, 1955) contains two sections standardized for children (administrations A and D). Administration A, which was discussed in chapter 8, is useful as a test of visual memory because the child is asked to reproduce the figures from memory after a 10-sec display. In administration C, the design is copied by the subject while it remains in his view. (See Figure 8.7 for an example of a typical design.) Although Benton includes administration C as a test of visual memory, I do not think it qualifies as such an instrument. Rather, it is a good test of visuoconstructive ability and certain aspects of visual processing (organization, differentiation, and Gestalt).

When administering the test, the child is shown the 10 plates and instructed to copy each in turn. If the test had been given to assess visual memory, the examiner does well to use another set of the 3 series of 10 plates that are supplied. Otherwise, the child will have already been familiar with the particular designs and this may provide him with some advantage over those who were utilized in the collection of the normative data. The child is allowed to take any reasonable amount of time to copy the design. Erasures and corrections are permitted.

The scoring procedure is the same as that described for administration A in chapter 8. Briefly, the examiner scores for correct responses by giving one point for each card that has been copied in an entirely correct way. No partial credit is given. Errors (omissions, distortions, perseverations, rotations, misplacements, and size errors) are scored in accordance with criteria outlined in the manual. A child may make as many as four or five errors per card. However, it is rare for a child to get an error score over 24 points. Means and standard deviations are provided for ages 7 through 13 for two categories of children: those with average IQs (85–115) and those with superior IQs (116–147). Separate tables are provided for correct scores and error scores.

A 9½-year-old girl with a 108 IQ gets a correct score of 8 and an error score of 3. Referring to the table of correct scores, we note that the average score for children her age is 7.28 ± 1.86. She is, therefore, above average and within 1 standard deviation of the normal. Going to the table of error scores, we see that the average error score for children her age is 3.08 ± 2.15. Again, she is very much in the average range. A 10¼-year-old boy, with a 103 IQ, gets a correct score of 4 and an error score of 6. On the table of normal values for correct scores, we note that the average child his age gets a score of 8.13 ± 1.32. The boy's score, therefore, is about 3 standard deviations below the average for his age and IQ. We also note on the correct score table that the critical score for his age is 5 and that 100% of the children in the normal group exceeded this score. This child's correct score of 4 is below the critical level. Looking at the error score table, we see that the average child of his age and IQ obtains 2.13 ± 1.65 errors. He has made over 2 standard deviations more errors than normal children. The critical score for his age bracket and IQ is 5, with 91% of the normal group getting 4 errors or fewer. This child's error score of 6, then, is beyond the critical level. One can conclude that this child exhibits pathology in either visual processing and/or in the graphomotor area. If there is no other evidence for defective visual processing, then he either has a fine-motor-coordination deficit or is dyspraxic. From other tests to be found in chapter 5 and this section of this chapter, the examiner should be able to determine which type of pathology is more likely.

My primary aim in this chapter was to describe the relationship between the traditional 3 A's (aphasia, agnosia, and apraxia) and some of the signs and symptoms of MBD. I hope the reader has come to appreciate that there is much overlap here and that specialists in each area have much to offer one another.

10

Intelligence

It is very difficult to define intelligence and it may be impossible to measure it accurately. Dictionary definitions usually refer to intelligence as the capacity to acquire and apply knowledge, the faculty of thought and reason, and the power of understanding. Piaget considers the individual's capacity to adapt in a novel situation to be central to intelligence (Flavell, 1961). I find the emphasis on this element in intelligence to be appealing because it focuses on the more demanding and difficult aspects of human mental functioning, namely, one's ingenuity and creativity. However, it is still selective. Yet if one were to broaden one's definition, which elements should one include and which should be ignored, and by what criteria should such differentiations be made? Generally, societies have selected those qualities that are of premium value in that culture and have labeled as "smart" those individuals who possess and/or have acquired these specific traits. A smart Eskimo is one who knows how to catch fish well. A smart Indian is a good hunter. A smart general is one who is skilled at warfare. A smart physician is a skilled diagnostician and therapist. A smart surgeon is good with his scalpel. And a smart criminal is one who is clever at his job.

Whatever one's definition of intelligence, most MBD children in Western industrialized society are not considered smart. Of course, there are some who score high on certain IQ tests, but most do not.

Those who claim that MBD children are usually of average intelligence are either providing platitudes to assuage the grief of these children's parents or are selectively inattending to obvious deficits that most MBD children exhibit. In my experience, the average child who has been diagnosed as having MBD is in the 85 to 95 IQ range. This average, like all averages, does not preclude an occasional child who is functioning at the superior level. It does preclude high IQ children's appearance with a high degree of frequency in the MBD group.

As mentioned, testing intelligence objectively is a difficult if not impossible task. One must first select, from the broad range of traits in the human repertoire, certain specific functions for evaluation. It is important for the person who refers to such a test as an *intelligence test* to appreciate that he or she is, at best, only measuring a small segment of all the qualities that one could assess. Even the broadest IQ tests evaluate only a limited fraction of human capability. Most of the standard tests of intelligence do not measure to any significant degree artistic talent (What would Da Vinci or Rembrandt's scores have been?), musical ability (How would Bach or Mozart have done?), athletic ability (Would Babe Ruth have done well?), crafts (How would Michelangelo have performed?), adaptability (What about concentration camp survivors, political leaders, and heroes?), psychotherapists (Freud? Jung?), leadership ability (Caesar? Alexander the Great? Winston Churchill? Adolf Hitler? Stalin?). Garcia (1972) deals with this issue in depth.

MBD children are likely to do poorly on tests that happen to include traits in which they are deficient. The Stanford-Binet Intelligence Scale (Terman and Merrill, 1960) does not include nearly as many manual skill items as the Wechsler Intelligence Scale for Children-Revised (Wechsler, 1974). Accordingly, MBD children with motor problems are likely to appear more intelligent on the Stanford-Binet than on the WISC-R. MBD children's impaired ability to sustain concentration is likely to reduce their scores on most IQ test items, both timed and untimed. Some examiners consider the attentional impairment to be the primary factor in MBD children's low scores on most standard IQ tests, and they assume that if this impairment were not present, these children would score in the normal range. Although I agree that the attentional deficit is extremely important, I believe that their low scores are the result of many other deficits, unrelated to impaired concentration, which have been discussed in the various chapters of this book. Similarly, these children's hyperactivity and impulsivity can certainly lower their IQ test scores, but I would not explain their low IQ to be primarily the result of such behavior.

Many schools test pupils' intelligence in groups, rather than individually. Most agree that IQs obtained in a group tend to be lower than those obtained when the tests are administered individually. This is especially the case for MBD children. Their distractibility is likely to interfere with their concentration on the tasks at hand. In the group situation, they are less compelled by an observing examiner to concentrate on the test. The child has less opportunity to question the examiner to gain clarification about test instructions. And MBD children typically have trouble following instructions, especially when they are complex. Lastly, their many experiences with defeat and failure make them more fearful of such tests than the average child. In a group situation they are deprived of the reassurances and calming effect that a single examiner can provide throughout.

The main thrust of my comments so far has been that IQ tests do not test enough to warrant their being called general tests of intelligence. I also believe, at the same time, that they do not provide as much information as they might. Most end up giving a simple number which is a kind of statistical average of scores on a wide variety of functions. The child's specific strengths and weaknesses are not identified. Everything gets buried under that one number. And, as discussed in chapter 8, even the subtests are composites of many functions and capacities. I am not suggesting that we dispense with the IQ number entirely. I am suggesting that no report be simply confined to presenting that number and that the scores on various sections (even if that requires reformulation and restandardization of the test) be presented. And I am also suggesting that research be done to subdivide the various sections so that there is greater specificity regarding the particular function that is being assessed. This, of course, will require the creation of new or modified subtests and the collection of extensive normative data.

THE WECHSLER INTELLIGENCE SCALE FOR CHILDREN-REVISED

The WISC (Wechsler, 1949) and the WISC-R (Wechsler, 1974) have been the most widely used tests of intelligence in recent years. The test consists of 12 subtests, 6 verbal (Information, Similarities, Arithmetic, Vocabulary, Comprehension, and Digit Span) and 6 performance (Picture Completion, Picture Arrangement, Block Design, Object Assembly, Coding, and Mazes). In the original WISC (Wechsler, 1949) one summed the scaled scores of any 5 of the 6 subtests within each group to obtain (via a conversion table) the Verbal IQ and the Performance IQ. One summed the 10 scaled scores to obtain the Full Scale IQ. At Wechsler's suggestion the Digit Span and the Mazes subtests were the ones that were usually omitted because he considered them to have the lowest correlation with general intelligence. One could, however, substitute the Digit Span or Mazes for one of the other tests in the same category if for some reason one of the standard tests was not properly administered or the child's lack of cooperation made the score suspect. One could also administer all 6 tests and prorate them (by multiplying the sum by a factor of 5/6) and then use that number as if only 5 subtests were administered. In the WISC-R all of the aforementioned instructions hold with one exception: the examiner is not permitted to prorate 6 tests into 5. The Digit Span and Mazes subtests can be substituted for another one of the subtests in its section (verbal or performance) if warranted.

There was a time when many psychologists believed that MBD children tended to do poorly on the performance tests as compared to the verbal. This was considered to be related to the common observation that MBD children do poorly on visuo-constructive tests such as Block Design, Object Assembly, and Picture Arrangement. Many psychologists considered there to be a maximum numerical gap (the figure varied among examiners) which if met or exceeded was strongly suggestive of the MBD diagnosis. Many held, for example, that if the performance score were 15 points below the verbal that MBD was very probable. In recent years most examiners have come to appreciate how simplistic this view was (Ackerman et al., 1971). An MBD child may do poorly on any one of the subtests in that each one may reveal a possible impairment that MBD children may manifest. Children with language problems may score low on some of the verbal subtests such as Vocabulary, Comprehension, and Similarities. Such children, then, may have a much lower Verbal than Performance IQ. Others may have isolated deficiencies on subtests in both major categories, giving them no great discrepancy between Verbal and Performance IQ scores.

Another common view was that MBD children exhibited greater "scatter" than normals. The ideal "normal" child is supposed to have most of his scores fall in the 9–11 scaled score range. MBD children are believed to exhibit greater variation, with some scores going quite low (3–6 range, for example) and others quite high (14–16, for example). Such great variations among the scores is referred to as *scatter*. I believe that this concept has validity. However, rigid criteria are not generally used to define scatter. Usually the examiner comes to this conclusion on the basis of subjective impressions regarding the MBD child's scatter as compared to his or her general impression about what the normal degree of scatter is. Ackerman et al. (1971)

found that their MBD group did not exhibit more scatter than controls. My own opinion is that MBD children probably do exhibit more scatter than normals. However, I do not think the concept is particularly useful. One is mainly interested in the information that each individual subtest can provide, not whether there is scatter. And one should not even be too concerned with the Full Scale IQ (I am not saying it should be ignored entirely). It is the subtests that give us our most important data and hopefully the time will come when the sub-subtests will give us even more specific information.

We have recently seen a new trend with regard to the significance of differences between the Verbal and Performance IQs. Many hold that a low score on the performance section may result from right-hemisphere dysfunction and that low scores on the verbal section are a manifestation of left-hemisphere impairment (Russell et al., 1970; Rudel, et al., 1974). This appears reasonable to me in that many language functions are left-hemisphere functions and linguistic impairment is likely to reduce a child's score on such verbal section subtests as Vocabulary, Similarities, and Information. Appreciation of spatial relationships is more a right-hemisphere function and this may interfere with the child's functioning on such performance section subtests as Block Design, Picture Arrangement, Picture Completion, Object Assembly, and Mazes. Although I am in general agreement that this concept is useful, one runs the danger of oversimplifying and too quickly classifying too many MBD children into right- and left-brain-damaged children. There are some children for whom this designation is useful. Many, however, appear to have bilateral deficits.

Many examiners have tried to select a specific constellation of subtests on which MBD children are likely to do poorly. I have never found any of these studies convincing. I believe that one does better to recognize that an MBD child may do poorly on any of the 12 subtests and that he may do well on any of them as well. He is not likely, however, to do extremely well on all 12. In fact, if he were to do well, I would not consider it likely that the diagnosis is valid. It is important for the examiner to appreciate that the concentration impairment of these children can reduce an MBD child's score on any of the subtests. Some subtests (like Arithmetic and Digit Span) are more sensitive to concentration impairments than others. But there is no subtest score that cannot be lowered if the child is not attending. Accordingly, one must always consider this to be a factor in a low score, no matter how compelling other contributing factors may be. Also, the impulsivity of MBD children may artificially lower their scores. Although this is more likely to be the case for tests such as Mazes and Coding, other test scores can be reduced by this factor as well because such children commonly blurt out answers and act without proper forethought. Lastly, we would do well to have more information about the process by which the child arrives at his answer. I am sure that there are differences between MBD children and normals in this regard. However, the WISC-R is not designed to evaluate this factor. It concerns itself with the final response and well objectifies that element. Perhaps the time will come when we can measure objectively these important processes and use such tests as part of our general battery.

In various sections of this book I have discussed the individual subtests. Each subtest was described in the section where it appeared to be most relevant to the topic under discussion. For example, the Digit Span subtest was discussed in the sections on auditory and visual memory (chapters 7 and 8). The Picture Completion subtest appeared in my discussion of Visual Memory (chapter 8). And the Comprehension and Picture Arrangement subtests will be discussed in chapter 11 in my discussion of the social problems of MBD children. Here I will focus upon the four subtests that are most sensitive to what is referred to as general intelligence: vocabulary, information, similarities, and arithmetic.

Vocabulary

The Vocabulary subtest of the WISC-R is generally considered to be more highly correlated with general intelligence than any other subtest. Cohen (1959) factor analyzed each subtest regarding its contribution to general intelligence (often referred to as G) and found Vocabulary to be first among the 12 subtests. Although most examiners agree that cultural elements could play an important role in a child's performance, this factor does not appear to be significant enough to deprive vocabulary of its rank as the single best indicator of intelligence.

In administering the test the child is simply told, "I am going to say some words. Listen carefully and tell me what each word means." The total list contains 30 words, ranging from the simple (e.g., knife, umbrella) to the most difficult (e.g., imminent, dilatory). Credit points of 2, 1, or 0 (the first four items provide 1 or 0 credits only) are given for each response in accordance with strictly defined criteria described in the test manual. Not all children start with the simplest words; the older the child, the further down the list the examiner begins. If a child does not correctly define the words at the starting point for his age, the examiner reverses the order of presentation until the child has two full-credit (2 point) successes. The examiner discontinues presenting words after 5 consecutive failures.

The Vocabulary subtest provides information about a child's learning ability in the linguistic area. Visual and auditory remote memory (storage and retrieval) are assessed as well. The words selected are those that most children will be exposed to in our society in the normal course of growth and development. The subjects on whom the WISC-R was standardized were white, black, and other nonwhite groups in the same proportions as reported in the 1970 census. Children from socioeconomically deprived neighborhoods were also included. This was not true in the standardization of the original WISC. Therefore, WISC-R vocabulary scores are less likely than WISC scores to be artificially lowered by socioeconomic disadvantage. For the same reasons, WISC-R scores are less affected by impaired educational exposure than WISC scores. These considerations notwithstanding, one cannot completely disregard the socioeconomic and educational influences on a child's score on this subtest. This is especially the case for the extremely deprived who may receive such a limited educational exposure that they will appear less intelligent than they are. Similarly, children brought up in homes where parents are highly verbal and educated, are likely to appear more intelligent than they might really be.

The test also measures the child's ability to interchange and manipulate words, to substitute one for another, and to express himself verbally. All these qualities have generally been considered to be hallmarks of what we regard to be general intelligence (Glasser and Zimmerman, 1967). The test provides more credit for more sophisticated, abstract answers than the more simple and concrete responses. The child who defines *alphabet* as "the letters of a language" gets 2 points credit; the one who responds "you say your ABC's with it" gets 1 point credit. In the Peabody Picture Vocabulary Test (chapter 7) the child is merely asked to point to the one of four pictures that best corresponds to the word presented by the examiner. In the WISC-R Vocabulary test the child is asked to define a word, to come forth with a verbal answer that is distinctly his own. The Vocabulary subtest, then, requires more sophisticated cognition and language capability and is therefore a more sensitive test of intelligence. Although the PPVT is described as highly correlated with a number of tests of general intelligence, most examiners agree that it does not provide the kind of rich information about the quality of language development that the WISC-R Vocabulary subtest offers. There is nothing particularly creative about being able to point one's finger at a picture, but devising a good definition of a word can be a highly challenging and creative experience.

A 10-year-6-month-old boy obtains a raw score of 30 points. Referring to the conversion table for children his age we note that this corresponds to a scaled score of 10. We can conclude that this child is functioning in the normal range on this test. A 9½-year-old caucasian, middle-class girl obtains a raw score of 18. This corresponds to a scaled score of 6. Referring to the age-equivalent table we note that a raw score of 18 is the average for children aged 7 years 2 months. This girl's vocabulary score is more than 2 years below what would be expected for her age. It is highly likely that she has an intellectual impairment. Were she to have been socioeconomically disadvantaged and to have had an inadequate educational exposure, then we could not be so sure about a basic intellectual deficit. Scores on some of the other WISC-R subtests could be helpful here. Many of the other tests are more "culture free," e.g., Block Design, Object Assembly, Coding, Digit Span, Picture Completion, and Mazes. These tests are less likely to be affected by cultural and educational factors. The middle-class, caucasian child who does well on all six of these subtests and poorly on vocabulary is likely to have a language disorder. And because our concept of intelligence is so heavily weighted with the capacity to utilize certain linguistic operations, we would say that an intellectual impairment is present as well.

Information

The Information subtest is thought second only to Vocabulary as a test of general intelligence (Cohen, 1959). The test consists of 30 questions in ascending order of difficulty, from the simple ("How many ears do you have?") to the most difficult ("What does turpentine come from?") One point is given for each correct answer and the manual provides criteria for scoring.

The test assesses the child's fund of general information that is generally acquired if one experiences the usual opportunities in society. Accordingly, the same drawbacks described for the Vocabulary subtest are valid for the Information subtest. Similarly, the WISC-R attempts to reduce the disadvantage to children with cultural and educational deprivation by including such children in the population used for standardization. Nevertheless, children with severe disadvantage or unusual opportunity may appear less or more intelligent than they actually are. This drawback, however, is not great enough to deprive the Information subtest of its high rank among the WISC-R subtests as an indicator of general intelligence. The intelligent person is more curious than those of lower intellectual abilities and gathers much more information about the world around him, even when there is some environmental hindrance. The intelligent generally have broader interests and derive more from their educational exposures. The intelligent person seeks more mental stimulation and so is more likely than the less bright to acquire knowledge about the world. The test also measures visual and auditory remote memory, associative memory, as well as intellectual ambition. Lastly, there are some children who are not very bright, but who are pedantic. They acquire information in order to impress. The more minutiae they collect the smarter they think they are. Such children may do well on Information and Vocabulary, but this high level of performance is not achieved on other tests that are sensitive to general intellectual capacity such as Arithmetic and Similarities.

Similarities

Wechsler (1949, 1958) himself considered Similarities to be an excellent test of general intelligence. Although Cohen (1959) did not rate it as high as Vocabulary and Information as a measure of G, most examiners agree that the Similarities subtest assesses functions we generally consider to be specifically related to intellectual capacity. The test consists of a series of word pairs and the child is simply asked in what way the two words are alike. There are a total of 17 pairs of words, ranging from the simplest (wheel—ball) to the most difficult (salt—water). In order to avoid the kinds of potential socioeconomic and educational contaminations that one sees with the Vocabulary and Information subtests, the words selected are extremely common and likely to be familiar to even the most deprived child. For the first four word pairs the child can receive either a 0 or 1 point. For items 5 through 17, the child can receive 0, 1, or 2 points, depending upon the sophistication of the child's response. The manual provides specific criteria for scoring. For example, with regard to the question "In what way are an *apple* and *banana* alike?" the child gets 2 points if his response indicates that they are both *fruits*. He gets 1 point if he responds that they are both *sweet* or that both are *foods*.

Similarities assesses the child's ability to classify. Generally lower-order concepts receive 1 point and higher-order abstractions receive 2 points. Responses that demonstrate that the child appreciates a superficial likeness receive 1 point. Answers in which the child exhibits sophisticated and complex relationships receive 2 points. The capacity to appreciate such classificatory relationships is central to what most consider to be general intelligence. The more intelligent a person is, the more creative and perceptive his thinking, and the greater the likelihood he will be able to discern these relationships. The test also assesses remote auditory and visual memory.

The words conceptualization and abstraction are often loosely defined. I prefer to use the word conceptualization to refer to the capacity to appreciate a relationship between objects that have a physical reality. For example, a child is shown a picture of a blue hat with a badge, a pair of handcuffs, and a night stick, and asked what these things bring to mind. Most children will respond with the word "cop" or "policeman." The child is not shown a policeman, but his appreciation of the concept enables him to see the relationship between the objects he is viewing and to recognize that they are all part of the concept of policeman. The term policeman is a concept. It has a physical reality that can be seen and touched. In further discussion with the child we may elicit from him his recognition that policemen provide *protection* and are involved in a process that attempts to insure that *justice* is done. Protection and justice are abstractions. There is no way to actually visualize them in a concrete way as one can a concept. At best, we can form a concrete entity that symbolizes an abstraction; for example, a blindfolded woman holding a balance can represent justice.

The child develops the capacity for conceptualization before he can appreciate abstractions. It is much more difficult to appreciate the meaning of abstractions than to understand concepts. On the Similarities subtest, the child is generally given 1 point for concepts, and 2 points for abstractions. When the child says that an apple and a banana are both *fruits*, he is demonstrating his capacity to abstract and receives 2 points. There is no actual object called fruit. At best we can visualize various kinds of fruits. When the child says that both an apple and a banana are *sweet*, he is referring to a physical reality because sweetness can be tasted. He is also demonstrating conceptualization capacity in that there is a whole class of objects that possess this quality. Accordingly, he receives 1 point. When the child says that both an apple and a banana are *foods*, he is using an abstraction. However, for this particular question the food response is a lower order abstraction than fruit, in that fruit is one small category of foods and the response that is more specific to this question. He, therefore, gets 1 point for the *foods* response.

Goldstein (1952) observed that his adult patients with known brain damage often exhibited difficulty in forming abstractions, but did well with concrete concepts. Many children with MBD will have trouble when, for example, first learning the word *chair* they will consider the word to refer only to the particular chair that is being focused upon. They will not appreciate that the term refers to a wide category of objects with similar but not necessarily identical attributes. The impairment in the ability to abstract may interfere with MBD childrens' appreciation of jokes, riddles, proverbs, rules of games, and sportsmanship (I will discuss these impairments in greater detail in chapter 11). The examiner does well, therefore, to look carefully at the MBD child's Similarities score. It can provide valuable information about a child's intellectual level as well as alert the examiner to the presence of an important impairment commonly seen in MBD children, namely, difficulty in formulating concepts and abstractions.

Arithmetic

This WISC-R subtest has previously been mentioned in chapter 3 as a test of concentration. It is also a good test of intelligence. However, its reliance on educational experiences is so formidable that it is less valuable than Similarities as a measure of G. Although the WISC-R standardization lessens this contamination via the utilization of some deprived children in collecting the normative data, this drawback is still present for those who have been significantly disadvantaged in the socioeconomic and educational areas.

As mentioned, the child is presented with a series of 18 arithmetical questions, each of which has a time limit. Questions 1-4 are based on a picture of 12 trees that is presented to the child. Questions 5-15 are verbalized by the examiner. Similar questions are shown in Figure 10.1. The child is asked to read questions 16-18; however, if he cannot read them the examiner is instructed to do so. The child is given 1 point for each question answered correctly within the time limit. No credit is given for correct answers given after the time limit. Pencil and paper are not provided and all problems must be done mentally.

The test measures the child's ability to add, subtract, multiply, and divide—functions that are considered by most to reflect intellectual capacity. It assesses the ability to manipulate numerical abstractions and to translate word problems into numerical operations. Remote memory is involved in that the child must call upon learned mechanisms (generally from the schoolroom) for performing arithmetic procedures. In addition, recent auditory memory is involved

Figure 10.1
The Arithmetic Subtest of the WISC-R

1. Sam had three pieces of candy and Joe gave him four more. How many pieces of candy did Sam have altogether?
2. Three men divided eighteen golf balls equally among themselves. How many golf balls did each man receive?
3. If two apples cost 15¢, what will be the cost of a dozen apples?

in that the child has to recall the questions presented by the examiner and repeat them (usually subvocally) one or more times in the process of responding. Lezak (1976) holds that patients with impaired right-hemisphere functioning may do poorly on the first four questions that involve counting trees presented in a visual array. They may do better on the remaining questions that tap primarily left-hemisphere functioning. Because there is a time limit, MBD children may receive no credit for correct responses they might have obtained had they been given more time. One might want to let the child have more time to see whether he can answer the question correctly, but this should not be a reason for giving the child credit if he ultimately does so. We have learned something about the child if he can get many correct answers with more time, namely, that slowness is a characteristic of his disorder, but basic competence may not be.

My one criticism of the test is that it is really three separate tests. The first four items test arithmetical ability with regard to a visual stimulus (the picture of 12 trees) and verbal questions and instructions. The second series of questions relates only to verbal questions presented by the examiner. In the third series, the child is requested to read the questions. Here a different kind of visual processing element is being introduced. The test would have been "purer" if these visual elements had not been included. This drawback notwithstanding, I consider the test a good measure of general intelligence. It can also detect the kind of specific arithmetic difficulties sometimes seen in MBD children. One does well in such cases to administer a written arithmetic test such as the Wide Range Achievement test to ascertain more accurately the nature of the arithmetic impairment. Lastly, one must be ever aware of the fact that most of the test assesses what children learn in school. Even though the WISC-R was standardized on some educationally deprived children, children with significant deprivation in this area are likely to appear less intelligent than they really may be.

SLOSSON INTELLIGENCE TEST

Slosson (1963) has devised an intelligence test that can usually be administered in 15–20 minutes. Many of the questions are similar to those found in the Stanford-Binet Test of Intelligence (Terman and Merrill, 1960). The questions are presented in order of increasing complexity and each question is preceded by an age level (Figure 10.2) at which the normal child should be able to respond successfully to the question. There are a total of 194 questions in the complete test, but most children require only a small fraction of the questions. All questions are presented verbally. Most are responded to verbally, but eight

Figure 10.2
Sample Questions from the Slosson Intelligence Test

Years and months

＊5-0 　How many apples am I drawing now? (On back of score sheet, while child is watching, slowly draw 6 circles about ½ inch in diameter. Don't tell the child to count them, just say: "How many?"

＊5-2 　Draw a block for me like this. (Found on the back of score sheet. The square should have well formed angles and the lines should be relatively straight. It may be a bit lop-sided and may be rectangular but the longer sides should never be more than twice the length of the shorter sides. Score leniently. Give two trials if necessary and one of them must be correct.)

5-4 　Which is bigger, a cat or a mouse? (Cat)

5-6 　What number comes after 8? (Nine)

5-8 　If I cut an apple in half, how many pieces will I have? (Two)

5-10 　Must pass both.

　　a. How is a crayon different from a pencil? (One is colored and the other is black, one is big and the other is little, one is made of wax and the other of lead, etc. Any sensible answer is scored plus.)

　　b. In what way are a crayon and a pencil the same or alike? (They both write, both can make marks, etc. If a child gives another difference, say: "Yes, that's how they are different but can you tell me how they are the same or alike."

6-0 　A lemon is sour. Sugar is____. (Sweet, sweetish.)

6-2 　What is a forest made of? (Trees, woods, pine trees, woodland, a place with trees and birds and animals, etc.)

6-4 　Must pass both.

　　a. How is milk different from water? (Milk is white and water is clear, milk comes from cows and water from the tap, they taste differently, etc.)

　　b. In what way are milk and water the same or alike? (You can drink them, we need both to live, they are liquids, both are wet, etc. If a child gives another difference, say: "Yes, that's how they are different but can you tell me how they are the same or alike?")

6-6 　Must pass both.

　　a. How is a cat different from a dog? (A dog barks and a cat says meow, a cat can climb trees and a dog can't, a dog is usually bigger than a cat, etc.)

　　b. In what way are a cat and a dog the same or alike? (Both are animals, both have fur, both can run, both are alive, both have tails, both have feet, etc. If a child gives another difference, say: "Yes, that's how they are different but can you tell me how they are the same or alike?")

6-8 　A carrot is a vegetable. An apple is a____ (Fruit)

6-10 　What does brave mean? What would you do to show you were brave? (I would not be afraid, an Indian warrior, not scared, someone who does not cry when they get hurt, someone who is not "chicken," etc.)

(5-0) - (6-10)

questions require the child to draw a geometric configuration. For many of the arithmetic questions, the child is shown printed numbers that are crucial to the problem that the examiner is presenting.

The examiner begins the test with the question that is at the child's chronological age level. If the examiner suspects that the child is of lower than average intelligence, then he or she begins with lower-age-level questions. Similarly, if the examiner suspects that the child is bright, he or she begins at higher-age-level questions. The basal age is the highest in a series of 10 correct questions in succession. After the basal level has been established, the examiner presents increasingly more difficult questions until the child has failed 10 questions in succession. Scores are expressed in months (of age) with questions in the first year of life being granted 1/2 month credit; the second through fourth years, 1 month credit; the fifth through fifteenth years, 2 months credit; and the sixteenth through twenty-sixth years, 3 months credit. The examiner adds up the credit months to obtain the mental age. The mental age (in months), divided by the chronological age (in months), is multiplied by 100 to obtain the IQ.

The scores obtained on the Slosson Test of Intelligence correlate well with the Standford-Binet Form L-M (the correlation coefficients for ages 4–17 vary from .90 to .98). I have found the Slosson test useful in situations where time limitations require a quick test of the child's general level of intelligence. The test, however, does not provide the kinds of specific information about the various aspects of intelligence that one can obtain from the WISC-R. When administering the test, the examiner may get a general impression about certain areas of weakness, but the test does not provide data that allows for the quantification of the particular areas of deficit that might be contributing to a low IQ score. Therefore, when time permits (the usual situation) I use the WISC-R and get much more information.

THE PEABODY PICTURE VOCABULARY TEST

In chapter 8 I discussed the Peabody Picture Vocabulary Test (Dunn, 1965) in assessing long-term visual memory. As mentioned, the test was originally devised to serve as a method of assessing general intelligence when a limited amount of time was available. The traditional view that a child's vocabulary level is a very sensitive index of general intelligence has been upheld in studies of the Stanford-Binet (Terman and Merrill, 1960) and the WISC (Wechsler, 1949) in which the vocabulary subtest, more than any other, was found to correlate with general intelligence. The Stanford-Binet and WISC require the child to verbally define words. The PPVT requires only that the child point to the one of four pictures that is closest to the word verbalized by the examiner. In spite of these differences, Dunn (1965) considered the PPVT to be similar to the Stanford-Binet and WISC in that all assess the patient's comprehension of the spoken word. It is the mode of decoding that is different.

Dunn (1965) found a median correlation coefficient of 0.83 between Stanford-Binet (1960) mental ages and those obtained by the same children on the PPVT. For the WISC full scale IQ, the correlation was 0.61. The PPVT correlation with the WISC verbal IQ was 0.67, whereas for the WISC performance IQ the correlation coefficient was only 0.39. Similar findings were obtained with the Wechsler Adult Intelligence Scale (Wechsler, 1955), the correlation coefficients being: full scale IQ, 0.79; Verbal IQ, 0.84; and Performance IQ, 0.62. Again, the highest correlation was, not surprisingly, with the Verbal IQ.

My own experience with the PPVT has been that it gives an artificially high IQ for children whose parents are highly educated and articulate. Children from homes where the opposite has been the case may often obtain artificially low IQs on this test. Accordingly, I find it more useful as a test of long-term visual memory than one of intelligence. When time limitations interfere with my administering a WISC-R, I generally choose the Slosson over the PPVT. With very obstructionistic children, however, or those with little inclination to apply themselves, the PPVT may be the best test to utilize because so little effort is required of the child.

THE DRAW-A-PERSON TEST

The sophistication of a child's drawing can be used to assess intellectual level. The child begins to draw recognizable figures between ages three and four. Most often the most primitive figures include a head with some facial characteristics and the extremities typically emanating from the face. The head and body are generally depicted together as one circle or oval. With increasing age the child's drawing of the human figure becomes ever more complex and accurate. Goodenough (1926) published the first commonly used system for scoring the child's drawing in order to provide IQ level and age-equivalent. Harris (1963) refined Goodenough's scoring system. Because his method is the most widely used today, it is the one I will discuss in detail here.

Administering the test is quite simple. The child is simply requested to draw three pictures, a man on one page, a woman on the second, and a picture of him- or herself on the third. In each case the child is told to draw the complete figure, not just the head and shoulders. There is no time limit because the examiner wants to ascertain the child's maximum knowledge of the parts of the human body. In the Draw-A-Person projective test (Mackover, 1949; Koppitz, 1968) the child is simply told to "draw a whole person" and no request is made regarding which sex. In the projective test one gains information from the choice of sex and the characteristics of the parts included or omitted. In the Harris test one is not primarily concerned with psychodynamics; rather, one wants to be sure to obtain a full figure of each sex that is as detailed as the child is capable of executing. The male and female figures are scored separately. The scoring system is quite specific and detailed (Figure 10.3). Seventy-three items are scored on the male figure and 71 on the female. No half credit is given, each item being scored as either 1 or 0 points. No scoring of the self-portrait is done, nor are tables provided. However, one can certainly score it using the male or female tables. Harris is not clear in his manual as to why this drawing is included in the test. I, myself, find it useful for psychological purposes as well as helping me decide whether a child should earn credit for a questionable item. Specifically, if there is some question of score on one of the other two drawings, the self drawing can help me determine whether the child indeed does have the competence to draw the part well enough to earn a point score. In addition, it can provide a third maturity level and this may be useful information to have when there is a great discrepancy between the male and female scores.

Raw scores are converted to standard scores for both the male and female figures. Separate tables for each figure are provided for both boys and girls. The mean standard score is 100 with a standard deviation of 15. Accordingly, a child with a standard score of 120 is one and one-third standard deviations above normal children of his age and sex. One can also convert the standard score to a percentile rank by referring to the proper table. For example, the aforementioned 120 standard score is at the eighty-fourth percentile, the level that one would expect for a normal bell-shaped distribution curve. Koppitz (1968) has also devised a scoring system for ascertaining the intellectual maturity of a child from his or her drawings. However, one's final conclusions are expressed in more general terms than the specific numerical scores provided by the Harris charts. For each drawing one describes the number of items "expected," "common," "not unusual," or "exceptional" for the child's age. One can conclude that a child's drawing is typical of a child of a particular age, not necessarily the chronological age of the drawer. The Harris method appeals more to those like myself who feel more accurate when expressing findings in numbers. But I recognize that such numbers may be pseudoscientific and that the more general comments used by Koppitz may be more con-

Figure 10.3

Sample Scoring Criteria for the Harris Draw-A-Person Test

16. **Line of jaw indicated**	**Full Face:** Line of jaw and chin drawn across neck but not squarely across. Neck must be sufficiently wide, and chin must be so shaped that the line of the jaw forms a well-defined acute angle with the line of the neck. Score *strictly* on the simple oval face.

Credit

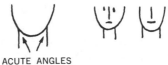

ACUTE ANGLES

No Credit

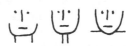

Profile: Line of jaw extends toward ear.

Credit

17. **Bridge of nose**	**Full Face:** Nose properly placed and shaped. The base of the nose must appear as well as the indication of a straight bridge. Placement of upper portion of bridge is important; must extend up to or between the eyes. Bridge must be narrower than the base.

Credit

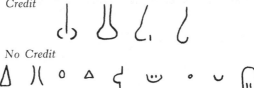

No Credit

Profile: Nose at angle with face, approximately 35–45 degrees. Separation of nose from forehead clearly shown at eye.

Credit

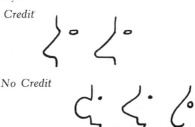

No Credit

sistent with the low degree of refinement that we really can provide for this test.

I have always felt that the Harris test does not pay enough attention to the psychological factors that can contribute to a child's performance. Resistant and inhibited children, those who perform the test in a slipshod manner, or those who passive-aggressively do not perform up to their capacity are going to obtain artificially low scores. Harris agrees that the test's value as an index of intelligence has not been firmly established. Numerous studies are described in Harris' manual which have attempted to ascertain correlations between scores on the Harris test and tests of intelligence. Correlation coefficients have ranged from the low 20s to the high 80s. He claims, however, that the test still measures intellectual level more successfully than it measures esthetic or personality factors. In other words, the conclusions that one can derive regarding a child's personality are even less validated than the conclusions that one can gain about intelligence. Owen et al. (1971) found that the Harris scores correlated more highly with WISC performance IQs than Verbal IQs. This is reasonable in that the functions being assessed with the Performance IQ subtests are similar to those involved in drawing a picture whereas the functions evaluated on the Verbal IQ section appear to be more in the linguistic category. One does well then to view the PPVT as better correlated with the WISC-R Verbal IQ and the Harris Draw-A-Picture Test as better correlated with the WISC-R Performance IQ.

11

Socialization
Problems

The socialization problems of MBD children may be among their most crippling. It is common for parents of children with minimal brain dysfunction to comment, "You know, Doctor, I somehow feel that he'll ultimately learn enough of the 3 R's to get by in life and be self-sufficient. The thing my husband and I are worried about is his problem in social relationships. He just can't make friends. He just doesn't know how to relate to people. He always seems to be saying and doing the wrong things. He's always turning people off." This parent's comment is not only a statement about her priorities regarding her goals for her child, but about the degree of help parents have been offered by professionals who deal with children with MBD. We speak often of these children's hyperactivity, poor concentration, and impulsivity (for which we can often provide useful medication) and their visual and auditory processing problems (for which we provide special education). Although we who deal with MBD children are ever aware of their socialization problems, we have not studied those problems in the same depth as their other difficulties; accordingly we have not been able to provide these children with as much help with their interpersonal difficulties as we have in other areas of their functioning. Newland (1957) points out that the social-behavior problems of these children are among their more crippling, yet they have not been given the attention they deserve. In this chapter I will delineate some of the neurological factors that contribute to the social problems of children with MBD. Such clarification is the first step toward devising techniques that might prove useful in the alleviation of these children's socialization problems. I will not discuss here the psychogenic aspects of MBD children's problems, having given some attention to such problems in previous publications (Gardner, 1968, 1970, 1971a, 1972, 1973a, 1973b, 1974a, 1974b, 1975a, 1975b, 1975c, 1975d, 1975e). In addition, a book devoted to this subject is in preparation.

Some anecdotal accounts can describe better than a more formal description the nature of the socialization problems with which these children suffer. James, an 11-year-old boy with minimal brain dysfunction, visits the home of a new acquaintance for the first time. He immediately notices the fine new house in which his friend lives and upon meeting his friend's father says to him, "Wow, what a great big beautiful house. Thus must have cost a lot of money. How much money do you make?"

Another example: I was talking with Robert, a 10-year-old boy with MBD, and his mother (who had joined us in the session). Suddenly Robert passed gas—loud and odiferous—and continued talking as if nothing had happened. I consider it part of my role as therapist to point out to my patients, as benevolently as possible, their socially alienating behavior. Others may say nothing about such behavior and merely avoid further contact, leaving the patient wondering why he is so frequently rejected by others. If the therapist does not provide such information, there may be no one who will apprise the patient of this important information. Such confrontations are best done at the time when the patient has just exhibited the undesirable behavior. At such time alienating qualities are clear in memory and less subject to the distortions of time. Furthermore, the repression that serves to remove such experiences from conscious awareness, thereby reducing embarrassment and anxiety, will have had less chance to operate if the confrontation is made early. Accordingly, I interrupted Robert: "I'm sorry to interrupt you Robert, but something just happened that I think is important for us to discuss. Do you know what I'm talking about?" Robert meekly nodded in the affirmative. I did not consider it judicious to require him to confirm verbally his indiscretion; his ashamed response to my query convinced me that we were thinking about the same thing. I then continued: "You know, that's not the kind of thing you're supposed to do in front of other people. When you feel you have to pass gas, you're supposed to either hold it back or leave the room and do it outside where there's no one around or in the bathroom. Do you understand what I've just said?" Robert nodded that he had understood and so I suggested we return to the previous subject.

In the middle of his next joint session with his mother, Robert suddenly got up and proudly announced, "Excuse me everyone. I have to go to the bathroom and pass gas! I'll be right back." He then strutted out the door. Upon his return I slowly and calmly stated, "Robert, I'm very pleased that you remembered what I said last week about passing gas in front of others, because we know you sometimes have trouble remembering things. However ... " I then went on to a discussion of the rules regarding the passing of flatus, when and where, under what circumstances, the way people feel when they smell other people's gas, etc.

The following week, in the middle of a discussion, Robert once again stood up and proudly announced, "Excuse me everyone. I've got to leave the room to do something. I'll be right back." I let this one pass, deciding that Robert had suffered enough embarrassment and concluded that the new criticisms I had would be a little too subtle for him to comprehend.

A last example. Ruth, a 6-year-old who is repeating kindergarten because of her neurologically based learning impairments, is in the supermarket shopping with her mother. Susan, a classmate who is also shopping with her mother, spies Ruth and excitedly runs toward her "Ruth. Ruth. Hi, Ruth!" Then turning to her mother, Susan exclaims, "That's Ruth. She's in my class at school." Ruth stares at Susan, quite confused. It is clear that she does not recognize Susan, even though they have been classmates for many months.

Why do these children behave as they do? What is the nature of the impairments that result in such behavior? It is my purpose here to clarify some of the causes of these three children's socialization problems and I will return to these three examples at various points in my discussion in order to provide some explanations for these as well as other children's socialization impairments.

PHYSICAL APPEARANCE

Although the abnormalities one observes in the MBD child's physical appearance are not strictly or primarily neurological, I mention them because they can play an important role in the socialization problems of these children. (In chapter 12 I will discuss these deficits in greater detail.) These children may be short and/or underweight for their age (especially those who were born prematurely). Children of atypical size for their age, expecially those who are smaller (the more likely height problem for MBD children), are often excluded and may even be ridiculed with pejorative epithets ("shorty," "shrimp," "midget," "dwarf"). A child's small stature may be one manifestation of generalized neurophysiological immaturity. Such a child will score as younger on a wide variety of measures: psychometric, physical, neurological, and developmental. With such children one is often tempted to deal with the problem by treating them totally as if they were one or more years younger. In a few cases I know of, the parents did this to the point of withholding from their children knowledge of their true ages, told them they were younger, and even enlisted the aid of neighbors, physicians, and school authorities to go along with the conspiracy. Retaining such small MBD children one or two academic years is often judicious and therapeutic. But hiding their age from them, and enlisting the aid of others to maintain the conspiracy of silence, is asking for trouble. When the child learns what has been happening, his distrust and disillusionment more than outweigh any benefits he may have derived from the scheme.

The child's head may be atypically large or small. When such deviation of head size is proportional to body size abnormalities, it may have little special significance (aside from the problems causing the general body deviation). However, when the head size is out of proportion to the body then one should consider entities such as microcephaly, premature or atypical fusion of the bones of the skull, or hydrocephalus (arrested or active). In addition to the physical problems that such disorders entail, the child may be subject to ridicule from his peers ("pinhead," "balloon head").

Other head and facial anomalies often called *stigmata* may result in the child's being taunted. Some of these children have epicanthal folds that give their eyes and eyelids an atypical appearance. Hypertelorism may result in an abnormally large separation between the eyes. The child with strabismus (not uncommon in MBD children) is almost invariably labeled "cross eyes." And ears set somewhat inferior to their normal position can give the child a comic-book-like appearance. Waldrop and Halverson (1970), Waldrop and Goering (1971), and Durfee (1974) describe these and other anomalies that can contribute to such children's social alienation.

HYPERACTIVITY

Hyperactivity is one of the most common manifestations of MBD, so much so that the term hyperactivity is often used instead of minimal brain dysfunction as the name of this group of disorders. In the classroom such children's excessive activity may irritate their teachers and interfere with their classmates' learning. Instead of sitting still in their seats, they are constantly up and about, flitting from one aimless activity to another, rarely remaining for long at one activity. Their constant activity interferes with their classmates' learning and frequently alienates them. In cooperative activities with classmates they do not stick to their tasks long enough to be a contributing member of the group. Rather, their coworkers find them much more a liability than an asset.

At home, as well, they fidget at the meal table, knock things over, rock in their seats, and give everyone at the table "knots in the stomach." They may be the last to go to sleep and the first to awaken, thereby disrupting the sleeping pattern of others in the family. In conversation with others they speak incessantly. The other party does not feel he or she is being listened to (and the speaker is right), that the MBD child is not interested in his or her opinion (correct again), and so soon wishes to part company. Lastly, there is an infectious quality to the hyperactivity that makes others tense ("He makes me nervous just to look at him") and few wish to associate themselves with those who make them feel uncomfortable.

IMPAIRED CONCENTRATION AND DISTRACTIBILITY

As discussed in chapter 3, the attentional problem of children with MBD is not simply one of attending well, but of *sustaining* attention. Accordingly, these children may exhibit little difficulty in watching television cartoons (in which the turnover of stimuli is very rapid), but may have great trouble with reading (where prolonged focusing of attention is crucial for success). In conversations they do not attend for long to what others are saying and so quickly alienate. They do not concentrate well on what parents, teachers, and other adults have to teach them about correct social behavior and so they learn less than other children about how to get along in society. In games with peers they do not concentrate enough to plan ahead and so are undesirable teammates or even opponents.

Although distractibility and poor attention are often clumped together, their differentiation is useful. The traditional view, early proposed by Strauss and Lehtinen (1947), was that the distractibility of these children is a manifestation of their figure-ground problem. Inability to differentiate foreground from background results in poor appreciation of the difference between important and unimportant stimuli. Accordingly, in conversations they do not listen more intently to the important communications, are distracted by irrelevant and extraneous stimuli, and so their comprehension of what is being told to them is significantly impaired. (The pencil dropped at the back of the classroom assumes greater importance than what the teacher is saying.) Douglas (1975) considers the distractibility of MBD children to be the result of their responding to the most compelling stimulus, regardless of its importance. Because the most salient stimulus may not be the most crucial, they often misinterpret and misunderstand (e.g., the picture in the book is more important than the text).

Many, such as Douglas (1974b) and Cantwell (1977), hold that the hyperactivity of MBD children may not be a primary manifestation at all, but secondary to the impairment in sustaining attention. They consider hyperactive children to be no more active than normals regarding the *quantity* of their activity. It is the *quality* of their activity that is different. They cannot sustain attention on one activity, flit from goal to goal, and so *appear* to be more active. When they are able to attend better they become less hyperactive.

Strong support for this theory comes from drug research. One need not attribute a "paradoxical effect" to the psychostimulants to explain their capacity to reduce hyperactivity. By improving attention (just as they do in normals) they enable MBD children to concentrate longer on a stimulus, to stick with a goal longer, and so the shifting and aimless quality to their activity is reduced. Recently Rapoport (1978) has demonstrated that normal children responded to a single dose of dextroamphetamine with decreased motor activity and reaction time, and improved performance on cognitive tests, thereby lending support to the thesis that there is nothing paradoxical about MBD children's reaction to psychostimulant medication. As mentioned in chapter 2, I believe that this explanation is true for some of these children, especially those who respond to psychostimulant medication. However, there are others, those who are "driven from within" and are not improved by psychostimulant medication, whose hyperacitivty is not related to an attentional deficit.

Conners (1976) goes further and claims that not only hyperactivity but most, if not all, of the impairments that MBD children exhibit on the WISC-R are not the result of visual-motor, visual-perceptual, and cognitive problems, but secondary to the inability to sustain attention. MBD children do poorly on the Arithmetic subtest because they do not concentrate on the computations, on Digit Span because they do not attend well to the examiner's recitation of the numbers, on Block Design because they do not look long enough at the model that they are copying, on Mazes because they do not focus fully on each of the alternative paths, on Coding because they do not focus attention on the symbols, etc. Although I do not go as far as Connors in attributing so much to the attentional problem, I believe his emphasis has merit. I believe that independent difficulties related to symbolization capacity (language), various types of auditory and visual processing problems, aphasias and apraxias, cognitive impairments, and other factors described in this book are often operative. Their emphasis is useful, however, and has important implications for these children's socialization problems. Because of the mounting evidence that the primary action of the psychostimulants in helping MBD children is that of improving attention (Douglas, 1972; Conners, 1974; Dykman et al., 1974; Fish, 1975; Ross and Ross, 1976), and because impaired attention is so important a factor in these children's learning correct socialization, their work is crucial with regard to the treatment of the socialization problems of MBD children.

IMPULSIVITY

Impulsivity is one of the more common manifestations of MBD and can play a significant role in the socialization difficulties of children with this disorder. They blurt out what is on their minds, without censoring between thought and verbalization (like James who asked his new friend's father how much he earned). In conversations they interrupt frequently, hardly giving the other person a chance "to get a word in edgewise." They do not wait their turns in play with friends and are so compelled "to get what they want when they want it" that they quickly alienate their peers who resent their rights being so ignored. Their impulsivity causes them to be "bossy" with friends, who soon withdraw because they resent being so ordered around. When they lose a game of checkers, for example, they may pick up the board and throw everything at the opponent. In the classroom they have great difficulty holding up their hands while waiting to be called upon by the teacher. Rather, they blurt out the answer, irritating teachers and classmates. They cannot restrain themselves from striking out at others, at an age when their peers have learned the judiciousness of such self-control. Further alienating is the inability to restrain aggressive outbursts (not that normal children are so characteristically restraining, just that these children are less so). And when picked upon by bullies they cannot seem to hold back crying and primitive outbursts, even though they may appreciate that such reactions only encourage their tormentors even more. Accordingly, they are singled out by bullies as especially vulnerable targets, exhibit just the kinds of responses their taunters crave, and encourage, thereby, even further scapegoating.

One manifestation of impulsivity is the desire for the quick, easy solution. This contributes to lying and stealing, which are often attempts to take the path of least resistance out of a difficult situation. Once their duplicity becomes known to peers (almost inevitably the case) they suffer the scorn and rejection that is so often the lot of those who engage in such behavior. Kinsbourne (1975) describes well how the impulsivity problem of these children results in their rejection: "They do not play the courtship game of approach, look, hesitate, gather signals and cues. They crash in and are rejected from the group just as fast."

IMPAIRMENTS IN AUDITORY PROCESSING

As mentioned in chapter 7, the term *auditory processing* covers a number of functions related to the brain's utilization of auditory stimuli. These include localization and identification of the sound source; discrimination among different sounds; differentiation between significant and insignificant auditory stimuli; understanding the meaning of sounds; reproduction of pitch, rhythm, and melody; and combining speech sounds into words (Chalfant and Scheffelin, 1969).

Auditory discrimination refers to the process by which the individual differentiates between auditory stimuli. The problem is not one of auditory acuity since the audiometric examination may be normal. Rather, the patient has trouble discriminating between two auditory stimuli, especially when they are similar. It is rare, for example, that the MBD child has difficulty differentiating between such disparate sounds as a bell and a car horn. When sounds resemble one another, however, the MBD child may have particular difficulty discriminating between them, for example, words like *book* and *brook, moon* and *noon, soon* and *spoon*, etc. The child who does not hear the spoken word accurately is going to miss important verbal communications and thereby be compromised in social interaction. If the child does not differentiate properly between the subtle but nevertheless different speech intonations, he will miss important auditory cues and may misconstrue entirely many spoken communications.

The child with auditory distractibility tends to focus attention on auditory stimuli that may not be as important as those to which he or she had originally been attending. As mentioned, this problem should be differentiated from an impairment in concentration in which the child primarily has difficulty in *sustaining* focus on auditory stimuli. When the teacher speaks, the MBD child shifts attention to the birds outside, whose chirps attract him but no one else. When a camp counselor is explaining the rules of a game the MBD child is compelled to attend to each new sound emanating from the playing field. When children do not listen to those who speak to them, conversation becomes difficult if not impossible. Not listening, they do not learn those things that are so vital to learn if one is to adapt socially.

MBD children may have defects in the capacity to appreciate the meaning of auditory stimuli. They have difficulty matching an auditory stimulus with the specific meaning that social convention has ascribed to it. There is nothing intrinsic to the ring of a classroom bell that means *recess,* nor in the schoolyard teacher's whistle that means *give me your attention.* The child who has trouble appreciating the relationships between such stimuli and their meanings will have difficulty functioning in society. Probably the area in which such a deficiency will produce the greatest difficulty is in spoken language. If one cannot link the spoken word with the meaning assigned to it by society, one is going to have great difficulty relating properly to others. If one does not understand the significance of the subtle vocal intonations and stresses that add to the meaning of the spoken word, one is going to be significantly impaired in one's social relationships (Brutten et al., 1973). If one cannot understand the emotional qualities so communicated by spoken words, one is going to be impaired in developing sympathy and empathy for others (Kronick, 1973).

In learning to read, the child is usually exposed simultaneously to the visual symbol of an entity (the written word that denotes the entity) and the auditory symbol (the spoken word that represents it). The two processes complement and reinforce one another in the process of learning to read. Accordingly, the child with such an audio-visual integration deficit will generally have trouble learning to read and will be deprived thereby of many of the socialization benefits to be derived from the reading skill. Similarly, such children may have trouble using the telephone where they are deprived of the visual cues that might have served to help them compensate for their auditory deficit. They therefore shy away from, and may even refuse, use of the telephone, thereby depriving themselves of this powerful instrument of communication and socialization.

Auditory memory deficit refers to the impairment in storing and retrieving auditory stimuli. We learn much about the world around us from what parents, teachers, and other significant individuals say to us. Especially in the younger years, before we have learned to read, is this source of information particularly important. Sometimes an auditory memory problem may be worsened by language becoming negatively conditioned. Because so much of what is told to MBD children relates to criticism, they may automatically "tune out" most verbalizations (Siegel, 1974). Receiving less auditory input, there is less to remember. If we do not recall well the lessons to be learned from legends, myths, and Bible stories, we will be less equipped to deal with life's problems.

Children who do not remember well the advice and admonitions of their parents are less likely to cope outside their homes.

Sometimes auditory sequential memory is impaired so that the child is not able to remember a sequence of auditory stimuli, but may be able to recall each item in the sequence. This deficiency interferes with such children's heeding a series of instructions or directions. When Mother says, "When supper is over I want you to take out the garbage and then go up to your room and do your homework. When that's done, then you can watch TV," these children are not likely to recall the requests in the correct order. When the coach describes a series of football plays, they may become hopelessly confused.

Deficient auditory memory causes impairment in auditory blending in which the child has trouble recognizing a word when it is broken down into its phonetic components when presented verbally. It appears that the pattern or model against which the new form (in this case, words broken down into their phonetic components) is compared is either not well stored, or not readily available for comparison and identification. When children are taught to read by the phonetic process, in which words are broken down into their phonetic components (as opposed to the "Look-Say" method in which children are taught to recognize words as whole units), the teacher is likely to associate the written phonemes with their auditory counterparts in order to facilitate the learning process. Children with a problem in auditory blending are deprived of this contribution to their learning to read and are likely to be deprived thereby of the socialization benefits enjoyed by those who read more adequately.

Deficient auditory closure capacity is probably also related to auditory memory impairment. If a phonetic component is dropped from a word, the MBD child may have much more trouble identifying the word from what remains than does the normal child. We all develop the capacity to understand messages when segments are either not transmitted or not received. We somehow surmise the meaning from the other bits of information that get through to us. MBD children who have problems in this area probably have auditory memory problems that make the model words unavailable for comparison. They therefore understand less of what is said to them and suffer socially because of the interpersonal difficulties that such an impairment produces.

Clinically, it may often be difficult to separate impaired retrieval from impaired storage of information. When a child, for example, cannot repeat verbally an auditory message that one is convinced has been heard, one may not be able to determine with certainty whether the message didn't "stick" for long (stored) or whether the message is stored but there is trouble "finding" (retrieving) and then verbalizing it. When the problem is definitely one of retention the term auditory memory impairment is warranted. When the difficulty is one of retrieving the word from storage, *aphasia* is then the correct term to apply. Patients with retrieval problems are slow in naming a series of pictures, letters, and numbers presented to them (Denckla and Rudel, 1974), are slow thinking, slow acting, and thereby far less effective than normals in social situations. If, however, a peripheral (that is, not in the brain) articulatory defect is present, the child may be unable to utter what has been adequately stored and retrieved. Then, differentiation between storage and retrieval problems may become even more difficult.

When auditory memory is impaired one does not learn well from experience, because the auditory components of the experience (what the various people said, for example) are not well retained. And those who do not learn from their experiences are likely to repeat them—a severe hindrance in the socialization process.

A discussion of auditory processing problems would not be complete without a discussion of *amusia*, the impairment in discrimination and recall of musical pitch, loudness, rhythm, timbre, and tone (usually the result of right-hemisphere damage [Heilman et al., 1975]). Although usually considered uncommon, it may be more common than is generally appreciated. Because it is not often considered in the battery of diagnostic tests given to MBD children, we may be missing many cases. Recognition of popular music is important in the social involvements and acceptability of most teenagers. The child who has trouble differentiating one song from another, who cannot recall lyrics and music, and who cannot sing along with the rest is likely to be less acceptable to many teenage groups.

IMPAIRMENTS IN VISUAL PROCESSING

The term *visual processing* is a rubric under which are subsumed a number of functions related to the ways in which the brain receives, scans, identifies, integrates, classifies, and utilizes visual information (Chalfant and Scheffelin, 1969).

Visual discrimination refers to the process by which the individual differentiates one visual stimulus from another. A color-blind person has a problem in visual discrimination in that he or she may not be able to differentiate between hues that others may readily distinguish. Orton (1937) noted that children with neurological learning disabilities may have trouble differentiating between letters that are reversals of one another. This deficiency may be one of the contributing factors (but certainly not the total cause) of the reading disability so common to these children. Reading less efficiently, they learn less about how to cope in the world and acquire less of a repertoire of the knowledge so vital to have if one is to relate successfully with others. Children with MBD may have trouble discriminating distances. So they stand too close to or too far away from those with whom they are speaking. The same problem may contribute to their speaking too softly or loudly as they misjudge the distance between themselves and their listeners (Kronick, 1973).

Differentiating between the faces of those whom we encounter is a capacity that most take for granted; it must, however, be learned. When we look at a cage of monkeys in a zoo we may have trouble differentiating one monkey's face from another; yet the monkeys probably don't have any trouble. (Perhaps the monkeys peering out on us may view us as indistinguishable and wonder how we differentiate ourselves from one another.) Infants must gradually learn to make such differentiations among the people they encounter. The one-year-old may call many men "Da Da," clumping together as identical all those who bear even the remotest resemblance to his or her father. The child with MBD takes longer to learn such facial discriminations. The deficiency in which one has difficulty differentiating among familiar faces is sometimes referred to as *prosopagnosia* or *facial agnosia* (Benton and Van Allen, 1972). Some investigators believe that this deficiency is likely to occur when there has been right-hemisphere damage (Benson and Geschwind, 1968; Rudel et al., 1974), especially in the right-tempoparietal region (Critchley, 1953). Perhaps Ruth, the 6-year-old kindergartner who did not recognize her classmate Susan, was suffering with such a deficit in visual discrimination. Some children with MBD have difficulty differentiating between different facial expressions such as sadness, happiness, anger, politeness, impoliteness, etc. (Johnson and Myklebust, 1967). When shown pictures of different facial expressions, they cannot differentiate among them or correctly identify the emotion being depicted. It is not difficult to appreciate how such a deficiency could significantly impair one's interpersonal relationships. Not only could such an inadequacy produce communication difficulties between the MBD child and others, but could impair significantly the child's capacity to develop intimate involvements with others. If one cannot ascertain what other people are feeling, one cannot possibly be sympathetic or empathetic to their situation, which is a capacity vital to the development of intimate relationships.

Visual distractibility refers to an impairment in which the child's capacity to focus on the most important stimulus is deficient because attention is too readily shifted to competing stimuli of less significance. When doing the traditional hidden-picture puzzle game, in which the child tries to find various figures camouflaged in a complex scene, visual distractibility interferes with the child's performance. More important, when reading, the child's eyes tend to wander away from the line being read to other words on the page. Clearly, under such circumstances, speed and comprehension are impaired, the knowledge gained from reading is reduced, and the socialization benefits of reading are compromised. In addition, the capacity to learn from other visual experiences in life is reduced, further impairing the socialization process.

MBD children often suffer impairment in the capacity to ascribe meaning to a visual sensation. The MBD child may readily be able to identify red and green and easily differentiate these from other colors. However, he or she may have trouble learning that a red light means *stop* and a green light means *go*. There is nothing intrinsic to these colors to suggest that they should mean *stop* and *go*. Social convention adds special meanings to these sensations. The linkage between the color and its meaning may seem obvious and easily learned, but this is not the case for children with MBD. They are puzzled by such associations and do not readily make them. This impairment can truly be crippling. The aforementioned children who do not readily distinguish between different facial expressions certainly have their difficulties. In the visual impairment discussed here the child may recognize the difference between facial expressions, but may not be able to appreciate that the sad facial expression *means* that the person is feeling sadness inside. This inability to make the proper associations between facial expressions and their meanings significantly impairs the MBD child's socialization capacity (Critchley, 1970).

This problem is related to one of the central impairments of the MBD child: the difficulty in linking a visual stimulus with its culturally determined symbol. Gestures and body position lose their capacity to provide the extra messages that not only enrich communication, but may be vital to accurate interpersonal understanding (Brutten et al., 1973). Playing games such as *charades* becomes almost impossible, because verbal clues are absent, clues that help such children (if they do not, in addition, have auditory problems) understand the game's multiple symbolic gestures. Difficulty in appreciating the significance of clothing styles (authority, rebellion, conformity), position in space (head of table vs. side, dais vs. audience seat), and hair style (youth vs. age) interferes with adequate understanding of other people's functioning.

This capacity is central to the phenomenon of what we refer to as *language*. A *knife* is a concrete object that may be recognized visually as such by the MBD child and easily differentiated from a fork, for example. The word knife, however, and the letters k - n - i - f - e that are used to refer to the object, are not intrinsically a part of the object nor is there anything particular about these five letters that should warrant their being used to refer to the object knife. The Germans do quite well with the letters M - e - s - s - e - r and the French with c - o - u - t - e - a - u. Convention dictates the utilization of these particular letters for this purpose for social convenience, to enhance communication, and to prevent the confusion that would result if such labels were not employed. The MBD child may have significant difficulty making these connections. When such a child sees the letters k - n - i - f - e he has trouble associating them with the object that they signify. When viewing these letters, he does not readily envision a knife. This is clearly a severe handicap in understanding written language and a significant determinant in enjoying the social benefits to be derived from being able to read.

The term visual memory refers to the capacity to store and retrieve visual stimuli. Often differentiation is made between short-term and long-term visual memory but, as mentioned, the two impairments represent extremes on a continuum. Children with impairments in short-term visual memory may have difficulty recalling direction signs, paragraphs read only a few seconds previously, and even events that were observed only a few minutes earlier. Impairments in long-term visual memory may also be present. Obviously, if there is a deficiency in short-term visual memory there is going to be less material available for long-term retention. When long-term memory is impaired, things that were retained for a short time are not recalled over longer periods. A related impairment involves visual sequential memory—the child has difficulty recalling visual stimuli in proper sequence.

In short, things don't seem to "stick" in these children's minds as well as and as long as they do in normal children. De Hirsch (1975) refers to this impairment as the "fluidity" problem that these children have. She compares the process of impressing material into the memories of these children with writing in the sand with a stick. Their impressions are transient, blown away as easily as letters in the sand by passing breezes. If one does not remember what one sees, one is not likely to learn from observed experiences (one's own as well as those observed to have occurred to others). This is certainly one of the reasons why these children do not profit from their mistakes. And the ability to socialize properly cannot but be impaired if one does not profit well from one's errors, transgressions, faux pas, etc.

IMPAIRMENTS IN TACTILE PROCESSING

Tactile processing refers to those functions by which the brain makes use of sensory stimuli obtained through certain cutaneous sensory endings. The kinds of information so processed include geometric information concerning size, shape, area, etc.; texture; consistency such as hard-soft, resilient, viscous; pain; temperature; and pressure (Chalfant and Scheffelin, 1969). Impairments in tactile processing are not commonly described in children with MBD. It is rare for the report of the pediatric neurologist to describe an abnormal peripheral sensory examination. Although this may in part be the result of an inadequate examination (related to such children's typical lack of reliability and cooperation in such examination), it is not often that such modalities as pain, temperature, light touch, two-point discrimination, and recognition are impaired in these children.

Ross and Ross (1976) hold that these children usually have intact processing for the *proximal* sensory modalities (touch, taste, and smell), that is, those sensory modalities that involve close contact between the body, sensory receptor sites, and close external stimuli. It is the *distal* modalities (vision and hearing), in which there is some distance between the body receptor sites and the external stimuli, that one usually sees difficulty. The infant utilizes primarily proximal receptors in learning about the world (unknown objects are smelled, fondled, and mouthed). As the infant grows older, the distal receptors are more frequently utilized to learn about the world (the child reads and listens to what others say). The infant is similar to lower animals in his preference for the proximal receptors. Perhaps the greater prevalence of auditory and visual processing problems in children with MBD relates to the fact that the elaboration of these modalities (as far as their more sophisticated cognitive and integrative aspects are concerned) is a relatively late evolutionary development and that MBD children are not as advanced as normals in their acquisition of these more elaborate mechanisms. Ross and Ross (1976) raise the possibility that these children do more touching in their interpersonal relationships than normal children in an attempt to compensate for their auditory and visual deficits. The extra touching alienates many people, especially in our culture, which tends to frown on such expression of familiarity.

IMPAIRMENTS IN INTERSENSORY INTEGRATION

In chapter 7 I discussed the theory that the evolutionary development from lower to higher animals is not characterized by an increase in the number of sensory modalities. Rather, the greater complexity and sophistication of the higher forms is the result of their greater *integration* of the basic sensory modalities.

Heilman et al. (1975) describe how patients with right-hemisphere lesions have great difficulty selecting that picture (from among a series presented) whose facial expression corresponds to a tape recorded sentence that expresses an emotion. (Patients with left-hemisphere lesions perform the function without difficulty.) They describe this impairment as an *affective agnosia* and state that the lesion in such cases is to be found in the nondominant temporoparietal region. They suggest that the problem may result from an inability to accurately discriminate the elements of pitch, tempo, inflection, and stress that provide information about the affective components of a verbal communication. Because their studies involve correlating an auditory stimulus (a tape-recorded voice) with a visual (a picture depicting a corresponding mood) one must consider the possibility that an impairment in sensory integration is contributing to these patients' disability.

Integrative impairments are certainly suggested by many other difficulties that MBD patients have—and many of these directly relate to their socialization problems. Appreciating the relationship between the spoken word and associated gestures and body movements requires the ability to combine auditory and visual stimuli into a meaningful composite. Eye-hand coordination requires (among other things) an integration of visual stimuli with information provided by proprioceptive fibers in the hand. Imitating a gesture (so that it can become part of one's own repertory) also requires such sensory integration. In fact, there are so many functions that involve such integration (learning to write words that the teacher recites, dancing to music, speaking, playing most games, carrying on a conversation, dressing, etc.) that such impairments, if extensive, can be especially crippling and may interfere significantly with one's functioning in society.

Related to problems in integration is the problem of organization. And organizational problems relate to problems of memory, especially sequential memory. Organizing a constellation of stimuli, differentiating among the important ones, and appreciating the relationship between them is especially difficult for many MBD children. In conversation one must be able to put together what is being spoken with facial expression, gesture, and body movement if one is to fully understand the speaker. The young man who attends only to the "no, no" coming from his girlfriend's lips and does not integrate this message with the "yes, yes in her eyes" and the "yes, yes" communicated by her verbal intonations will obviously not derive as much from this social situation as others who are more capable of organizing and integrating these various sensory stimuli.

PERSEVERATION

The term perseveration refers to the pattern of repetitious behavior often seen in children with neurological impairment. The child repeats the same message or engages in the same behavioral pattern over and over again, long after it seems to have served its purpose and in spite of the social alienation that such repetitions cause. These children appear to "get hooked" and seem unable to "unhook" themselves even though those around them repeatedly express their irritation with the seemingly endless repetitions. They just don't seem to know when to stop and do not heed readily those who encourage cessation. The impulsivity problem probably contributes to such repetitions as does psychogenic factors, in that one may often see some purpose served by the reiteration.

Steve, a 7-year-old boy with MBD spoke so often about Underdog, a character on one of his favorite TV programs, that he soon was given this name by classmates and friends. Although his identification with the underdog was facilitated by the reality of his situation (the psychogenic component), his inability to reduce his perseveration resulted in the stigma that he suffered from the epithet. Johnson and Myklebust (1967) describe a 13-year-old boy who was told to rise when an adult entered the room. He learned the lesson too well and indiscriminately applied it to all situations, no matter how inappropriate was his rising. A 10-year-old boy is preoccupied with sharks (the fantasy serves as an outlet for pent-up hostility). He doesn't seem to hear when parents tell him that he is "turning people off" with his incessant ramblings about the various habits of his favorite creature. Bob tells a joke, gets a laugh, and keeps telling the same joke over and over, ever trying to extract "more mileage" out of it. When playing with others these children don't seem to know when to stop. They continue with horseplay after others have indicated their wish to discontinue such play, and so they quickly become irritating. They remain goofy and silly after others have had their fill of such antics and wish to switch to more serious activities. It all ends with peers no longer wishing to play with them and adults wishing to remove themselves as soon as possible.

INTELLECTUAL DEFICITS

Many professionals claim that the MBD child is of average intelligence. I believe that many who claim this do not really believe what they profess, but make the statement in order to provide parents with reassurance that their child is basically "normal." The statement, of course, is not consistent with the generally accepted observation that these children do poorly on many of the WISC-R subtests (in fact, such poor performance may have been the most conclusive evidence for making the diagnosis). In my experience the average child in whom the MBD diagnosis is definitely warranted is generally in the 85 to 95 range on the WISC-R. Some claim that these children are basically of normal intelligence, but that tests such as the WISC-R do not measure basic intelligence because they focus so much on what is learned in the classroom. It behooves those who hold such a view to define more accurately what this basic intelligence is and how one can best measure it. Piaget holds that a central element in intelligence is the ability to adapt to the environment, especially the novel environment (Flavell, 1961). This seems like a reasonable criterion. If one uses it with children with MBD they are not likely to do well. They have particular difficulty in the novel situation. I think, then, that it is reasonable to conclude that these children are generally of lower intelligence than normals (this does not preclude some children with very high WISC-R IQs in whom the diagnosis is still warranted) and such deficiency contributes to their socialzation impairments. The intellectual deficit becomes an even greater liability for children attending schools where the majority of their classmates have above-average IQs.

The problem in conceptualization and abstraction that contributes to MBD children's poor performance on IQ tests can impair them significantly in social situations. They do not understand well the rules of games and concepts like sportsmanship. They have trouble keeping score in games. They do not get jokes and riddles, so commonly enjoyed by children. They may feign understanding of humor in order to gain social acceptance. But their failure to laugh at the appropriate times quickly reveals their bluff to others and results in further alienation. Their humorlessness also lessens their capacity for general enjoyment in life and can contribute to depression.

When a child is first told what a *chair* is, he or she may first learn that a particular chair in his or her room is so labeled. The child quickly learns that the one in his or her room is not the only object so designated, but all other objects that have basically similar, but not necessarily identical, characteristics are given the same name. The MBD child may have trouble with such generalizations and only use the word *chair* to refer to the one in his or her room. Such children do not appreciate well the nonconcrete, that is, those concepts that cannot be easily visualized. Accordingly, the meanings of abstractions such as *danger, fairness, justice, silence,* and *freedom* may completely escape them.

Such deficiencies in abstract and conceptualized thinking impair MBD children in learning more sophisticated modes of social interaction. They often have difficulty appreciating the appropriate time and place for various types of social behavior. They have trouble learning the situations in which profanity is acceptable and when and where it is not. They may speak of elimination at the meal table and crack jokes at funerals. They may attempt to compensate for their deficiencies by boasting, and the more they are rejected for their bragging the more they may resort to the maneuver. They seem not to realize that others appreciate that they are either grossly exaggerating or fabricating. They may not know when it is appropriate to touch another person and when not to. In the teens they make sexual advances at improper times or do not respect the privacy and intimacy of such experiences. Although teenage boys are not famous for their discretion and muteness about revealing their sexual experiences to others, MBD boys are even less so. One 15-year-old boy with MBD came to school one morning and loudly announced to his teacher that on the previous night he had "felt up" a classmate. The boast was not only heard by those near the teacher, but the girl herself. Problems in right-left differentiation may interfere with a teenager's learning to drive a car, depriving the youngster thereby of this important social asset. Lastly, in their craving to gain attention and affection they may try too hard and thereby suffer even greater rejection and social alienation. Again, they seem not to know how far to go, and where and when to stop.

Learning time concepts may be particularly difficult for children with MBD. They learn late the days of the week, months of the year, and the seasons. They may have particular difficulties with time sequences in these areas, so they may not know the correct order of the days, months, or seasons. They may have particular difficulty projecting themselves into the future. This deficiency may result in severe social difficulties as they do not appreciate well the future consequences of their actions. They are very much *here and now* people, with little concern for the future effects of their actions on both themselves and others. They may have little sense of the passage of time, so are often late for appointments. They do not seem to have well developed internal clocks that most utilize. They do not have the sophistication to appreciate when it is important to be precise (for a job interview, for example) and when one can be a little late without social consequences (for example, home social engagements).

Their intellectual impairments interfere with their academic as well as their social learning. (In fact, we would do well to use the term *learning disability* to refer to both types of impairment.) They do poorly academically and other children recognize this. Epithets such as "retard" or "ment" may be applied by their classmates. Those in special classes may be able to avoid such taunts while in the classroom, but in the hallways and schoolyard they enjoy no such protection.

MOTOR IMPAIRMENTS

The child with MBD may exhibit development lags that result in his not being able to perform as well as peers in various physical activities. He may find himself then faced with the choice of playing either alone or with younger children with whom he may be able to keep up. Problems in gross motor coordination may interfere with such a child's ability to ride a bicycle, throw a ball, swim, and run. He appears clumsy and is frequently so referred to by peers. Problems in fine motor coordination may result in poor handwriting and drawing, ball catching, and playing of musical instruments. Impairment in the ability to maintain muscular contraction well, often referred to as motor impersistence, may interfere with his capacity to run, stand, and sustain a hand grip over a period of time. He may thereby do poorly in games such as Indian leg wrestling, tug of war, and in contests of who can stand on one leg longer. MBD children with dyspraxias may have no muscular or coordination defect. Yet they cannot execute muscular activity adequately because their bodies do not seem to be able to follow what their minds want them to do. In the ideokinetic dyspraxias, children have trouble performing a single act like swinging a baseball bat. In the ideational dyspraxias children have difficulty performing a sequence of movements such as are necessary in swimming, playing football, and writing. In the constructional dyspraxias children have difficulty building things like models. Mention has been made previously of these children's inability to appreciate the subtle meaning of gestures. Dyspraxic children may be able to understand the meaning of a gesture well, but they may not be able to imitate it. Consequently it becomes lost to their communicative repertoire.

IMPAIRMENT IN THE ABILITY
TO PROJECT ONESELF
INTO ANOTHER PERSON'S SITUATION

This capacity is central to what we refer to as intimacy, empathy, and sympathy. Without this capacity one is seriously impaired in developing meaningful relationships. This is what the ancient Golden Rule ("Do unto others as you would have them do unto you") is all about. When one is incapable of appreciating what others want and need, of surmising what others are thinking and feeling, one is not going to have many friends. Deficiency in this area probably has both neurological and psychological components.

Piaget and Inhelder (1948), in an ingenious study, described the normal development of children's capacity to view a situation from a point outside of themselves. The child is shown a model scene of three mountains, each of which is different from the others. They are of different heights and colors and have other distinguishing characteristics (one has a house, another a red cross on the top, and the third an icecap). The mountains are set on a board one meter square and the child is asked to construct from shaped cardboard the view that would be seen by a 2–3 cm. figurine from four different positions, namely, the middle point on each of the four edges of the board. In another phase of the study the child is shown 10 pictures and asked to select those that correspond to the views the man would have from various positions. Piaget found that up to about 8 years of age the child considers the figurine to have the same view that he has in reality, regardless of where the figurine is set. Ages 8 to 9 represent a transition stage for the development of the capacity to make correct discriminations. After 9, and especially by 10, children are able to ascertain the scene visualized from the various points of view of the figurine. Benton (1968), in his studies of the development of right-left discrimination, has found that children are usually able to point out various parts of their own body ("Touch your left eye with your right hand") by age 9. However, the capacity to ascertain right and left on another person ("Point to my right eye") does not appear until 11 and the ability to consider simultaneously one's own and an outsider's orientation ("Put your right hand on my left ear) does not occur until 12. Although these studies pertain to a concrete capacity (Piaget's is part of a study of geometric perspective), it is reasonable to consider the findings relevant to the child's capacity to appreciate the more complex phenomenon of another person's thoughts and feelings. It may be that the children with MBD are defective in their ability to view a situation from another person's vantage point because of lags in the development of cerebral centers involved in this capacity. However, psychological factors related to immaturity and egocentricity are probably also operative.

Robert, the boy who passed gas during our session, clearly had a problem in appreciating how alienating this practice is to others. These children do not seem to appreciate others' reactions to their picking their noses, drooling, scratching their genitalia, and interrupting. The inability to project oneself into another's situation may play a role in the cruelty to animals often seen in MBD children (Gardner, 1973b).

Parents will often complain that the MBD child hurts his dog unmercifully, to the point where the animal flees the child whenever possible.
Peers cannot but be alienated by such insensitivity, especially because
animals play such an important role in the lives of many children. MBD
children may not feel the need to say anything when they don't wish to
answer a question. They may sit silently, without any change in facial
expression, not recognizing that the questioner is waiting for a response.
They do not feel the need to compliment others because they fail to
appreciate how good such statements make the other person feel. When
they hit other children they are surprised that the recipient of their
blows reacts with anger and cannot understand why those who observe
such bullying are also alienated (Gardner, 1975a). Goldstein (1952), in
his studies of adults with brain damage, describes how these patients
do not appear to understand situations not directly related to themselves. When they hear a story about events occurring to someone
else, and the story is not at all relevant to themselves, they neither
understand nor show interest in the story. When, however, the story is
about a person whose situation is very similar to their own, such patients may be able to understand. Such egocentricity cannot but interfere with one's capacity for meaningful involvements with others and
it is likely that children with MBD suffer similarly.

EMOTIONAL REACTIONS

All emotions, like all thoughts, basically have a neurological substrate.
However, the psychogenic component in emotional reactions is formidable. I will not focus here on these psychological factors; rather, I will
confine myself to the neurological. The latter contribute to emotional
expression and play an important role in the way the individual will
react to stimuli that are likely to induce emotional responses. The neurological factors probably determine the intensity of emotional reactions
and may even play a role in determining the quality of the emotional
response as well.

Many of the findings of Goldstein (1952), who studied adults with
brain damage, may be applicable to MBD children as well. Goldstein
was struck by the fact that many of his patients did not respond emotionally to stimuli that would normally evoke strong affective responses
in others. In many patients he considered this to be related to the fact
that the patient did not fully understand the nature of the provoking
stimulus. The cognitive defect was the primary problem, and the emotional flattening was secondary to this neurological deficit. Sometimes
the patient only understood part of the situation that would tend to

evoke emotional reactions. The patient did not have enough information to warrant an emotional reaction, or he or she may have seen the situation concretely without appreciation of the abstract aspects vital to the emotional response. Many of Goldstein's patients needed a real rather than an imagined stimulus in order to respond emotionally. For example, when loved ones were out of sight there was little, if any, affection displayed; but when such individuals appeared, strong loving feelings could be expressed. Perhaps an impairment in visual memory or in the capacity to form visual imagery might have been present in these patients.

Goldstein also remarked on the emotional liability so often observed in patients with brain damage. He considered this to be the result of damage to higher inhibitory centers. At such times Goldstein's patients exhibited what he referred to as a "catastrophic reaction" in which the patient would cry pathetically or exhibit angry outbursts with little or no ostensible provocation. On investigation, however, Goldstein concluded that such outbursts were related to the patients' awareness of their deficits and the frustration they felt over their helplessness to deal with life's challenges with their previous efficiency. The most minor deficiencies become almost intolerable to accept. All of these reactions can be seen in children with neurological impairment and it is not difficult to imagine how each can be a social detriment.

Wender (1971) describes an anhedonia in these children that he considers to have a neurological basis, and he believes that this is one of the central problems of children with MBD. One manifestation of the anhedonia is hyporeactivity to painful stimuli. These children often deal with painful accidents with impunity and punishment (even physical) does not seem to change their behavior. In addition, they exhibit a general incapacity to experience pleasurable responses and an absence of grateful feelings for what is given to him. Wender considers the anhedonia to be related to a neurophysiological impairment in responding to both positive and negative reinforcement. This contributes to their poor response to punishment and discipline and plays a role in their antisocial behavior and delinquency problems. Douglas (1975) does not consider these children necessarily hyporesponsive to reinforcement. She has found that they can be conditioned as well as normals when reinforcement is provided after every desired response. When the reinforcement is noncontingent, that is, partial or aperiodic, they become less responsive to conditioning techniques. The clinical implications of her findings suggest that these children are best conditioned when there are opportunities to reward them after every desired response. Wender also describes the hyperreactivity and lability, the greater capacity to swing either up or down, so often seen in these children (the type sometimes referred to as "merry monkeys").

Although it would be difficult to refute Wender's theory of a neuro-physiological basis to these children's anhedonia, it is not difficult to attribute it to other factors. Cognitive impairments alone might result in such absence of pleasurable response. If a child does not appreciate the pleasurable implications of a communication he is not going to rejoice. An MBD child's distractibility might produce an anhedonic response. The child may be so distracted that he reacts neither to painful nor pleasurable stimuli. The MBD child has fewer experiences that provide pleasure and so he is likely to be depressed, a state that Wender agrees is closely associated with anhedonia. Defects in the ability to project oneself into the future can also impair pleasurable response. In addition, many MBD children build up a wall of psychological defenses in order to protect themselves from the multiple social rejections that are often their lot. This state of chronic psychological insensitivity to the environment may also impair pleasurable responses. Lastly, these children's protective withdrawal may also remove them from pleasurable stimuli, and because they have fewer experiences with pleasure they could be considered to have "forgotten" how to react.

A. Wechsler (1972) studied adult neurological patients and found that they recalled more neutral than emotionally charged segments of two stories (one neutral and one emotionally charged) that were read to them. He concluded that the memory impairment caused by brain damage is greater for emotionally charged than for neutral material and that this may explain the unemotionality of many of these patients. However, when one reads the emotionally charged story that was read to these patients, one cannot help but consider psychological factors to have been operative (either alone or in combination with the neurological). In short, the story is of a sick man who hopes for a magic cure. The story ends with his hopes being dashed as the means by which the cure was to have been effected are not successful. Even the author admits that the neurological patient would have good reason to repress memory of such a story, purely on a psychological basis.

Gainotti (1972) found that adult neurological patients with left-hemisphere lesions tended to exhibit the catastrophic reaction described by Goldstein in which the patient experiences severe anxiety and feelings of helplessness to deal with tasks. Patients with right-hemisphere lesions, however, did not manifest such reactions. Rather they were most often indifferent to noxious stimuli. Such indifference seemed to be part of the unilateral neglect syndrome often seen in patients with right-hemisphere lesions. Typically such patients are indifferent to their failures, joke about them, and minimize significantly their neurological defects. One can only wonder whether the hyperreactive, labile MBD children may be the ones with left-hemisphere involvement (similar to Goldstein's patients who exhibited catastrophic reactions) and the indifferent, hyporeactive MBD children may be the ones with right-sided lesions (similar to Wender's anhedonic patients and Gainotti's patients with indifference reactions).

The socialization problems of children with neurological learning disabilities may be a greater source of psychological pain than the educational problems. Yet these problems have not been given the attention they deserve in the professional literature. Therapeutic programs for these difficulties must be based on a deeper understanding of both the neurological and psychological factors that contribute to these impairments. In the service of this goal I have attempted to delineate how each of the common neurological impairments can result in specific types of difficulties in socialization. Such data is, in my opinion, the best point of departure for devising treatment programs for these children's socialization problems. Further work is needed in delineating these neurological factors and utilizing such information in the formulation of therapeutic programs.

Considering the vast array of problems that can contribute to MBD children's socialization difficulties, there is no single test for assessing their socialization problems. Here I describe those instruments that provide general clues that socialization deficits are likely to be present. Abnormal scores on any of these should lead the examiner to attempt to ascertain the more specific defects that have brought about the low score on the test.

The Comprehension Subtest of the WISC-R

The test consists of 17 questions that assess a child's knowledge of a variety of social phenomena. Many relate to knowing what to do when one is confronted with a common problem. For example, the child is asked what to do when "you cut your finger?" "you find someone's wallet?" and "you lose a ball that belongs to one of your friends?" Other questions ask the child why certain things are done. For example, the child is asked "Why are criminals locked up?" "Why should a promise be kept?" and "Why do we put stamps on letters?" The questions can be viewed as assessing the child's ability to use facts in a meaningful and practical way, a quality that is generally referred to as "common sense." The child who has been involved meaningfully with others and exposed to the usual experiences in life is likely to obtain an age-level score if there are no impairments that have interfered with the acquisition of this practical knowledge.

Each question is scored 2, 1, or 0 points depending upon the sophistication of the response. The manual contains specific scoring criteria. The test does not differentiate children whose impairments are neurophysiological from those whose impairments are psychological. There are children who will do poorly because their neurological impairments have interfered with their acquisition of the knowledge necessary to obtain a good score. There are others who have the intellectual capability, but have been so withdrawn, disinterested, or uninvolved in the world around them that they have not gained the knowledge necessary for adequate performance on the test. And there are children whose low score may be the result of a combination of deficits in both areas. The child with a basic neurological impairment may withdraw from social involvements in order to protect himself from the humiliations he so often suffers in his relationships with peers. He may thereby deprive himself of learning social techniques that he is capable of comprehending but does not do so because of lack of exposure. The subtest only reflects the total deficit; it does not enable one to determine which of these three possible situations has caused the low score. The subtest also assesses the child's social judgment and his conscience or moral sense. Although psychogenic factors can certainly play a role in the development of this faculty, there are neurodevelopmental factors as well that contribute [Piaget (1932) has studied these levels in detail]. A related function assessed by the test is the child's capacity to project himself into another person's situation. This quality is central to the development of conscience.

A 9½-year-old boy, for example, obtains a raw score of 9. Referring to the conversion table we note that this corresponds to a scaled score of 6. From the age-equivalents table we note that this is the average score for a child 6 years 2 months. Clearly, this child's social awareness is significantly impaired. Inquiry into the child's history and examination of the child's scores on other tests in this battery should help the examiner ascertain whether the social impairment is related to neurological factors, psychological factors, or a combination of both.

It is important for the reader to appreciate that psychological problems that cause social withdrawal are likely to reduce a child's score on this subtest. On many of the other WISC-R subtests as well, psychogenic factors can contribute to a child's low performance. The child's score on the Vocabulary and Information subtest can be reduced by psychogenic social withdrawal. The Arithmetic score can be reduced by inattentiveness in school caused by psychological problems. The Similarities score can be artificially lowered by a lack of intellectual curiosity, a failure on the child's part to rise to the challenge of "figuring out" the answer. In this book I have emphasized the neurological factors that may cause impaired performance on WISC-R subtests. The reader should not let this emphasis lead him or her to the conclusion

that WISC-R assesses exclusively "organic" deficits. And the Comprehension subtest is one that is sensitive to such psychogenic impairments,
especially in the area of social naiveté, and withdrawal.

The Picture Arrangement Subtest
of the WISC-R

Social judgment is one of the primary functions assessed by the Picture
Arrangement subtest of the WISC-R. The child is presented with a
series of pictures which, if placed in proper sequence, would tell a
coherent and reasonable story. The examiner presents the cards in a
mixed-up sequence in accordance with specific instructions indicated
by a numerical order on the back of the cards. The child is requested to
rearrange the cards "in the right order so they tell a story that makes
sense." The child is timed for each item, with bonus points being given
if the item is correctly completed before the time limit. One of the simple
sequences consists of four pictures. One shows a child playing with
matches while his mother is admonishing him. Another depicts the
curtains of the child's house beginning to burn while the child is running off with a smoking match in his hand. Another shows a fire truck
racing through the streets. And the fourth shows firemen fighting a fire
while the same child is outside the house crying. These four cards are
presented in the wrong sequence and the child is timed while he attempts to organize them into the order just described.

One could consider the Picture Arrangement subtest to be a visual
rendition of the Comprehension subtest. Knowledge of social situations
is required if one is to be successful on Picture Arrangement. The test
also assesses the child's sequential planning ability and the capacity to
anticipate, comprehend, and judge the causes and consequences of
common events. Such capacity is central to social sensitivity. The test
also assesses what is usually referred to as "common sense." Many
examiners consider this subtest to be the best measure of G of all the
performance subtests. Visual sequential memory as well as visual
Gestalt (the ability to synthesize visual stimuli into an intelligible whole)
is also measured. Some of the items relate to punishment and morality
themes, so that a child's development of conscience is also being assessed. Lastly, the impulsive child or the one who does not concentrate
well, even without any of the aforementioned defects, may do poorly.

An 8-year-2-month-old girl obtains a raw score of 9. This corresponds to a scaled score of 6 and an age-equivalent of 6-2. One must
consider it likely that this girl has a socialization deficit. From this
subtest alone, one cannot come to any definite conclusions regarding
whether the impairment is organic or psychogenic. Nor can one make

any specific statement as to whether any of the other functions that the test assesses are impaired. One must consider this score in the context of others if one is to come to definite conclusions. Consider, for example, the child whose clinical behavior is impulsive with low frustration tolerance, frequent interrupting, and difficulty waiting his turn with peers. If he is observed to complete the test items in a short time with many errors, then one may conclude that there is an impulsivity problem present. However, one may not be able to say much more (especially with regard to social judgment) because the child has not really done the test. Another child completes each test item in a reasonable period but does not appear to be concentrating well. His scores on the Steadiness Tester, the Coding subtest of the WISC-R, and the Visual Closure subtest of the ITPA all suggest an attentional deficit. His good response to psychostimulant medication also lends support to this conclusion. Again, we can only say that a concentration impairment has contributed to the child's low score, but we cannot conclude that a social sensitivity deficit is present. Another child with a low score has done average to above average on all other WISC-R subtests with the exception of Comprehension. There is no evidence for organic deficit on any other tests sensitive to MBD manifestations. We can conclude that this child has a psychogenic defect, most likely in the area of social comprehension. However, one should consider as well the possibility that some of the other aforementioned functions may also be impaired. The child who does poorly on Picture Arrangement and who exhibits evidence of MBD on other instruments may very well have a socialization problem on an organic basis. I hope that the reader appreciates how risky it is to come to any definite conclusions on the basis of simply considering one score in isolation from all others. It is only trends and patterns that really count. Single items only raise suspicions; only repeated deficiencies provide the basis for definite conclusions.

The Vineland Social Maturity Scale

The child we refer to as "immature" is generally one who is not functioning at age level. The term provides no information regarding whether the immaturity is organic or psychogenic. When we are simply told that a child is immature we do not know whether there is a neurologically based developmental lag or whether psychological factors have produced the regression and/or fixation at earlier levels of development. In addition, when neurological factors have caused the immaturity, superimposed psychogenic factors are most often also contributing. Such children may fear exposing their neurological deficits and so withdraw from peer involvement. They may thereby be less mature than their neurological condition warrants since they do not gain competence in areas that they otherwise might have been quite capable of mastering.

The Vineland Social Maturity Scale (Doll, 1965) provides the examiner with information about a child's general level of development. It does *not* differentiate psychogenic and neurological impairments. One unique aspect of the scale is that the information is obtained entirely from the parent, although the examiner may wish to observe the child if he or she doubts the validity of a parental response. As can be seen from Figure 11.1, the scale consists of a series of developmental capabilities listed in age-hierarchal order. Age levels are represented by Roman numerals, e.g., III-IV, and the average fraction of a year at which the average child attains the particular level is recorded in Arabic numerals, e.g. 4.80, placed to the right of each item. The letters to the left of each item represent the various categories of developmental capacities assessed by the scale: self-help general (SHG), self-help eating (SHE), self-help dressing (SHD), self-direction (SD), occupation (O), communication (C), locomotion (L), and socialization (S). I have not found attention to these categories especially useful especially because they are not separately considered in ascertaining the general maturity level. Although only one of the categories specifically refers to socialization problems, just about all of the other items in the Vineland test relate to socialization difficulties, although some do so indirectly. Accordingly, for the purposes of evaluating a child's level of socialization attainment, one need not concern oneself significantly with the categories abbreviated to the left of each item.

A detailed inquiry is conducted so that the examiner is certain that he or she knows whether or not the child should be given a pass (+) or a fail (−) for the particular item. The manual describes other possible scores for special situations, e.g., F + score for a patient who has previously developed a specific capacity but has lost it through physical illness (this still receives a + 1 score).

A child's score is obtained by first ascertaining the basal score, which is the highest of all the continuous pluses. To this is added the scattered credits beyond the basal. This sum provides the social maturity level. For example, an 8-year-old boy achieves continuous credits up to item 55 (see Figure 11.1). His scattered additional plus credits amount to 8 points. His total then is 63 points. Referring again to Figure 11.1, we note that the 63-point level is one-half way between ages 6 and 7. Accordingly, we can conclude that this boy is one and one half years below age level in general social maturity. This score alone gives no information about whether such deficit is organic or psychogenic. If other information supports the conclusion that the child has MBD then

Figure 11.1

Vineland Social Maturity Scale

Categories	Items		Life Age Mean
S H E	39.	Gets drink unassisted	2.43
S H D	40.	Dries own hands	2.60
S H G	41.	Avoids simple hazards	2.85
S H D	42.	Puts on coat or dress unassisted	2.85
O	43.	Cuts with scissors	2.88
C	44.	Relates experiences	3.15

III – IV

L	45.	Walks downstairs one step per tread ..	3.23
S	46.	Plays cooperatively at kindergarten level	3.28
S H D	47.	Buttons coat or dress	3.35
O	48.	**Helps at little household tasks**	3.55
S	49.	"Performs" for others	3.75
S H D	50.	Washes hands unaided	3.83

IV – V

S H G	51.	Cares for self at toilet	3.83
S H D	52.	Washes face unassisted	4.65
L	53.	Goes about neighborhood unattended	4.70
S H D	54.	Dresses self except tying	4.80
O	55.	Uses pencil or crayon for drawing ..	5.13
S	56.	Plays competitive exercise games ...	5.13

V – VI

O	57.	Uses skates, sled, wagon	5.13
C	58.	Prints simple words	5.23
S	59.	Plays simple table games	5.63
S D	60.	Is trusted with money	5.83
L	61.	Goes to school unattended	5.83

VI – VII

S H E	62.	Uses table knife for spreading	6.03
C	63.	Uses pencil for writing	6.15
S H D	64.	Bathes self assisted	6.23
S H D	65.	Goes to bed unassisted	6.75

VII – VIII

S H G	66.	Tells time to quarter hour	7.28
S H E	67.	Uses table knife for cutting	8.05
S	68.	Disavows literal Santa Claus	8.28
S	69.	Participates in pre-adolescent play ...	8.28
S H D	70.	Combs or brushes hair	8.45

Reproduced from the Vineland Social Maturity Scale by Edgar A. Doll, Ph.D. with the permission of the publisher, American Guidance Service, Inc., Circle Pines, Minnesota.

it is most likely that neurological impairments are contributing to the child's socialization deficiency. However, it is still probable that some of the failed items are psychogenic or at least have a psychological contributing factor.

12
General Body Characteristics

In this final chapter I describe some general physical abnormalities that one may see in children with MBD. Actually, this chapter goes further and includes deficits that do not fit neatly into any of the other categories described in this book. This should not be surprising, considering the wide variety of signs and symptoms that may result from, or be associated with, central nervous system impairment.

PHYSICAL APPEARANCE

Although most children with MBD do not appear different from normals, there are some who definitely do. Waldrop and Halverson (1970) and Waldrop and Goering (1971) have described some of the more common abnormalities of external appearance that are sometimes seen in MBD children. These anomalies are sometimes referred to as *stigmata*. Most of these abnormalities are the result of developmental pathology of the skin and subjacent tissues. The skin, we know, is ectodermal in origin, as is the central nervous system. It is reasonable to assume that the same early intrauterine influences that are detrimental to the fetus' central nervous system have also implicated the skin. In fact, it is probable that some of the pathological exposures occurred at the time before ectodermal differentiation into neural and dermal tissue. The most common skin pathology that one sees in these children are epicanthal folds, more than one hair whorl, café au lait spots, cross palmer fold (simian crease), and partial webbing of fingers and toes (syndactylia).

In addition, one sees stigmata that involve other tissues, especially bone. Here one must postulate that the detrimental intrauterine influences have been extensive. The most common stigmata in this category include strabismus, widely spaced eyes secondary to abnormalities of the sphenoid bone at the base of the skull (hypertelorism), high arched palate, low ears, adherent ear lobes, anteriorly oriented auricles, short inwardly curved fifth finger, wide gap between the first and second toes, and an abnormally long second toe.

ABNORMALITIES OF SIZE

One should measure a child's height and weight or obtain such data if the examiner does not have a measuring tape and scale readily available. The parent's questionnaire described in chapter 1 will generally provide the examiner with such data. If he suspects that the figures reported by the parents are inaccurate, he or she should verify the figures by his or her own observations or those of a reliable examiner (such as the child's pediatrician or school nurse). More important than the actual height and weight are the percentile ranks of these measurements. Most pediatric textbooks provide charts that will readily enable the examiner to determine the percentile level of a child's height and weight. I have found the charts published by the National Center for Health Statistics (1976) to be particularly useful. Along with their neurodevelopmental immaturity, many MBD children are small for their age. Such shortness of stature can be an asset if they are to be retained in school or placed in a class with younger children. Head circumference is also important to measure. As mentioned in chapter 1, mild cases of micro- and macrocephaly and arrested hydrocephalus are not uncommon among MBD children. Unfortunately, standard pediatric texts (in my experience) do not routinely publish head circumference data that provide percentile ranks. In Table 12.1, I have reproduced for the reader the very useful head circumference percentile data published by Paine and Oppé (1966).

Table 12.1

Head Circumferences, in Centimeters, in Children 1/2–10 Years of Age

Boys Age	10%	25%	Percentiles 50%	75%	90%
6 months	42.7	43.3	43.9	44.8	45.4
9 months	44.5	45.1	46.0	46.5	47.1
12 months	45.5	46.5	47.3	47.8	48.4
15 months	46.3	47.1	48.0	48.5	49.2
18 months	47.3	48.0	48.8	49.4	50.1
2 years	48.1	48.7	50.0	50.4	51.2
3 years	48.9	49.7	50.4	51.3	52.0
4 years	49.5	50.3	50.9	51.7	52.6
5 years	49.8	50.6	51.3	52.2	52.6
6 years	50.4	51.0	51.7	52.7	53.5
8 years	51.0	51.7	52.4	53.7	54.5
10 years	51.6	52.2	53.0	54.1	54.7

Girls Age	10%	25%	Percentiles 50%	75%	90%
6 months	41.4	42.0	42.8	43.6	44.5
9 months	43.2	43.8	44.6	45.4	46.3
12 months	44.3	45.0	45.8	46.7	47.7
15 months	44.9	45.6	46.5	47.4	48.4
18 months	45.8	46.5	47.3	48.3	49.1
2 years	46.3	47.1	48.1	49.1	50.2
3 years	47.6	48.3	49.3	50.3	51.2
4 years	48.1	49.1	49.8	50.8	51.7
5 years	48.4	49.5	50.3	51.3	52.2
6 years	48.9	49.7	50.9	52.0	52.8
8 years	49.9	50.4	52.0	52.8	53.6
10 years	50.8	52.1	52.9	54.2	54.8

Reproduced with the permission of the publishers from: Paine, R. and Oppé, T. (1966), *Neurological Examination of Children.* Spastics International Medical Publications. London: William Heinemann Medical Books, Ltd. and Philadelphia: J. B. Lippincott Co.

ABNORMALITIES OF BODY IMAGE

Body image is a term that has been used quite loosely and has a variety of meanings. Schilder (1950) paid particular attention to the concept and used the term *body schema* to refer to "an organized perceptual model of the body" which arises from the steady stream of interoceptive, proprioceptive, and tactual impulses that continually reach the brain. This "topographic configuration" is derived from both past and present stimuli. It "serves to impose an appropriate spatial quality on the parts of the body or on stimuli applied to it," i.e., it serves as a mental model of what the body is normally supposed to be like and recognizes abnormality or change by comparing the new state with the model pattern of the old. It is an active and organized mental model of the body. It is responsible for the appreciation of changes in body position, direction of body movement, accurate spot localization, and two-point discrimination. It is involved in right-left discrimination and finger localization. It is responsible for the feeling that one still has an extremity after an amputation and this is one of the most convincing confirmations of the body schema theory. Lastly, disorders of the cortex can result in malfunctioning of the body schema so that one may be impaired in localizing body stimulation, in identifying the position of various parts of the body, differentiating right from left. Such disorders may even be involved in the failure to be aware of the existence of certain parts of the body.

Benton (1959) similarly viewed the *body image* to be a mental representation of the body derived from the stream of interoceptive (internal organs), proprioceptive (muscles and joints), and tactile (skin) stimuli that are transmitted to the brain. He emphasized, however, the visual aspect of the body image. Not only do external visual stimuli play a role in the formation of the body image (we see our bodies and learn about their appearances in this way), but the mental representation is something that we internally visualize. The integrity of this visual image is necessary if one is to properly localize body parts. Benton studied two aspects of the body image concept that could be observed and measured: right-left discrimination and finger localization. I will present below his normative data on right-left discrimination. His studies on finger localization (the impairment of which is sometimes referred to as *finger agnosia*) are of interest, but the normative data he collected is not adequate enough to utilize as part of a standard MBD battery.

Money (1962) uses the term *body schema* to refer to the neurological pattern related to one's direct sensory awareness of one's body. He uses the term *body image* more broadly to include both the body schema and the emotional-psychological factors that contribute to one's view or feelings about one's body. Others have used the terms interchangeably. In recent years the term body image has been used much more frequently than body schema, but the confusion of whether one is talking about the neurological, the psychological, or a combination of both is still commonplace.

Johnson and Myklebust (1967) describe a variety of functions that relate to body image. The ability to identify the various parts of the body follows specific developmental patterns. Terman and Merrill (1937) and Ilg and Ames (1965) have provided normative data on this. I do not routinely include body part identification in my battery, because most of the children I see are over five and the overwhelming majority have already mastered this capacity, even though many have been late in doing so. Another manifestation of a body image disturbance is the impaired ability to construct models of the human body and to produce organized and readily identifiable drawings of the human figure (I will discuss the latter capacity below). Some children will be able to point to parts of their own body, but not to the same parts of the examiner. Others can identify such body parts on a doll or the examiner but not on themselves. The view that one has about one's body is determined by both neurological and psychological factors. The healthy person has a realistic view of his or her body, a view that generally coincides with that of the majority of others. Learning about one's body begins in infancy as the child explores his own body. Later, he gets information about it from significant figures in his milieu. The healthy person has no significant distortion about his body. Intact neuronal mechanisms must be present if one's body image is to be accurate. However, psychological factors commonly affect one's view of one's body. This is especially apparent during the adolescent period when the youngster may obsess about his or her body, is dissatisfied at times with almost every part, considers it unattractive, fears it is of abnormal size or shape, worries that it smells bad, etc. The psychotic may entertain delusions about the most gross distortions of the body, which may have both organic and/or psychological components.

Drawing of the Human Figure

In chapter 10 I discussed the Harris Draw-A-Person Test as useful in ascertaining a child's level of intelligence. I also made reference to its value as a projective test. Such use stems from the observation that the child tends to project his own feelings about himself onto the figure he has drawn. When he talks about the things that are happening to the figure, he is most often talking about himself (often without realization). Similarly, the actual drawing is a projection of the child's image of his own body. One might view it as external pictorial representation of the child's internal body image engram. Unfortunately, we have not reached the point where we can easily determine whether a particular distortion on a figure drawing is organic or psychogenic. When a child, for example, draws the figure as minuscule we tend to assume that he feels himself small, weak, and impotent, that he doesn't count for much in the world. We view this as a psychological phenomenon. A child with a physical deformity may accurately depict it in the figure drawing. On the other hand, he may omit the defect from the drawing. We would be likely to explain the omission as psychological denial, rather than to conclude that his body image does not contain the deficit. A child might draw a figure in whom there is unusual strength in the area of the child's impairment. We would say that he is psychologically compensating. When a deformity is accurately portrayed in the picture, we can say that the body image depicted by the picture is an accurate reflection of reality and that the person does not have an impairment in body image formation. We would also say that he does not manifest significant need to deny the deficit or to compensate pathologically for it. Usually, when a picture manifests a distortion, we more often conclude that a psychologic, rather than a neurologic, problem or factor is responsible for the distortion. Neither the Harris Test nor other human figure drawing instruments can, at this point, differentiate between neurologically based body image impairments and those that are psychogenic. Hopefully, future research will enable us to use figure drawing better as an instrument for ascertaining body image impairments.

Right-Left Discrimination

> Pooh looked at his two paws. He knew that one of them was the right, and he knew that when you had decided which one of them was the right, then the other one was the left, but he never could remember how to begin.
> "Well," he said slowly ...
>
> —House at Pooh Corner
> A. A. Milne

Like other vertebrates, we humans have fairly symmetrical bodies. And so many of us, like Pooh, have trouble at times differentiating our right from our left. Many learn in childhood some specific clues, a pimple or a mole, that can be useful. Some continue using such hints throughout life. Corballis and Beale (1976), however, hold that our bodies are not as symmetrical as we might initially think. They believe that there is a deep-seated right-left gradient that exists in all of us. It originates in the earliest phases of cell division, at the blastula level, before the stage of gastrulation. They believe that cytoplasmic coding affects cell division at the blastula level in such a way that a differential right-left gradient is set up between the two sides of the early embryonic cellular mass. This gradient results later in the left hemisphere developing earlier than the right. Later, the left hemisphere further distinguishes itself from the right by becoming the seat of linguistic functions, whereas the right becomes the center for spatial functions. The left hemisphere controls the right, stronger, more dominant hand. All these factors give the body an asymmetry that is subtle, but nevertheless present. And this asymmetry provides the same kinds of clues as the mole or pimple for differentiating right from left. They result in the two sides feeling different and this difference helps the normal person differentiate right from left.

Benton Right-Left Discrimination Test

Children with MBD may have more than the usual degree of difficulty in discriminating right from left. Benton (1968, 1976), who has been particularly interested in this subject, is not convinced of the general utility of normative data for right-left discrimination because of varying educational curricula as well as cultural attitudes regarding this function. In some areas the home and school may be particularly concerned with the child's making the proper differentiation and in other areas there may be little or no emphasis placed on this function. Accordingly, in his opinion, only local normative data is useful. He therefore suggests that only the most general criteria be utilized in objectively assessing lags in this area. The guidelines he proposes are summarized in Table 12.2. In short, the normal six-year-old should be

Table 12.2
Benton Right-Left Discrimination Test

Task	Age by Which Task Should Be Accomplished
1. Show me your *left* hand.	6
2. Show me your *right* eye.	6
3. Show me your *left* ear.	6
4. Show me your *right* hand.	6
5. Touch your *left* ear with your *left* hand.	7
6. Touch your *right* knee with your *right* hand.	7
7. Touch your *left* eye with your *left* hand.	7
8. Touch your *right* ear with your *right* hand.	7
9. Touch your *right* eye with your *left* hand.	8–9
10. Touch your *right* ear with your *left* hand.	8–9
11. Touch your *left* knee with your *right* hand.	8–9
12. Touch your *left* eye with your *right* hand.	8–9
13. Point to my *right* eye.	11
14. Point to my *left* leg.	11
15. Point to my *left* ear.	11
16. Point to my *right* hand.	11
17. Put your *right* hand on my *left* ear.	12
18. Put your *left* hand on my *left* eye.	12
19. Put your *left* hand on my *right* shoulder.	12
20. Put your *right* hand on my *right* eye.	12

Adapted from Benton, A. L., Right-Left Discrimination. *Pediatric Clinics of North America*, 15:747–758, 1968 and Benton, A. L., Personal Communication, 1976. Reproduced with the permission of the author and publisher, W. B. Saunders Co., Philadelphia.

able to identify single lateral parts of his own body ("Show me your left hand"). The normal seven-year-old should be able to execute uncrossed commands ("Touch your left ear with your left hand"). At that age he is likely to respond to a crossed command ("Touch your right eye with your left hand") in uncrossed fashion. By 8 or 9 years of age he should have no trouble with crossed commands, as long as they pertain to his own body. A majority of 9-year-olds will correctly identify parts on the confronting examiner's body ("Point to my right eye"), but it is not until 11 that all should be able to do this. By 12 a normal child should be able to use both systems (his own and the examiner's) in combination ("Put your left hand on my right ear").

A 7-year-old boy, for example, fails three of the four requests (items 1–4) to point to parts of his own body. This child should be suspect for a right-left discrimination problem. A 10-year-old girl is asked to point to various body parts on either the left or the right side of the examiner. Of the four questions (items 13–16) she gets three wrong. She may be in the normal range. However, by age 11, if she does not execute all these commands correctly one must consider a neurologically based impairment.

The Right-Left Discrimination Subtest of the Southern California Perceptual-Motor Tests

Ayres (1968) includes a right-left discrimination subtest in her perceptual-motor battery. This test is less concerned with developmental factors than Benton's; rather, it combines many developmental levels of right-left discrimination tasks into one series of 10 questions. Although this is a significant disadvantage, the test is timed and this, in my opinion, is one of its strengths. One determinant of whether the child receives 2, 1, or 0 points for each answer is the time it takes him to respond. A prominent factor in right-left discrimination tasks is the patient's speed of response. Thinking about various clues slows up response, as does changing one's decision. Raw scores are converted into standard scores (standard deviations from the mean) by reference to the proper table for the child's age. Unfortunately, normative data is only provided for ages 5-0 through 8-11. However, the test is so simple that in the 8-0 to 8-11 age bracket the mean raw score is 16 (20 is the maximum raw score).

A 7-year-2-month-old girl obtains a raw score of 6. The mean raw score for children her age is 14. Her score is 1.4 standard deviations below the mean and is strongly suggestive of a right-left differentiation problem. A 6-year-8-month-old boy obtains a raw score of 13. The mean raw score for children his age is 12. His score is 0.2 standard deviations above the mean. We can conclude that it is unlikely that this child has a right-left discrimination problem.

LATERALITY

Very little has been said in this book about laterality, the preferential use of one side in bilateral functions. In studies on MBD children, laterality considerations most commonly concern the preferential use of the hand, foot, eye, and ear. There are probably tens of thousands of articles in the literature on the subject of laterality. I believe that we have learned some useful things about the brain from studies involving laterality and we will no doubt learn much more. However, I do not believe that ascertaining whether the child prefers the right hand, foot, and eye is of diagnostic value at the present time. (Perhaps the recent studies on dichotic functions described in chapter 7 now warrant our utilizing laterality considerations for the ear.) Most agree that left handedness, for example, is more common among MBD children than normals. In my own studies (chapter 8) we found that approximately 90% of normal children and about 80% of those with MBD were right-handed. One could say that 1/10 of normal children and 2/10 of MBD children are left-handed, i.e., left-handedness is twice as common among MBD children than normal children. Or one could say that 9/10 of normal children are right-handed and 8/10 of MBD children are right-handed. When expressed in the second way, the examiner cannot really feel that handedness is a good differential criterion in making the MBD diagnosis. Accordingly, I do not ask questions about laterality in my questionnaire and I do not test for handedness in my battery. There are times when I am required to ascertain handedness in order to properly administer some of the tests in my battery. I am not, therefore, oblivious to the child's hand preference. I just do not think that the information is of significance for diagnostic purposes at the present time. I suspect that in the future, with greater understanding of its significance, laterality may prove to be of some diagnostic value.

We also find articles emphasizing the importance of mixed dominance and crossed dominance in MBD. Mixed dominance refers to the failure to establish strong laterality. Ambidexterity is an example of mixed dominance. Actually, one does well not to view a person as right-handed or left-handed; rather, one should consider degrees of handedness. Harris (1958) was well aware of this when he devised his *Tests of Lateral Dominance*. In Harris' battery, a series of tasks is presented in order to determine the *degree* of laterality that the child exhibits. All of us have some degree of ambidexerity. The crucial problem is that of differentiating the MBD child from the normal. There is a continuum among people: from the strongly right-handed, to the mildly right-handed, to those who are truly ambidextrous, to those who are mildly left-handed, to those who are strongly left-handed. At what point can one differentiate the normal from the MBD? We do not presently know. It is probable that more MBD children are closer to the mid-point than normals, but this does not warrant our automatically making ambidexterity an important diagnostic criterion.

Similar considerations are applicable with regard to crossed dominance, such as the preference for the *right* hand and the *left* foot. The literature here is even more confusing. The significance of hand and foot preference is probably different from eye preference. And ear preference is probably vastly different from all of these, considering the differences in the types of neurological pathways involved. To say that a normal person should prefer the *right* hand, *right* foot, *right* eye, and *right* ear is imposing what appears to me to be a very artificial and probably naive standard of "perfection" on people. At this point, then, I do not use mixed dominance as a criterion for MBD diagnosis. In fact, I do not test for it. This is not to say that we should not concern ourselves with such matters. As mentioned, these are important areas for research and there is much that we can still learn from studies in laterality.

In a way, ending this book on the subject of laterality provides us with a useful message. The field of MBD is in its present state of confusion because of the utilization of tests and criteria that have been poorly validated. Laterality criteria for MBD diagnosis are an excellent example of this phenomenon. We must clearly delineate the things we know from the things we do not. In this book I have attempted to provide some information about the things of which we are more certain. It is only by making this differentiation that we will be able to reduce the confusion in the field and help more efficiently and effectively those who suffer with minimal brain dysfunction.

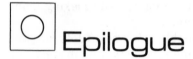# Epilogue

This book was written with two primary goals: First, to provide a comprehensive and detailed statement about the signs and symptoms of minimal brain dysfunction. Second, to enable the diagnostician to assess objectively such signs. It is my hope that these tasks have been accomplished. Such organization and assessment is crucial if we are to bring ourselves out of the present state of confusion that exists in the field. Delineation and objectification are important first steps toward identifying the various subcategories that surely exist under the rubric that we should refer to as *The Group of Minimal Brain Dysfunction Syndromes* and which we now more loosely call minimal brain dysfunction. When we have identified these separate syndromes, the term MBD will no longer serve its purpose and will most likely fall into disuse. As we become ever more sophisticated, each new syndrome will then, in all probability, become parent to a whole new family of disorders. The history of medicine is, in a sense, the history of such discriminations. Diagnostic progress depends upon such refinements; meaningful therapeutic progress is not likely to take place without them.

A ☐○ Appendix

Sample Evaluation of a Child with Minimal Brain Dysfunction[1]

Robert, who is 8 years 2 months old, is in a regular third-grade class. He was referred for psychiatric consultation with the chief complaints of disruptive behavior in the classroom, poor academic performance in spite of suspected above average intelligence, and uncooperative behavior at home.

In school, Robert is described as not sitting still for long, walking around the classroom without permission, refusing to wait his turn to be called upon, blurting out answers, not cooperating in group activities, and not paying attention to the teacher. He avoids doing his homework, but when it is done it is usually sloppy and done as quickly as possible. He often lies to his parents and tells them that he has no homework when assignments have been given or he tells them that he has done his homework in school when he has not. The teachers complain that he is not working up to his potential. He is functioning at below grade level in reading and spelling, but is approximately at grade level in arithmetic.

---

[1] Only that portion of the diagnostic evaluation that pertains to MBD is described here. No evaluation is complete without an assessment of the psychogenic problems that can be secondary to and/or concomitant with the neurologic. However, a report on the psychogenic problems, which are also invariably present, goes beyond the purpose of this book.

At home he is described as being messy at the table, so much so that by the end of the meal there is "more food on the floor than he has put into his mouth." He is cruel to the family dog and often kicks him when he is angry. When Robert comes home from school the dog runs from him and hides. The mother states, "He doesn't seem to appreciate that the dog has feelings and gets hurt." The family cannot take Robert to restaurants because "he only embarrasses us with his loud talking, messy manners, and getting up out of his seat all the time and running all around the place." He cannot join the family for church services because his noise would distract the minister and interfere with the services. He seems to have little appreciation of the sanctity of the situation. His brother (age 10) and sister (age 7) avoid bringing their friends into the house because he does not respect their privacy and interferes with their play. He is described as being hyperactive and "runs more than he walks." He is heedless to danger and has had many accidents and emergency room visits. He seems to learn little from these experiences.

A peer problem is also described. He does not respect the rights of other children, will not wait his turn in play, and is a poor sport. Coordination problems have resulted in his being the last to be chosen for competitive games. Peers do not seek him and he seeks primarily younger children with whom he can relate better, especially when he can make the rules and have his own way.

Inquiry into the past history reveals that Robert's mother had been a heavy smoker since her early teens and smoked an average of two-and-one-third packages of cigarettes per day during the pregnancy. During the fifth month she suffered for about a week with a "viral infection" associated with high fever. During this time the fetal heart sounds were at times inaudible. Delivery occurred spontaneously in the eighth month and his birth weight was four pounds three ounces. Incubator care lasted two weeks and he left the hospital after three weeks.

Unlike his siblings, Robert is described as never having enjoyed cuddling and generally could not be quieted down by being stroked. From the beginning he seemed to require little sleep and even when he would sleep, the slightest noise awakened him. Developmental milestones were generally late, but not severely so. He first walked at 15 months and his first words appeared at 18 months. He was bowel trained at three, but still wets the bed on an average of twice a week. He could not button his own clothing until age six and shoelace tying did not occur until eight and is still a cause of trouble for him. No unusual medical illnesses are described. His siblings were said to be normal in all major areas of functioning (school, home, social, etc.).

DIAGNOSTIC EVALUATION

Robert was generally cooperative throughout the evaluation, which involved seven one-hour interviews. At times, however, he was inattentive so that instructions had to be repeated. He was talkative, highly verbal, and appeared to have a good command of English. One got the general feeling that he was a "bright" and inquisitive child. When he did well on a task he was quite enthusiastic; when he felt he was doing poorly he would quickly lose interest and attempt to discontinue the task with comments such as, "This is boring," or, "This is a stupid test."

Hyperactivity

On the steadiness tester, Robert's score was 33.5 sec. The mean score for normal boys Robert's age is 8.23 ± 6.06 sec. Accordingly, Robert's score is 4.16 S.D. longer than the mean. His score is far below the tenth percentile level (20.32 sec) for normal boys. The mean score for MBD boys Robert's age is 43.04 ± 41.98. Robert's score is 0.23 S.D. below the mean, i.e., he does better (shorter total touch time) than the average MBD child, but is well within the normal range. His score also falls between the fortieth and fiftieth percentile levels for MBD children. Robert's score on the steadiness tester is much more like that of the MBD than the normal child.

There was no clinical evidence for choreiform movements and resting tremors. Also there was no evidence for motor impersistence as evidenced by Robert's normal score on the Standing Balance subtest of the Southern California Perceptual-Motor Tests. On the Eyes Open subtest of this instrument his score was 102 sec, which is + 0.1 S.D. His score on the Eyes Closed subtest was 14 sec, which is + 0.2 S.D. Accordingly, one can conclude that Robert's poor performance on the steadiness tester was the result of hyperactivity and/or impaired ability to sustain concentration. Robert's score, in my experience, was significantly higher than the levels (15–25 sec) seen in children with purely psychogenic hyperactivity/attentional problems.

In order to evaluate further Robert's hyperactivity/attentional deficit and to determine whether he would be a good candidate for psychostimulant medication, two more measurements were first made with the steadiness tester during subsequent evaluation sessions. His subsequent scores were 30.2 and 37.4 sec. His average score for the three trials was 33.7 sec. Immediately following the third trial Robert was given 10 mg methylphenidate. His steadiness tester score two hours later was 20.5 sec. Four hours later it was 9.2 sec. And five hours after administration it was 13.5 sec. These studies indicate that the attentional element is an important contributing factor in Robert's hyperacitivity. They also indicate that he is sensitive to psychostimulant medication. It is of note that his lowest score, 9.2 sec, is just above the thirtieth percentile level for normal boys and at the ninetieth percentile level for those with MBD. The medication then has brought Robert down to a level that is much more like that of normal children. Both his mother and I observed Robert to be much calmer while on the medication, and these observations provided clinical confirmation of the findings derived from his steadiness tester scores.

Concentration

On the Coding subtest of the WISC-R Robert's raw score was 26; scaled score, 8; age-equivalent, 6-2. On the Diamond Cancellation of Rapidly Recurring Target Figures Robert made 8 errors and took 80.5 sec. The normal scores for children Robert's age are 4 ± 3 errors and 66.26 ± 21.63 sec. Accordingly, Robert's error score is 1.3 S.D. greater than the average, whereas his time score is within the normal range ($+0.66$ S.D.). On the Number subtest of the Cancellation of Rapidly Recurring Target Figures Robert made 5 errors and took 140 sec. A normal boy Robert's age makes 2 ± 2 errors and takes 116.00 ± 33.71 sec. Robert's error score is 1.5 S.D. above the mean and his time score is within the average range ($+0.71$ S.D.). The findings on these tests suggest the presence of a concentration deficit and/or a visual processing impairment in the areas of short-term visual memory, visual discrimination, and visual-motor coordination.

Impulsivity

On the Mazes subtest of the WISC-R Robert's raw score was 14; scaled score, 8; and age-equivalent, 6-10. Clinically Robert was observed to draw his lines impulsively into blind alleys and his score suggests that an impulsivity problem is present. Concentration impairment, as well as visual memory and visual-motor coordination problems may also account for Robert's low score on this test.

Motor Coordination

On the Purdue Pegboard Robert's scores were as follows: preferred hand (right), 9 (normal = 12.70 ± 1.60, -2.3 S.D., below the tenth percentile); nonpreferred hand (left), 9 (normal = 12.17 ± 1.51, -2.1 S.D., below the tenth percentile); both hands, 7 (normal = 9.83 ± 1.51, -1.9

S.D., below the tenth percentile); assembly, 19 (normal = 23.20 ± 3.80, – 1.1 S.D., tenth percentile). On the repetitive finger-thumb opposition test Robert took 7.5 sec with his right hand (normal = 5.99 ± 0.98, 1.5 S.D. longer than the mean) and 8.2 sec with his left (normal = 6.31 ± 0.64, 2.9 S.D. longer than the mean). On the successive finger-thumb opposition test he took 13 sec with his right hand (normal = 10.41 ± 2.03, 1.2 S.D. longer than the mean) and 14 sec with his left (normal = 10.84 ± 2.70, 1.2 S.D. longer than the mean). It is reasonable to conclude from this data that Robert has a fine-motor-coordination problem.

On the Balls and Basket Test Robert successfully threw 8 of the 21 balls into the basket. The average normal boy Robert's age gets 11.40 ± 3.21 balls into the basket. Robert's score is 1.06 S.D. below that of the average boy his age and below the twentieth percentile level. On the foot tally counter Robert's average score with the dominant foot (right) was 26.3 taps in 10 sec. The mean score for children Robert's age is 31.7 ± 4.5 taps. Robert's score is 1.2 S.D. below the mean. With the nondominant foot (left) Robert score average was 25.0 taps in 10 sec. The mean for normal children is 29.9 ± 4.5 taps. Robert's score here is about 1.1 S.D. below the mean. On the basis of these two tests one can conclude that it is likely that Robert has a gross-motor-coordination problem.

Auditory Processing

Auditory Acuity

Clinically, Robert showed no evidence for auditory acuity deficit. He heard whispers adequately in both ears tested separately when seated sideways 15 ft from the examiner.

Auditory Discrimination

Robert correctly identified all same-word pairs and all different-word pairs on the Auditory Discrimination Test, suggesting that there is no deficit in this area.

Auditory Memory

On the Digits Forward section of the Digit Span subtest of the WISC-R Robert's score was 8. The average boy his age scores 5.81 ± 2.05. Robert's score here is 1.1 S.D. above the mean and at the ninetieth percentile level. These findings make it unlikely that a problem in short-term auditory sequential memory is present.

On the Sound Blending subtest of the ITPA Robert's raw score was 20. This corresponds to a scaled score of 36 (the mean for all subtests of the ITPA is 36 ± 6), and an age equivalent of 8-2. On the Auditory Closure subtest of the ITPA Robert's raw score was 22; scaled score, 36; age equivalent, 7-11. We can conclude here that Robert's long-term auditory memory for linguistic material is intact and that he is functioning in the normal range for this function.

Auditory Language

On the Peabody Picture Vocabulary Test (Form A) Robert's raw score was 72, which corresponds to an IQ of 111, a mental age of 9-2, and a percentile rank of 80. The findings indicate that Robert does not have an impairment in understanding auditory linguistic symbols and integrating them with their visual counterparts. On the Listening Comprehension Test of the Standard Reading Inventory, Robert successfully satisfied all criteria for questions at the third-grade level. A problem in the processing of auditory linguistic material does not appear to be present.

Visual Processing

Visual Acuity

Robert passed all sections of the Visual Screening Test, indicating that myopia, hyperopia, lateral phoria, vertical phoria, or binocularity impairment are not present. It is reasonable to conclude that occular problems are not contributing to Robert's difficulties.

Visual Discrimination

On the Colored Progressive Matrices Robert's raw score was 23, which places him at the seventy-fifth to ninetieth percentile. On the Form Constancy (III) subtest of the Developmental Test of Visual Perception, Robert's raw score was 13, which corresponds to an age equivalent of 9-0. On the Matching (III) subtest of the Reversals Frequency Test Robert made no errors. The average boy Robert's age makes 0.33 ± 0.69 errors. It is reasonable to conclude that Robert does not have problems with visual discrimination for either nonlinguistic or linguistic material. His high score on the Colored Progressive Matrices suggests, as well, that there is no impairment in visual conceptualization.

Visual Figure-Ground Discrimination

On the Southern California Figure-Ground Visual Perception Test Robert's raw score was 10. This corresponds to a standard score of − 2.0 S.D. On the Figure-Ground Discrimination (II) subtest of the Developmental Test of Visual Perception his raw score was 18, which corresponds to an age equivalent of 7-0. The findings suggest either a problem in visual figure-ground discrimination or visual concentration. Robert appeared clinically to be having trouble concentrating on these tasks (especially on the Southern California test). Accordingly, one can conclude that a visual concentration impairment contributed to Robert's low scores here. A visual figure-ground deficit is also suggested, but one cannot be certain.

Visual Memory

On the Administration A subtest of the Revised Visual Retention Test, Robert made 3 correct responses. The expected number of correct responses for children his age with IQs over 105 is 4. He made 11 errors; the expected number is 8 to 9. On the Picture Completion subtest of the WISC-R Robert's raw score was 12, which corresponds to a scaled score of 8 and an age equivalent of 6-6. On the Object Assembly subtest of the WISC-R his raw score was 11, which corresponds to a scaled score of 7 and an age equivalent of 6-2. The findings here suggest impairments in visual concentration and/or visual memory for nonlinguistic symbols. The low Object Assembly score suggests, also, the possibility of an impairment in visual organizational capacity and visual Gestalt.

On the Execution (I) subtest of the Reversals Frequency Test Robert made 3 execution reversals and 2 unknown errors. The average boy his age makes no execution reversals errors and .02 ± .012 unknown errors. The average MBD boy Robert's age makes 1.21 ± 2.01 execution errors and 1.78 ± 2.23 unknown errors. Clearly, Robert's performance on this test is much more like the MBD than the normal child. On the Recognition (II) subtest of the Reversals Frequency Test Robert made 14 errors. The average normal boy his age makes 3.73 ± 4.07 errors. The average MBD child makes 13.10 ± 11.01 errors. Robert's score is 2.44 S.D. above the mean for normal boys and well within 1 S.D. from the mean for MBD boys. His score is significantly below the tenth percentile for normal boys and at the thirtieth to fortieth percentile level for those with MBD. His scores then on this test are much more like those of MBD children than normals. It is reasonable to conclude that Robert has a problem in visual memory for linguistic symbols. His poor performance on the execution subtest suggests the possible presence of a dyspraxic problem as well. (His low scores on the tests for dyspraxia to be described below confirm that such a problem is present.)

Robert's score on the Digits Backward subtest of the WISC-R was 3. The average score for boys his age is 3.69 ± 1.43. Robert's score then is 0.48 S.D. below the mean for boys his age and is at the thirtieth to fortieth percentile level. As mentioned, Robert's performance on the Digits Forward section was above average (1.1 S.D. above the mean), indicating that a problem in short-term auditory sequential memory is not present. His performance on the Digits Backward section suggests an impairment in either short-term auditory sequential memory or short-term visual sequential memory and visual scanning. Considering his good performance on the Digits Forward section, it is reasonable to conclude that the impairment on the Digits Backward section was the result of visual processing (sequential memory and/or scanning for linguistic symbols) and not an auditory processing problem. Using the Wechsler scoring criteria, Robert's raw score was 11 (8 + 3) and his scaled score was also 11. Apparently, Robert's high score on the Digits Forward section has so offset his low score on the Digits Backward that the combined score suggests that neither an auditory nor a visual sequential memory problem is present. The visual problem is only speciously absent; it has been "buried" by the high auditory score.

On the ITPA Visual Sequential Memory subtest Robert's raw score was 17. This corresponds to a scaled score of 30, which is 1 S.D. below the mean. The age equivalent for this raw score is 6-2. This finding adds further support to the aforementioned conclusion that Robert has a visual sequential memory problem, in this case for nonlinguistic material.

On the Spelling (Level I) subtest of the WRAT Robert's raw score was 21, which is the average score for the child at the one-year-three-month grade level. This raw score corresponds to a scaled score of 4 (10 is the average scaled score for all subtests of the WRAT) and places Robert at the third percentile level. Considering all the aforementioned evidence for a problem in visual sequential memory (for both linguistic and nonlinguistic material) it is reasonable to conclude that Robert's poor spelling performance is related to a visual sequential memory deficit rather than to auditory problems or an impairment in audio-visual integration.

Visual Organization and Gestalt

On the Block Design subtest of the WISC-R Robert's raw score was 9, which corresponds to a scaled score of 8 and an age equivalent of 6-6. The findings suggest the presence of impairments in one or more of the following visual functions: analysis, synthesis, organization, and Gestalt. In addition, dyspraxia can contribute to a low score on this test. On the Spatial Relations (V) subtest of the Developmental Test of Visul Perception Robert's raw score was 8, which corresponds to an age equivalent of 8-3. Although this implies normal functioning in the areas of visual discrimination, organization, and Gestalt, I consider this test to be a simple one and would rely more on the Block Design (a more comprehensive test) scores in assessing these areas of visual functioning. Considering the findings on these two instruments together I consider problems in visual organization and Gestalt to be present, but to a mild degree. Also suggested is the possibility of an apraxic problem.

Visual Language

On the Comprehension subtest of the Gilmore Oral Reading Test Robert's raw score was 13. This corresponds to the 1.8-grade level, the fourth to tenth percentile level, and the "below average" range for third-grade students. On the Silent Reading Comprehension subtest of the Standard Reading Inventory, Robert scored 5 points (of a possible 10) at the third-grade level, 6 points at the second-grade level, and 9 points at the first-grade level. In both of these tests of reading comprehension Robert scored at the first-grade level. So his understanding of visual linguistic symbols is deficient.

Dysphasia and Dyspraxia

Dysphasia

Three tests of Rapid "Automatized" Naming were adminstered. On the color naming section Robert took 68 sec to name the 50 colors, and he made 3 errors. The normal child his ages takes 54.7 ± 6.9 seconds. Robert's time was 1.92 S.D. longer than the average. Approximately 75% of normal children his age make no errors at all. On the use objects section Robert took 90 sec to name the objects. The average time for boys his age is 61.6 ± 12.6 sec. Therefore, Robert took 2.3 S.D. longer than the average. Robert made 3 errors. Only 3.3% of normal children make 3 or more errors and 86.7% make no errors. On the numbers section Robert took 37 sec. The average time for boys his age is 30.8 ± 5.8 sec. Robert's score is 1.07 S.D. above the mean. He made one error; 86.7% of children his age do not make any errors on this section. Throughout the testing one could observe Robert struggling to "find" and "get out" words that seemed to be on the tip of his tongue. The evidence is strong that Robert is dysnomic.

Dyspraxia

On the Manual Expression subtest of the ITPA Robert's raw score was 21 and his scaled score was 29, which is 1.12 S.D. below the mean for children his age and corresponds to an age equivalent of 6-1 years. The findings here are suggestive of the presence of ideational and ideokinetic dyspraxias. Robert's reproductions on the Visual Motor Gestalt Test were scored by Koppitz criteria. He made 8 errors. The mean score for children his age is 4.2 ± 2.5. Robert's score then is 1.52 S.D. above the mean. His score is normal for the child in the 6-0 to 6-5 age bracket. Considering the previous findings that Robert does not have a problem in visual discrimination, it is likely that Robert's poor performance on this test is related to the presence of a constructional dyspraxia. On the Administration C section of the Revised Visual Retention Test Robert scored 5 points for correct responses and made 12 errors. The mean correct points for children his age in the normal IQ range is 7.16 ± 2.06. Accordingly, Robert's correct score is 1.05 S.D. below the mean. The average error score for children at his age and IQ level is 3.41 ± 2.77. Robert's error score then is 3.10 S.D. greater than the mean. The findings on this test are strongly suggestive of the presence of a constructional dyspraxia. In addition, the findings on these two tests suggest the presence of problems in visual organization and Gestalt, problems also suspected from findings on previous tests described above.

Intelligence

Robert's scores on the WISC-R subtests were as follows:

	Raw Score	Scaled Score		Raw Score	Scaled Score
Information	13	13	Picture Completion	12	8
Similarities	15	15	Picture Arrangement	16	9
Arithmetic	11	13	Block Design	9	8
Vocabulary	30	15	Object Assembly	11	7
Comprehension	17	14	Coding	26	8
(Digit Span)	11	11	(Mazes)	14	8

Verbal IQ: 124; Performance IQ: 86; Full Scale IQ: 106

Robert's overall IQ is in the high average range. Clinically he appears to be brighter and this, without doubt, is related to his excellent command of language. In a sense Robert is brighter than his total IQ score would suggest because he does very well on those subtests most highly correlated with general intelligence. The pattern we find here is the kind that one sometimes sees in patients with right-hemispheric impairment, where spatial impairments are compromised but left-hemispheric functions involving language remain intact. His high scores on the Vocabulary, Information, and Similarities subtests indicate that, in spite of his difficulties, both at home and at school, Robert is still acquiring significant amounts of information from the world around him. His intact auditory memory is probably of great help to him in these areas and compensates for the difficulties he has in learning visually. His above average score on the Arithmetic subtest also relates to his strong auditory memory. Were this a written test, he probably would have done more poorly. This is substantiated by his poorer performance on the Arithmetic (Level I) section of the Wide Range Achievement Test where his raw score was 26, which corresponds to a scaled score of 9, a grade equivalent of 2.8, and the forty-second percentile. Robert's adequate performance in arithmetic in school is probably due to the fact that his good performance on auditory arithmetic helps him compensate for his poor performance on visual arithmetic.

Harris norms were utilized in scoring the human figure drawing he executed. His point score was 20, corresponding to a standard score of 89. This is 0.73 S.D. below the mean. Twenty is the average raw score for the child between 6 and 7. Robert had great difficulty executing the drawing. This, I believe, was due to his dyspraxic and visual problems, rather than an overall intellectual deficit.

SOCIAL FUNCTIONING

It is of interest that there is an apparent disparity between Robert's scores on the two WISC-R tests of social functioning: Comprehension and Picture Arrangement, where his scaled scores were 14 and 9, respectively. This disparity becomes understandable when one appreciates that visual problems probably interfered with Robert's performing well on the Picture Arrangement subtest, whereas the Comprehension subtest is an auditory one. I believe that Robert does have a clinical problem in social functioning. However, his high score on the Comprehension subtest indicates that he has somehow acquired basic social knowledge and judgment, but that other problems (hyperactivity, impulsivity, poor concentration, etc.) have interfered with his properly exhibiting such judgment. I believe that he has the knowledge to appreciate the basic social issues being depicted in the Picture Arrangement subtest, but his visual organization problems have interfered with his performing optimally on this subtest. His poor performance on overall social functioning is not revealed by his performance on the Vineland Social Maturity Scale where he scored at the 8.53 level. This suggests that there is developmental adequacy, but the test is not assessing the kinds of social problems that Robert exhibits (disruptive behavior in the classroom, poor peer relationships, etc.).

General Body Characteristics

Robert's physical appearance was normal. No stigmata or anomalies were apparent and no such abnormalities were described by the patient or his parents. He was 51″ tall (fiftieth to seventy-fifth percentile) and his weight was 60 pounds (fiftieth to seventy-fifth percentile). His head circumference was 53.0 centimeters, which is between the fiftieth and seventy-fifth percentile levels. On the Right-Left Discrimination Test, Robert successfully performed all four of the uncrossed commands referring to his own body. Seven-year-olds generally can accomplish this. Of the four crossed commands pertaining to his own body, he succeeded in only one. This is just about normal for children in the 8–9 age bracket. He was not capable of performing correctly any of the uncrossed commands pertaining to the examiner's body (an 11-year-old function) nor was he able to accomplish any of the crossed commands pertaining to the examiner's body (a 12-year-old function). Although Robert's score was just about average here, he did have definite trouble accomplishing the tasks. There were long pauses, ambivalence, and uncertainty about many of his answers. On the Right-Left Discrimination subtest of the Southern California Perceptual-Motor Tests, Robert did not do as well. Robert's raw score was 10, which is 1.1 S.D. below normal for his age. The main reason for his poorer performance on this test was that it is timed, whereas the aforementioned Right-Left Discrimination Test is not. I believe that Robert does have a mild right-left discrimination problem. It is probable that he will ultimately make such distinctions to the normal degree; however, he is much slower in accomplishing such tasks than the normal child and therein lies his deficit.

SUMMARY AND CONCLUSIONS

Robert exhibits a constellation of signs and symptoms that are associated with mild generalized neurophysiological impairment commonly referred to as minimal brain dysfunction. The main clinical manifestations of his disorder are disruptive behavior at home and in the classroom, poor academic performance (especially in reading and spelling), and poor peer relationships. Diagnostic evaluation reveals the following manifestations of MBD: hyperactivity, impairment in the ability to sustain attention; impulsivity; fine and gross motor coordination deficits; dysnomia; dyspraxia; and right-left discrimination impairment. In addition, visual processing deficits in organization, figure-ground discrimination, Gestalt, and short- and long-term visual memory for linguistic and nonlinguistic material are present.

414

The etiology of Robert's disorder cannot be ascertained with certainty. His mother has been a heavy smoker since her teens and smoked an average of over two-and-a-third packages of cigarettes per day during the pregnancy. Smoking of this degree has been implicated as a possible cause of MBD. In addition, during the fifth month of pregnancy the mother suffered with a "viral infection" for one week which was associated with intermittently inaudible fetal heart beat. We cannot be certain whether the fetus was affected by this illness and/or whether the infection was of etiological significance in Robert's disorder. Delivery took place in the eighth month (according to the mother's calculations) and his birth weight was 4 pounds 3 ounces. Incubator care was provided for two weeks and the baby was discharged after three weeks. This is the kind of baby that we would today designate as small for gestational age (SGA). Such babies are more likely than those whose weights are appropriate for gestational age (AGA) to have MBD and other disorders associated with low birth weight.

RECOMMENDATIONS

Robert has demonstrated sensitivity to methylphenidate. His performance on the steadiness tester indicates that a good starting dose would be 10 mg b.i.d. Robert's class placement presents a special problem. His problems are mild in most categories and his overall intelligence is in the high average range. In the verbal-auditory area he is above average to superior. His neurophysiological status then is probably better than that of most youngsters placed in special classes for MBD children. However, Robert is not functioning at this point in his regular classroom. Perhaps his positive response to psychostimulant medication will enable him to remain in a regular classroom situation. If that proves to be the case, then I would suggest that he be given special tutoring by someone specifically trained to teach children with neurologically based learning disabilities. Although secondary psychogenic problems are contributing to Robert's behavioral difficulties, I would not recommend psychotherapy at this point. Perhaps his positive response to psychostimulant medication will obviate the need for psychotherapy. If this does not prove to be the case, it is still preferable to wait and see what symptoms remain before proceeding with psychotherapy.

B Appendix

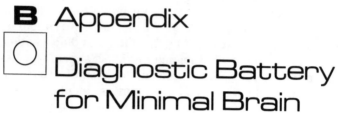

Diagnostic Battery
for Minimal Brain
Dysfunction

Diagnostic Instrument	Primary Information Provided	Additional Information Provided
Steadiness Tester (Gardner)	Hyperactivity Concentration	Motor impersistence Choreiform movements Resting tremors
WISC-R: Coding (Digit Symbol) (Wechsler)	Concentration	Visual memory Visual discrimination Visual-motor coordinati Dyspraxia
Cancellation of Rapidly Recurring Target Figures: Geometric Forms (Rudel et al.)	Concentration	Visual discrimination Visual memory
Cancellation of Rapidly Recurring Target Figures: Numbers (Rudel et al.)	Concentration	Visual discrimination Visual sequential memo
ITPA: Visual Closure (Kirk et al.)	Concentration	Visual Gestalt Visual memory
WISC-R: Mazes (Wechsler)	Impulsivity	Concentration Planning and foresight Visual memory Visual-motor coordinati
Matching Familiar Figures Test (Kagan, Messer)	Impulsivity	Visual discrimination

Diagnostic Instrument	Primary Information Provided	Additional Information Provided
▪nd tally counter (Knights and Moule)	Fine motor coordination	
▪rdue Pegboard (Gardner)	Fine motor coordination	
▪velopmental Test of Visual Perception: Eye-Motor Coordination (Frostig)	Fine motor coordination	Dyspraxia
▪ger-thumb opposition: repetitive and sequential (Denckla)	Fine motor coordination	
▪ot tally counter (Knights and Moule)	Gross motor coordination	
▪petitive foot taps (Denckla)	Gross motor coordination	
▪petitive heel-toe alternating movements (Denckla)	Gross motor coordination	
▪pping on one foot (Denckla)	Gross motor coordination	
▪petitive hand pats (Denckla)	Gross motor coordination	
▪nd flexion-extension movements (Denckla)	Gross motor coordination	
▪rm pronation-supination movements (Denckla)	Gross motor coordination	
▪lls and Basket Test (Gardner)	Gross motor coordination	
▪ncil grasp	Fine motor coordination	Gross motor coordination Grasp development
▪eech articulation (Shank)	Articulation	
▪ysician's Handbook: Screening for MBD: Articulation Screening Test (Peters et al.)	Articulation	
▪lancing on one foot (Denckla)	Motor impersistence	
▪cCarron Assessment of Neuromuscular Development: Foot Balancing (McCarron)	Motor impersistence	
▪uthern California Perceptual-Motor Tests: Standing Balance (Ayres)	Motor impersistence	
▪sts of motor impersistence (Garfield)	Motor impersistence	
▪outh-opening finger-spreading phenomenon (Towen and Prechtl)	Motor overflow	
▪nger stick test (Kinsbourne)	Motor overflow	

Diagnostic Instrument	Primary Information Provided	Additional Information Provided
Tests of motor overflow (Cohen et al.)	Motor overflow	
Screening test for auditory acuity	Auditory acuity	
G-F-W Auditory Selective Attention Test (Goldman, Fristoe, and Woodcock)	Auditory attention	Auditory distractibility
Auditory Discrimination Test (Wepman)	Auditory discrimination	
WISC-R: Digit Span (Digits Forward) (Weschler, Gardner)	Auditory sequential memory	Concentration
ITPA: Sound Blending (Kirk et al.)	Auditory memory	Auditory Gestalt
ITPA: Auditory Closure (Kirk et al.)	Auditory memory	Auditory Gestalt
Denver Developmental Screening Test: Language (Frankenburg and Dodds)	Auditory language	Auditory memory
Peabody Picture Vocabulary Test (Dodds)	Auditory language	Intelligence Auditory memory Visual memory Audio-visual integration
Physician's Handbook: Screening for MBD: Receptive Language (Peters et al.)	Auditory language	Auditory memory
Standard Reading Inventory: Listening Comprehension (McCracken)	Auditory language	Auditory concentration
Audio-Visual Integration Test (Kahn and Birch)	Audio-visual integration	Concentration
Schrier Visual Screening Test (Schrier)	Myopia Hyperopia Phorias Binocularity	Anisometropia Aniseikonia
Colored Progressive Matrices (Raven)	Visual discrimination	Visual conceptualization
Developmental Test of Visual Perception: Form Constancy (Frostig)	Visual discrimination	Concentration
Reversals Frequency Test: Matching (Gardner)	Visual discrimination	
Southern California Figure-Ground Visual Perception Test (Ayres)	Visual figure-ground discrimination	Visual concentration

Diagnostic Instrument	Primary Information Provided	Additional Information Provided
evelopmental Test of Visual Perception: Figure-Ground Discrimination (Frostig)	Visual figure-ground discrimination	Visual concentration
vised Visual Retention Test: Administration A (Benton)	Visual memory	Visual sequential memory
ISC-R: Picture Completion (Wechsler)	Visual memory	Visual concentration Visual Gestalt
ISC-R: Object Assembly (Wechsler)	Visual memory	Visual concentration Visual Gestalt Visual conceptualization Visual organization Persistence
versals Frequency Test: Execution (Gardner)	Visual memory	Dyspraxia
versals Frequency Test: Recognition (Gardner)	Visual memory	
ISC-R: Digit Span (Digits Backward) (Wechsler, Gardner)	Visual sequential memory Auditory memory	Concentration
PA: Visual Sequential Memory (Kirk et al.)	Visual sequential memory	Concentration
ide Range Achievement Test: Spelling (Jastek et al.)	Visual sequential memory	Auditory memory Audio-visual integration
ISC-R: Block Design (Wechsler)	Visual analysis Visual synthesis Visual organization Visual Gestalt	Dyspraxia
evelopmental Test of Visual Perception: Spatial Relations (Frostig)	Visual discrimination Visual organization Visual Gestalt	Dyspraxia
ilmore Oral Reading Test: Comprehension (Gilmore and Gilmore)	Visual language	Visual memory
tandard Reading Inventory: Oral Reading Comprehension and Silent Reading Comprehension (McCracken)	Visual language	Visual memory
ldfield-Wingfield Picture-Naming Test (Oldfield and Wingfield)	Dysnomia	Auditory memory Visual memory Audio-visual integration
apid "Automatized" Naming (Denckla and Rudel)	Dysnomia	Visual memory
PA: Manual Expression (Kirk et al.)	Ideational dyspraxia Ideokinetic dyspraxia	

Diagnostic Instrument	Primary Information Provided	Additional Information Provided
Visual Motor Gestalt Test (Bender, Koppitz)	Constructional dyspraxia	Visual Gestalt Visual discrimination Visual-motor coordinat Visual organization
Revised Visual Retention Test: Administration C (Benton)	Constructional dyspraxia	Visual Gestalt Visual discrimination Visual-motor coordinati Visual organization
WISC-R: 10 subtests (Wechsler)	Intelligence	
WISC-R: Vocabulary (Wechsler)	Intelligence Linguistic learning ability	Auditory memory Visual memory
WISC-R: Information (Wechsler)	Intelligence Fund of information	Intellectual curiosity Auditory memory Visual memory
WISC-R: Similarities (Wechsler)	Intelligence Conceptualization Abstraction	Auditory memory Visual memory
WISC-R: Arithmetic (Wechsler)	Intelligence Conceptualization Abstraction	Auditory memory Visual memory Concentration
Wide Range Achievement Test: Arithmetic (Jastek et al.)	Intelligence Conceptualization Abstraction	Auditory memory Visual memory Concentration
Slosson Intelligence Test (Slosson)	Intelligence	
Draw-A-Person Test (Harris)	Intelligence Body image	Dyspraxia
WISC-R: Comprehension (Wechsler)	Social judgment Common sense	Conscience Auditory memory Visual memory
WISC-R: Picture Arrangement (Wechsler)	Social judgment Common sense Intelligence Visual organization Visual Gestalt Visual sequential memory	Conscience Visual memory
Vineland Social Maturity Scale (Doll)	Social maturity	
Inspection for stigmata and anomalies (Waldrop, Halverson, and Goering)	Stigmata Anomalies	
Height measurement (National Center for Health Statistics)	Height	
Weight measurement (National Center for Health Statistics)	Weight	

Diagnostic Instrument	Primary Information Provided	Additional Information Provided
۰d circumference ۱easurement ۰aine and Oppé)	Head circumference	
۱t-Left Discrimination Test 3enton)	Right-left discrimination	Body image
thern California Perceptual- 1otor Tests: Right-Left ۰iscrimination (Ayres)	Right-left discrimination	Body image

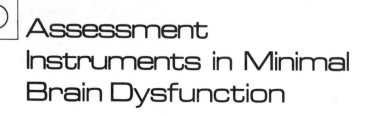

C Appendix

O Assessment Instruments in Minimal Brain Dysfunction

Listed below are the individuals, publishers, manufacturers, and organizations that produce and distribute the tests and other assessment instruments described in this book. These sources, plus the descriptions and data provided in this book, will enable the examiner to administer the complete battery described herein.

G-F-W Auditory Selective Attention Test
Peabody Picture Vocabulary Test
Vineland Social Maturity Scale
    American Guidance Service, Inc.
    Publishers' Building
    Circle Pines, Minnesota 55404

Physician's Handbook: Screening for MBD
    CIBA Medical Horizons
    556 Morris Avenue
    Summit, New Jersey 07901

McCarron Assessment of Neuromuscular Development
    Common Market Press
    Suite 255
    2880 LBJ Freeway
    Dallas, Texas 75234

Developmental Test of Visual Perception
   Consulting Psychologists Press
   577 College Avenue
   Palo Alto, California 94306

Reversals Frequency Test
   Creative Therapeutics
   155 County Road
   Cresskill, New Jersey 07626

Wide Range Achievement Test
   Guidance Associates of Delaware, Inc.
   1526 Gilpin Avenue
   Wilmington, Delaware 19806

Gilmore Oral Reading Test
   Harcourt Brace Jovanovich, Inc.
   757 Third Avenue
   New York, New York 10017

Matching Familiar Figures Test
   Jerome Kagan, Ph.D.
   William James Hall
   Harvard University
   33 Kirkland Street
   Cambridge, Massachusetts 02138

Standard Reading Inventory
   Klamath Printing Co.
   Klamath Falls, Oregon 97601

Gardner Steadiness Tester (Cat. No. 32019)
Purdue Pegboard (Cat. No. 32020)
   Lafayette Instrument Co.
   P.O. Box 1279
   Lafayette, Indiana 47902

Auditory Discrimination Test
   Language Research Associates, Inc.
   P.O. Box 2085
   Palm Springs, California 92262

Denver Developmental Screening Test
   Project and Publishing Foundation, Inc.
   East 51st Avenue and Lincoln
   Denver, Colorado 80216
   Also:
   Mead Johnson Laboratories
   2404 West Pennsylvania Street
   Evansville, Indiana 47221

Coloured Progressive Matrices
Revised Visual Retention Test
Wechsler Intelligence Scale for Children-Revised
   The Psychological Corp.
   757 Third Avenue
   New York, New York 10017

Schrier Vision Screening Test
    Dr. Melvin Schrier
    11 East 74th Street
    New York, New York 10021

Slosson Intelligence Test
    Slosson Educational Publications
    140 Pine Street
    East Aurora, New York 14052

Balls and Basket Test (basket only, cat. no. 1056)
    Sterlite Corp.
    Townsend, Massachusetts 01469

Southern California Figure-Ground Visual Perception Test
Southern California Perceptual-Motor Tests
    Western Psychological Services
    12031 Wilshire Boulevard
    Los Angeles, California 90025

Illinois Test of Psycholinguistic Abilities
    University of Illinois Press
    University of Illinois
    Urbana, Illinois 61801

☐ References

Abbott, C. (1882), The intelligence of batrachians. *Science*, 3:66–67.

Abercrombie, M., Lindon, R., and Tyson, M. (1964), Associated movement in normal and physically handicapped children. *Developmental Medicine and Child Neurology*, 6:573–580.

Abraham, K. (1927), *Selected Papers on Psychoanalysis*. London: Hogarth Press.

Ackerman, P. T., Peters, J. E., and Dykman, R. A. (1971), Children with specific learning disabilities: WISC profiles. *Journal of Learning Disabilities*, 4:150–166.

American Academy of Ophthalmology and the American Academy of Pediatrics (1972), The eye and learning disabilities: a joint organization statement. *Journal of School Health*, 42:218.

Anapolle, L. (1971), A profile of a visual dyslexic. *American Journal of Optometry and Archives of American Academy of Optometry*, 48(5):390.

Apgar, V. (1953), A proposal for a new method of evaluation of the newborn infant. *Anesthesia and Analgesia*, 32:260.

———— Holaday, D. A., James, L. S., Weisbrot, I. M., and Berrien, C. (1958), Evaluation of the newborn infant: second report. *Journal of the American Medical Association*, 168:1985–1988.

Ayres, A. J. (1968), *Southern California Perceptual-Motor Tests*. Los Angeles: Western Psychological Services.

Barsley, M. (1970), *Left-handed Man in a Right-handed World*. London: Pitman.

Bell, R. Q. (1968), Adaptation of small wrist watches for mechanical recording of activity in infants and children. *Journal of Experimental Child Psychology*, 6:302–305.

——— Waldrop, M. F., and Weller, G. M. (1972), A rating system for the assessment of hyperactive and withdrawn children in preschool samples. *American Journal of Orthopsychiatry*, 42:23–34.

Belmont, L. and Birch, H. G. (1965), Lateral dominance, lateral awareness, and reading disability. *Child Development*, 36:57–71.

Bender, L. (1938), *A Visual Motor Gestalt Test and Its Clinical Use*. Research Monograph No. 3. New York: American Orthopsychiatric Association.

——— (1946), *Bender Motor Gestalt Test: Cards and Manual of Instructions*. New York: American Orthopsychiatric Association.

——— (1947), Clinical Study of 100 schizophrenic children. *American Journal of Orthopsychiatry*, 17:40–56.

Benson, D. F. and Geschwind, N. (1968), Cerebral dominance and its disturbances. *Pediatric Clinics of North America*, 15:759–769.

Benton, A. L. (1955), *The Revised Visual Retention Test: Clinical and Experimental Applications*. New York: Psychological Corporation.

——— (1959), *Right-Left Discrimination and Finger Localization*. New York: Harper & Brothers.

——— (1966), Language disorders in children. *The Canadian Psychologist*, 7:298–312.

——— (1968), Right-left discrimination. *Pediatric Clinics of North America*, 15:747–758.

——— (1970), Neuropsychological aspects of mental retardation. *The Journal of Special Education*, 4:3–11.

——— (1973), Minimal brain dysfunction from a neuropsychological point of view. *Annals of the New York Academy of Sciences*, 205:29–37.

——— (1976), Personal communication.

——— and Van Allan, M. W. (1972), Prosopagnosia and facial discrimination. *Journal of the Neurological Sciences*, 15:167–172.

Bernstein, J. E., Page, J. G., and Janicki, R. S. (1974), Some characteristics of children with minimal brain dysfunction. In: *Clinical Use of Stimulant Drugs in Children*, ed. C. K. Conners. Amsterdam: Excerpta Medica, pp. 24–35.

Birch, H. and Lefford A. (1964), Two strategies for studying perception in "brain-damaged" children. In: *Brain Damage in Children*, ed. H. G. Birch. New York: The Williams & Wilkins Co., pp. 46–60.

Birnbaum, M. H. (1973), The therapeutic use of lenses—functional prescribing. *Optometric Journal and Review of Optometry*, 110(21):23–29.

Blair, F. X., *Blair Language Evaluation Scales*. Milwaukee, Wisconsin: Department of Exceptional Education, The University of Wisconsin-Milwaukee.

Blakemore, C. B. (1969), Binocular depth discrimination and the nasotemporal division. *Journal of Psychology*, 205:471–497.

Blakiston's New Gould Medical Dictionary (1951). Philadelphia: The Blakiston Co.

Boies, L. R. (1954), *Fundamentals of Otolaryngology*. Philadelphia: W. B. Saunders Co.

Bortner, M. and Birch, H. (1960), Perception and perceptual-motor dissociation in cerebral palsied children. *Journal of Nervous and Mental Diseases*, 130:49–53.

Brain, W. and Wilkinson, M. (1959), Observations on the extensor plantar reflex and its relationship to the functions of the pyramidal tract. *Brain*, 82:297-320.

Briggs, P. and Tellegen, A. (1971), Development of the manual accuracy and speed test (MAST). *Perceptual and Motor Skills*, 32:923-943.

Brock, S. (1945), *The Basis of Clinical Neurology*. Baltimore: The Williams & Wilkins Co.

Brown, G. L. (1977), Studies done at the Unit on Childhood Mental Illness, Biological Psychiatry Branch, National Institute of Mental Health. Bethesda, Maryland (personal communication).

Brutten, M., Richardson, S., and Mangel, C. (1973), *Something's Wrong with my Child*. New York: Harcourt Brace Jovanovich, Inc.

Burian, H. M., Walsh, R., and Bannon, R. E. (1946), Note on the incidence of clinically significant aniseikonia. *American Journal of Opthalmology*, 29(2):201-203.

Burman, M. L. (1959), Vision screening of preschool children in Prince George's County, Maryland, nursery schools. *Journal of the National Medical Association*, 61(4):352-353.

Burt, C. L. (1957), *The Backward Child*. London: University of London Press.

Betts, E. A. (1946), *Foundations of Reading Instruction*. New York: American Book Co., p. 187.

Cantwell, D. P. (1975a), A medical model for research and clinical use with hyperactive children. In: *The Hyperactive Child*, ed. D. P. Cantwell, New York: Spectrum Publications, Inc. (a division of John Wiley and Sons), pp. 193-205.

———(1975b), A critical review of therapeutic modalities with hyperactive children. In: *The Hyperactive Child*, ed. D. P. Cantwell. New York: Spectrum Publications, Inc. (a division of John Wiley and Sons), pp. 173-189.

———(1975c), Familial-genetic research with hyperactive children. In: *The Hyperactive Child*, ed. D. P. Cantwell. New York: Spectrum Publications, Inc. (a division of John Wiley and Sons), pp. 93-105.

———(1977), Hyperactive syndrome. In: *Recent Advances in Child Psychiatry*, ed. M. Rutter and L. Hersov. London: Blackwell. pp. 524-555.

Carter, D. (1967), Lecture on Learning Disabilities. San Diego, California: California Optometric Association Post-Graduate Courses.

Castner, B. M. (1940), Language development. In: *The First Five Years of Life*, ed. A. Gesell et al. New York: Harper and Row, p. 235.

Chalfant, J. and Scheffelin, N. (1969), *Central Processing Dysfunctions in Children: A Review of Research*. National Institute of Neurological Disease and Stroke, Monograph No. 9. Washington, D.C.: U.S. Government Printing Office.

Chamberlin, R. W. (1976), The use of teacher checklists to identify children at risk for later behavioral and emotional problems. *American Journal of Diseases of Children*, 130:141-145.

Charlton, M. (1973), *Clinical Aspects of Minimal Brain Dysfunction*. (one hour cassette tape). Behavioral Sciences Tape Library. Teaneck, New Jersey: Sigma Information, Inc.

Cohen, H., Taft, L., Mahadeviah, M., and Birch, H. (1967), Developmental changes in overflow in normal and aberrantly functioning children. The Journal of Pediatrics, 71:39–47.

Cohen, J. (1959), The factorial structure of the WISC at ages 7½, 10½, and 13½. Journal of Consulting Psychology, 23:149–154.

Colburn, T. R., Smith, B. M., Guarini, J. J., and Simmons, N. N. (1976), An ambulatory activity monitor with solid state memory. Instrument Society of America Transactions, 15(2):149–154.

Conners, C. K. (1969), A teacher rating scale for use in drug studies with children. American Journal of Psychiatry, 126:884–888.

—— (1970), Symptom patterns in hyperkinetic, neurotic, and normal children. Child Development, 41:667–682.

—— (1973), Parents' Questionnaire. Psychopharmacology Bulletin, pp. 231–234. Department of Health, Education, and Welfare Publication No. (HSM) 73-9002. Washington, D.C.: U.S. Government Printing Office.

—— (ed.) (1974), Clinical Use of Stimulant Drugs in Children. The Hague: Excerpta Medica. (Distributed by Abbott Laboratories, North Chicago, Illinois.)

—— (1976), CIBA Medical Horizons Conference on Minimal Brain Dysfunction. New York City, November 6, 1976.

Corballis, M. C. and Beale, I. L. (1976), The Psychology of Left and Right. New York: John Wiley and Sons.

Costa, L. D. (1975), The relation of visuospatial dysfunction to digit span performance in patients with cerebral lesions. Cortex, 11:31–36.

—— Scarola, L. M., and Rapin, I. (1964), Purdue pegboard scores for normal grammar school children. Perceptual and Motor Skills, 18:748.

Critchley, M. (1953), The Parietal Lobes. London: Arnold.

—— (1970), The Dyslexic Child. London: William Heinemann Medical Books Limited.

Cromwell, R. L., Baumeister, A., & Hawkins, W. F. (1963), Research in activity level. In: Handbook of Mental Deficiency, ed. N. R. Ellis. New York: McGraw-Hill, pp. 632–663.

Cruickshank, W. M., Bentzen, F. A., Ratzeburg, F. H., and Tannhauser, M. T. (1961), A Teaching Method for Brain Injured and Hyperactive Children. Syracuse, N.Y.: Syracuse University Press.

Curry, F.K.W. (1967), A comparison of left-handed and right-handed subjects on verbal and non-verbal dichotic listening tasks. Cortex, 3:343–352.

Dalton, M. M. (1943), A visual survey of 5000 school children. Journal of Educational Research, 37:81–94.

Davids, A. (1971), An objective instrument for assessing hyperkinesis in children. Journal of Learning Disabilities, 4:499–501.

Davidson, H. (1935), A study of the confusing letters b,d,p, and q. Journal of Genetic Psychology, 47:458–468.

Davis, K., Sprague, R., and Werry, J. (1969), Stereotyped behavior and activity level in severe retardates: the effect of drugs. American Journal of Mental Deficiency, 72:721–727.

Dearborn, W. F. and Anderson, I. W. (1938), Aniseikonia as related to disability in reading. *Journal of Experimental Psychology*, 23:559.

de Hirsch, K. (1965), The concept of plasticity and language disabilities. *Speech Pathology and Therapy*, 8:12–17.

———— (1974), Early language development. In: *American Handbook of Psychiatry*, ed. S. Arieti, 2nd edit., Vol. I. New York: Basic Books, Inc., pp. 352–367.

———— (1975), Language deficits in children with developmental lags. *Psychoanalytic Study of the Child*, 30:95–126.

Denckla, M. B. (1972), Performance on color tasks in kindergarten children. *Cortex*, 8:177–190.

———— (1973), Development of speed in repetitive and successive finger-movements in normal children. *Developmental Medicine and Child Neurology*, 15:635–645.

———— (1974), Development of motor coordination in normal children. *Developmental Medicine and Child Neurology*, 16:729–741.

———— (1976), Dyslexia: a neurologist's perspective. In: *Developmental Dyslexia*, ed. R. Spector. Springfield, Illinois: Charles C. Thomas.

———— (1976), Personal communication.

———— and Rudel, R. (1974), Rapid "automatized" naming of pictured objects, colors, letters, and numbers by normal children. *Cortex*, 10:186–202.

———— ———— (1976), Naming of object-drawings by dyslexic and other learning disabled children. *Brain and Language*, 3:1–15.

———— ————, Anomalies of motor development in hyperactive boys without traditional neurological signs. (unpublished manuscript)

Denton, F. W. and Dorland, H. G., Vertical latent deviations, *Optometric Weekly*, June 3, 1954, pp. 929–934; June 24, 1954, pp. 1043–1049; Aug. 5, 1954, pp. 1223–1227; Aug. 19, 1954, pp. 1305–1309, Aug. 26, 1954, pp. 1347–1351; Dec. 2, 1954, pp. 1931–1935; April 21, 1955, pp. 647–651.

Denhoff, E. (1973), Natural life history of children with MBD. *Annals of the New York Academy of Sciences*, 205:188–205.

Diagnostic and Statistical Manual (DSM-III). Washington, D.C.: American Psychiatric Association.

Diller, L. and Birch, H. (1964), Psychological evaluation of children with cerebral damage. In: *Brain Damage in Children*, ed. H. G. Birch. New York: The Williams & Wilkins Co., pp. 27–45.

Doll, E. A. (1965), *Vineland Social Maturity Scale*. Circle Pines, Minnesota: American Guidance Service, Inc.

Douglas, V. I. (1972), Stop, look and listen: The problem of sustained attention and impulse control in hyperactive and normal children. *Canadian Journal of Behavioral Science*, 4:259–282.

———— (1974a), Sustained attention and impulse control: Implications for the handicapped child. In: *Psychology and the Handicapped Child*, ed. J. A. Swets and L. L. Elliott. Washington, D.C.: U.S. Department of Health, Education, and Welfare. DHEW Pub. No. (OE)73-05000.

———— (1974b), Differences between normal and hyperkinetic children. In: *Clinical Use of Stimulant Drugs in Children*, ed. C. R. Conners, North Chicago, Illinois: Abbott Laboratories, pp. 12–23.

———(1975), Are drugs enough?—To treat or to train the hyperactive child. *International Journal of Mental Health*, 4:199-212.

Duke-Elder, W. S. (1935), *The Practice of Refraction*, 2nd edit. Philadelphia: P. Blakiston's Son & Co., pp. 177-178.

Duncan, D. B. (1955), Multiple range and multiple F-tests. *Biometrics*, 11:1-42.

Dunn, L. M. (1965), *Peabody Picture Vocabulary Test*. Circle Pines, Minnesota: American Guidance Service, Inc.

Dunphy, E. B., Stoll, M. R., and King, S. H. (1968), Myopia among American male graduate students. *American Journal of Ophthalmology*, 65(4):518-521.

Durfee, K. E. (1974), Crooked ears and the bad boy syndrome: asymmetry as an indicator of minimal brain dysfunction. *Bulletin of the Menninger Clinic*, 38:305-316.

Dvorine, I. (1953), *Pseudo-Isochromatic Plates*, ed. Section Two, 8 auxiliary plates (trails). New York: Harcourt, Brace and World, Inc.

Dykman, R., Ackerman, P. T., Clements, S. D., and Peters, J. E. (1971), Specific learning disabilities: An attentional deficit syndrome. In: *Progress in Learning Disabilities*, Vol. II, ed. H. Mykelbust. New York: Grune & Stratton.

——— ———, Peters, J. E., and McGrew, J. (1974), Psychological tests. In: *Clinical Use of Stimulant Drugs in Children*, ed. C. K. Conners. Amsterdam: Excerpta Medica, pp. 44-52.

Eames, T. H. (1938), The ocular condition of 350 poor readers. *Journal of Educational Research*, 32:10-16.

———(1955), The influence of hyperopia and myopia in reading achievements. *American Journal of Ophthalmology*, 39:375-377.

———(1964), The effect of anisometropia on reading achievement. *American Journal of Optometry and Archives of American Academy of Optometry*, 41(11):700-702.

Eisenberg, L. (1973), The overactive child. *Hospital Practice*, 8:151-160.

Ellis, N. R. and Pryer, R. S. (1959), Quantification of gross bodily activity in children with severe neuropathology. *American Journal of Mental Deficiency*, 63:1034-1037.

Escalona, S. and Stone, L. (1968), Normal development: personality and behavior. In: *Pediatrics*, ed. H. Barnett, New York: Appleton-Century-Crofts.

Farris, L. P. (1936), Visual defects as factors influencing achievement in reading. *Journal of Experimental Education*, 5:58-60.

Feinberg, R. (1959), Bifocals for children—a survey. *Optometric Weekly*, October 15, 1959, pp. 2055-2058.

Fink, Walter H. (1953), Etiological considerations of vertical muscle defects. *American Journal of Ophthalmology*, 36(11): 1551-1568.

Fish, B. (1975), Stimulant drug treatment of hyperactive children. In: *The Hyperactive Child*, ed. D. P. Cantwell. New York: Spectrum Publications, Inc. (a division of John Wiley & Sons), pp. 109-127.

Fisher, M. (1956), Left hemiplegia and motor impersistence. *Journal of Nervous and Mental Diseases*, 123:201-218.

Flavell, J. (1961), *The Developmental Psychology of Jean Piaget*. New York: Van Nostrand.

Fliess, R. (1956), *Erogeneity and Libido*. New York: International Universities Press, Inc.

Forness, S. (1975), Educational approaches with hyperactive children. In: *The Hyperactive Child*, ed. D. P. Cantwell. New York: Spectrum Publications, Inc. (a division of John Wiley & Sons), pp. 159–172.

Foshee, J. G. (1958), Studies in activity level. I. Simple and complex task performance in defectives. *American Journal of Mental Deficiency*, 62:882–886.

Frankenberg, W. K. and Dodds, J. B. (1969), *Denver Developmental Screening Test*. Denver, Colorado: Project and Publishing Foundation, Inc.

Friedman, N. (1971), Concepts of dyslexia and the role of fixation skills. *The Optical Journal and Review of Optometry*, 108(1):20–27.

Frostig, M. (1961), *Developmental Test of Visual Perception*. Palo Alto, California: Consulting Psychologists Press.

Gainotti, G. (1972), Emotional behavior and hemispheric side of the lesion. *Cortex*, 8:41–55.

Garcia, J. (1972), I.Q.: the conspiracy. *Psychology Today*, 6(4):40ff.

Gardner, R. A. (1968), Psychogenic problems of brain-injured children and their parents. *Journal of the American Academy of Child Psychiatry*, 7:471–491.

——— (1969), The guilt reaction of parents of children with severe physical disease. *American Journal of Psychiatry*, 126:636–644.

——— (1970), A four-day diagnostic-therapeutic home visit in Turkey. *Family Process*, 9(3):301–331.

——— (1971a), *Therapeutic Communication with Children: The Mutual Storytelling Technique*. New York: Jason Aronson, Inc.

——— (1971b), A proposed scale for the determination of maternal feeling. *The Psychiatric Quarterly*, 45:23–34.

——— (1972), *The Diagnosis and Treatment of Minimal Brain Dysfunction* (6 one-hour cassette tapes). Teaneck, New Jersey: Behavioral Sciences Tape Library.

——— (1973a), *MBD: The Family Book About Minimal Brain Dysfunction*. New York: Jason Aronson, Inc.

——— (1973b), Psychotherapy of the psychogenic problems secondary to minimal brain dysfunction. *International Journal of Child Psychotherapy*, 2:224–256.

——— (1974a), The mutual storytelling technique in the treatment of psychogenic problems secondary to minimal brain dysfunction. *Journal of Learning Disabilities*, 7:135–143.

——— (1974b), Psychotherapy of minimal brain dysfunction. In: *Current Psychiatric Therapies*, ed. J. Masserman, Vol. XIV. New York: Grune & Stratton, pp. 15–21.

——— (1975a), *Psychotherapeutic Approaches to the Resistant Child*. New York: Jason Aronson, Inc.

——— (1975b), Techniques for involving the child with MBD in meaningful psychotherapy. *Journal of Learning Disabilities*, 8:16–26.

——— (1975c), Psychotherapy in minimal brain dysfunction. In: *Current Psychiatric Therapies*, ed. J. Masserman, Vol. XV. New York: Grune & Stratton, pp. 25–38.

———(1975d), Dr. Gardner Talks to Children with Minimal Brain Dysfunction (one-hour cassette tape). Psychotherapy Tape Library. New York: Jason Aronson, Inc.

———(1975e), Dr. Gardner Talks to Parents of Children with MBD (one-hour cassette tape). Psychotherapy Tape Library. New York: Jason Aronson, Inc.

———(1978), Reversals Frequency Test. Cresskill, New Jersey: Creative Therapeutics.

———(1979), Throwing balls in a basket as a test of motor coordination: normative data on 1350 school children. Journal of Clinical Child Psychology (in press).

———and Broman, M. (1979a), The Purdue Pegboard: normative data on 1334 school children. Journal of Clinical Child Psychology (in press).

——— ———(1979b), Letter reversals frequency in normal and MBD children. Journal of Clinical Child Psychology (in press).

———Gardner, A. K., Caemmerer, A., and Broman, M. (1979), An instrument for measuring hyperactivity and other signs of minimal brain dysfunction. Journal of Clinical Child Psychology (in press).

Gardner, W. I., Cromwell, R. L., and Foshee, J. G. (1959), Studies in activity level: II. Effects of distal visual stimulation in organics, familials, hyperactives, and hypoactives. American Journal of Mental Deficiency, 63:1028–1033.

Garfield, J. C. (1964), Motor impersistence in normal and brain-damaged children. Neurology, 14:623–630.

———Benton, A., and MacQueen, J. (1966), Motor impersistence in brain-damaged and cultural-familial defectives. The Journal of Nervous and Mental Disability, 142:434–440.

Gates, A. I. (1949), The Improvement of Reading. New York: The Macmillan Co.

———and Bond, G. L. (1936), Relation of handedness, eyesighting, anxiety, and dominance to reading. Journal of Educational Psychology, 27:450–456.

Geschwind, N. (1965a), Disconnexion syndromes in animals and man, Part I. Brain, 88:237–294.

———(1965b), Disconnexion syndromes in animals and man, Part II. Brain, 88:585–644.

———(1971), Aphasia. New England Journal of Medicine, 284(12): 654–656.

———(1972), Language and the Brain. Scientific American, 226(4):76–83.

Gesell, A. (1940), The First Five Years of Life. New York: Harper and Row, Publishers.

———and Amatruda, C. S. (1947), Developmental Diagnosis. New York: Paul B. Hoeber, Inc.

———and Ilg, F. L. (1946), The Child From Five to Ten. New York: Harper and Row, Publishers.

——— ———and Bullis, G. E. (1950), Vision, its Development in Infant and Child. New York: Harper & Bros.

Gibson, E. J., Gibson, J. J., Pick, A. D., and Osser, H. (1962), A developmental study of the discrimination of letter-like forms. Journal of Comparative Physiological Psychology, 55:897–906.

Gilkey, B. and Parr, F. (1944), An analysis of the reversal tendencies of fifty selected elementary school pupils. *Journal of Educational Psychology,* 35:284-292.

Gilmore, J. V. and Gilmore, E. C. (1968), *The Gilmore Oral Reading Test.* New York: Harcourt Brace Jovanovich, Inc.

Ginsberg, G. P. and Hartwick, A. (1971), Directional confusion as a sign of dyslexia. *Perceptual & Motor Skills,* 32:535-543.

Glasser, A. and Zimmerman, I. (1967), *Clinical Interpretation of Wechsler Intelligence Scale for Children.* New York: Grune & Stratton.

Gold, A. (1976), The developmental neurologic examination. *Clinical Psychiatry News,* 4(11):8.

Goldman, R., Fristoe, M., and Woodcock, W. (1974), *Auditory Selective Attention Test.* Circle Pines, Minnesota: American Guidance Service, Inc.

Goldstein, K. (1952), The effect of brain damage on the personality. *Psychiatry,* 15:245-260.

Goodenough, F. (1926), *Measurement of Intelligence by Drawings.* New York: World Book Co.

Goodglass, H. and Kaplan, E. (1972), *The Assessment of Aphasia and Related Disorders.* Philadelphia: Lea and Febiger.

Haber, R. N. (1974), Visual perception. In: *Psychology and the Handicapped Child.* U.S. Department of Health, Education and Welfare Publication No. (OE) 73-05000. Washington, D.C.: U.S. Government Printing Office, pp. 40-72.

Hardyck, C. and Petrinovich, L. F. (1977), Left-handedness. *Psychological Bulletin,* 84:385-404.

Harris, A. J. (1957), Lateral dominance, directional confusion, and reading disability. *The Journal of Psychology,* 44:283-294.

———— (1958), *Harris Tests of Lateral Dominance.* New York: The Psychological Corp.

Harris, D. B. (1963), *Children's Drawings as Measures of Intellectual Maturity.* New York: Harcourt, Brace and World, Inc.

Harris, D. H. (1974), Accommodative-convergence control in myopia reduction. *Journal of the American Optometric Association,* 45(3):292-296.

Hayden, R. (1941), Development—prevention of myopia at the U.S. Naval Academy. *Archives of Ophthalmology,* 25:539.

Heilman, K., Scholes, R., and Watson, R. (1975), Auditory affective agnosia. *Journal of Neurology, Neurosurgery, and Psychiatry,* 38:69-72.

Herron, R. E. and Ramsden, R. W. (1967a), A telepedometer for remote measurement of human locomotor activity. *Psychophysiology,* 4:112-115.

———— ———— (1967b), Continuous monitoring of overt human body movement by radio telemetry: A brief review. *Perceptual and Motor Skills,* 24:1303-1308.

Hildreth, G. (1950a), The development and training of hand dominance: IV. Developmental problems associated with handedness. *Journal of Genetic Psychology,* 76:39-100.

———— (1950b), The development and training of hand dominance: V. Training of handedness. *Journal of Genetic Psychology,* 76:101-144.

Hinsie, L. E. and Shatzky, J. (1953), *Psychiatric Dictionary*. New York: Oxford University Press.

Ilg, F. and Ames, L. (1965), *School Readiness*. New York: Harper and Row.

Imus, H. A., Rothney, J. W., and Bear, R. M. (1938), *An Evaluation of Visual Factors in Reading*. Hanover, New Hampshire: Dartmouth College Publications.

Ingram, T. (1973), Soft signs. *Developmental Medicine and Child Neurology*, 15:527–530.

Ireland, W. W. (1881), On mirror-writing and its relation to left-handedness and cerebral disease. *Brain*, 4:361–367.

Irwin, O. C. (1930), The amount and nature of activities of newborn infants under constant external stimulating conditions during the first ten days of life. *Genetic Psychology Monographs*, 8:1–92.

————(1932), The amount of motility of seventy-three newborn infants. *Journal of Comparative Psychology*, 14:415–428.

Ivey, R. (1969), Test of central nervous system auditory function. Unpublished master's thesis. Fort Collins, Colorado: Colorado State University.

Jackson, T. and Schye, V. (1945), A comparison of vision and reading survey of ninth grade students. *Elementary School Teacher*, 46:33–35.

Jacques, L. (1957), Hyperphoria testing—A consistent inconsistency. *Optometric Weekly*, January 3, 1957, pp. 11–15.

Jansky, J. and de Hirsch, K. (1972), *Preventing Reading Failure*. New York: Harper & Row, Publishers.

Jastak, J. F. and Jastak, S. R. (1976), *The Wide Range Achievement Test*, revised ed. Wilmington, Delaware: Guidance Associates.

Jenkins, J. R., Gorrafa, S., and Griffiths, S. (1972), Another look at isolation effects. *American Journal of Mental Deficiency*, 76:591–593.

Jens, D. (1970), *Project Genesis Final Report*. U.S. Educational Resources Information Center, Document No. 049-820. Washington, D.C.: U.S. Government Printing Office.

Johnson, C. (1971), Hyperactivity and the machine: the actometer. *Child Development*, 42:2105–2110.

————(1972), Limits on the measurement of activity level in children using ultrasound and photoelectric cells. *American Journal of Mental Deficiency*, 77:301–310.

Johnson, D. and Myklebust, H. (1967), *Learning Disabilities: Educational Principles and Practices*. New York: Grune & Stratton.

Kagan, J. (1964), *The Matching Familiar Figures Test*. Cambridge, Massachusetts: Harvard University.

Kahn, D. and Birch, H. G. (1968), Development of auditory-visual integration and reading achievement. *Perceptual and Motor Skills*, 27:159–168.

Katz, J. (1977), The Staggered Spondaic Word Test. In: *Central Auditory Dysfunction*, ed. R. W. Keith. New York: Grune & Stratton, pp. 103–127.

Kawi, A. A. and Pasamanick, B. (1958), Association of factors of pregnancy with reading disorders in childhood. *Journal of American Medical Association*, 166:1420–1423.

———— ———— (1959), Prenatal and paranatal factors in the development of childhood reading disorders. *Monograph of the Society for Research in Child Development*, 24(4):1–80.

Keith, R. W. (1977), *Central Auditory Dysfunction*. New York: Grune & Stratton.

Kelly, C. R. (1957), *Visual Screening and Child Development*. Raleigh, North Carolina: Department of Psychiatry, North Carolina State College.

Kessen, W., Hendry, L. S., and Leutzendorff, A. (1961), Measurement of movement in the human newborn. *Child Development*, 32:95–105.

Kimura, D. (1963), Speech lateralization in young children as determined by an auditory test. *Journal of Comparative Physiological Psychology*, 56:899–902.

———— (1964), Left-right differences in the perception of melodies. *Quarterly Journal of Experimental Psychology*, 16:355–358.

Kinsbourne, M. (1973), School problems. *Pediatrics*, 52:697–710.

———— (1973), Minimal brain dysfunction as a neurodevelopmental lag. *Annals of the N.Y. Academy of Sciences*, 205:268–273.

———— (1975), The hyperactive and impulsive child. *Ontario Medial Review*, December 1975, pp. 657–660.

———— (1976a), Looking and listening strategies and beginning reading. In: *Aspects of Reading Acquisition*, ed. J. T. Guthrie. Baltimore: Johns Hopkins University Press.

———— (1976b), CIBA Medical Horizon MBD Conference. New York City, December 1976.

Kirk, S. A., McCarthy, J. J., and Kirk, W. D. (1968), *The Illinois Test of Psycholinguistic Abilities*, rev. edit. Urbana, Illinois: University of Illinois Press.

———— and Parastevopoulos, J. N. (1969), *The Development and Psychometric Characteristics of the Revised Illinois Test of Psycholinguistic Abilities*. Chicago: University of Illinois Press.

Klein, D. F. and Gittelman-Klein, R. (1974), Diagnosis of minimal brain dysfunction and hyperkinetic syndrome. In: *Clinical Use of Stimulant Drugs in Children*, ed. C. K. Conners. North Chicago, Illinois: Abbott Laboratories, pp. 1–11.

Knights, R. M. (1966), Normative data on tests for evaluating brain damage in children from 5 to 14 years of age. Research Bulletin No. 20, Department of Psychology. London, Canada: University of Western Ontario.

———— (1970), *Smoothed Normative Data on Tests for Evaluating Brain Damage in Children*. Publication of the Department of Psychology. Ottawa, Ontario: Carleton University.

———— (1973), *The Effects of Cerebral Lesions on the Psychological Test Performance of Children*. Final Report, Ontario Mental Health Foundation, Grant No. 53.

———— and Moule, A. (1967), Normative and reliability data on finger and foot tapping in children. *Perceptual and Motor Skills*, 25:717–720.

———— ———— (1968), Normative data on the Motor Steadiness Battery for children. *Perceptual and Motor Skills*, 26:643–650.

———— and Ogilvie, R. (1967), A comparison of test results from normal and brain damaged children. Research Bulletin No. 53. London, Canada: Department of Psychology. The University of Western Ontario.

Knobloch, H. and Pasamanick, B. (1966), Prospective studies on the epidemiology of reproductive casualty. *Merrill-Palmer Quarterly of Behavior and Development*, 12:27–43.

Koppitz, E. M. (1964), *The Bender Gestalt Test for Young Children*. New York: Grune & Stratton.

——(1968), *Psychological Evaluation of Children's Human Figure Drawings*. New York: Grune & Stratton.

——(1975), *The Bender Gestalt Test for Young Children*, Vol. II. New York: Grune & Stratton.

Krimsky, E. (1948), *The Management of Binocular Imbalance*. Philadelphia: Lea & Febiger.

Kronick, D. (1973), *A Word or Two about Learning Disabilities*. San Rafael, California: Academic Therapy Publications.

Lebensohn, J. E. (1957), The management of anisometropia. *American Orthoptic Journal*, pp. 121–128.

Lee, D. and Hutt, C. (1964), A play-room designed for filming children: a note. *Journal of Child Psychology and Psychiatry*, 5:263–265.

Leisman, G. (1976), *Basic Visual Processes and Learning Disability*. Springfield, Illinois: Charles C. Thomas, pp. 151–162.

Leuba, C. (1955), Toward some integration of learning theories. The concept of optimal stimulation. *Psychological Reports*, 1:27–33.

Leverett, H. M. (1955), A school vision health study in Danbury, Connecticut. *American Journal of Ophthalmology*, 39(4):527–540.

Lezak, M. D. (1976), *Neuropsychological Assessment*. New York: Oxford University Press.

Liberman, I., Shankweiler, D., Orlando, C., Harris, K., and Berti, F. (1971), Letter confusions and reversals of sequence in the beginning reader: implications for Orton's theory of developmental dyslexia. *Cortex*, 7:127–142.

Lipsitt, L. P. and DeLucia, C. (1960), An apparatus for the measurement of specific responses and general activity of the human neonate. *American Journal of Psychology*, 73:630–632.

Ludlam, W. M. (1961), Orthoptic treatment of strabismus. *American Journal of Optometry and Archives of American Academy of Optometry*, 38(7):369–388.

Lyle, J. and Goyen, J. (1968), Visual recognition, developmental lag, and strephosymbolia in reading retardation. *Journal of Abnormal Psychology*, 73:25–29.

McCarron, L. T. (1976), *McCarron Assessment of Neuromuscular Development*. Dallas, Texas: Common Market Press.

McCracken, R. A. (1966), *Standard Reading Inventory*. Klamath Falls, Oregon: Klamath Printing Co.

McKee, G. W. (1972), Vision screening of preschool and school age children: the need for re-evaluation. *Journal of the American Optometric Association*, 43(10):1062–1073.

Mackover, K. (1949), *Personality Projection in the Drawing of the Human Figure*. Springfield, Illinois: Charles C. Thomas.

Makita, K. (1968), The rarity of reading disability in Japanese children. *American Journal of Orthopsychiatry*, 38:599–614.

Melkin, M. (1960), The controversial subject of bifocals in myopia. *The Optical Journal and Review of Optometry,* May 1, 1960, 35–36.

Messer, S. B. (1976), Reflection-impulsivity: a review. *Psychological Bulletin,* 83:1026–1052.

Money, J. (1962), Dyslexia: a postconference review. In: *Reading Disability,* ed. J. Money. Baltimore: Johns Hopkins Press.

Montagu, J. D. and Swarbrick, L. (1974), Hyperkinesis: The objective evaluation of therapeutic procedures. *Biological Psychology,* 2:151–155.

National Center for Health Statistics: NCHS Growth Charts (1976), *Monthly Vital Statistics Report,* Vol. 25, No. 3, Supp. (HRA) 76–1120. Rockville, Maryland: National Center for Health Statistics. (These charts may also be obtained from Ross Laboratories of Columbus, Ohio.)

Newcombe, F., Oldfield, R. C., Ratcliff, G. G., and Wingfield, A. (1971), Recognition and naming of object-drawings by men with focal brain wounds. *Journal of Neurology, Neurosurgery, and Psychiatry,* 34:329–340.

Newland, J. (1972), Children's Knowledge of Left and Right. Unpublished master's thesis. Auckland, New Zealand: University of Auckland.

Newland, T. E. (1957), Psychosocial aspects of the adjustment of the brain injured. *Exceptional Child,* 23:149–153.

Nielson, J. F. (1962), Some visual problems of retarded as revised by analytical examination. *Optometric Weekly,* January 25, 1962, 53(11):149–153.

Nolan, J. A. (1974), An approach to myopia control. *Optometric Weekly,* February 7, 1974, pp. 33–38.

Oldfield, R. and Wingfield, A. (1965), Response latencies in naming objects. *Quarterly Journal of Experimental Psychology,* Vol. XVII, part IV.

Orton, S. T. (1925), "Word-blindness" in school children. *Archives of Neurology and Psychiatry,* 14:581–615.

———(1929), A physiological theory of reading disability and stuttering in children. *New England Journal of Medicine,* 199: 1046–1052.

———(1931), Special disability in reading. *Bulletin of the Neurological Institute of New York,* 1:159–192.

———(1937), Reading, Writing and Speech Problems in Children. New York: W. W. Norton & Co., Inc.

Owen, F. W., Adams, P. A., Forrest, T., Stolz, L. M., and Fisher, S. (1971), Learning disorders in children: sibling studies. *Monographs of the Society for Research in Child Development,* 36(4):1–75, Serial No. 144.

Paine, R. and Oppé, T. (1966), *Neurological Examination of Children.* Clinics in Developmental Medicine, Vol. 20/21. Spastics International Medical Publications. London: William Heinemann Medical Books Ltd.; Philadelphia: J. P. Lippincott Co.

Palmer, J. O. (1970), *The Psychological Assessment of Children.* New York: John Wiley & Sons, Inc.

Paraskevopoulos, J. N. and Kirk, S. A. (1969), *The Development and Psychometric Characteristics of the Revised Illinois Test of Psycholinguistic Abilities.* Urbana, Illinois: University of Chicago Press.

Pasamanick, B. and Knobloch, H. (1960), Brain damage and reproductive casualty. *American Journal of Orthopsychiatry,* 30:298–305.

Penfield, W. and Roberts, L. (1959), Speech and Brain Mechanisms. Princeton, N.J.: Princeton University Press.

Peters, H. B., Blum, L., Bettman, J. W., Johnson, F., and Fellows, V. (1959), The Orinda vision study. American Journal of Optometry and Archives of American Academy of Optometry, 36(9):455–469.

Peters, J. E. (1974), Minimal brain dysfunction in children. Archives of General Practice, 10(1):115–123.

——— Davis, J. S., Goolsby, C. M., Clements, S. D., and Hicks, T. J. (1973), Physician's Handbook: Screening for MBD. Summit, New Jersey: CIBA Pharmaceuticals, Inc.

——— Dykman, R. A., Ackerman, P. T., and Romine, J. S. (1974), The special neurological examination. In: Clinical Use of Stimulant Drugs in Children, ed. C. K. Conners. The Hague: Excerpta Medica, pp. 53–66. (Distributed by Abbott Laboratories, North Chicago, Illinois.)

Piaget, J. (1932), The Moral Judgment of the Child. Glencoe, Illinois: The Free Press.

——— and Inhelder, B. (1948), The Child's Conception of Space. New York: W. W. Norton & Co., Inc. (1967).

Pierce, J. (1968), Lecture on Learning Disabilities. Beverly Hills, California: American Academy of Optometry Post-Graduate Courses.

Pincus, J. H. and Glaser, G. H. (1966), The syndrome of "minimal brain damage" in childhood. The New England Journal of Medicine, 275(1):27–35.

Pontius, A. A. (1973), Conference on minimal brain dysfunction. New York Academy of Sciences, March 20–22, 1972. Annals of the New York Academy of Sciences, Vol. 205, pp. 61–63.

Pope, L. (1970), Motor activity in brain-injured children. American Journal of Orthopsychiatry, 40:783–794.

Porter, R. J. and Berlin, C. I. (1975), On interpreting developmental changes in the dichotic right-ear advantage. Brain and Language, 2:186–200.

Prechtl, H.F.R. and Stemmer, J. (1962), Choreiform syndrome in children. Developmental Medicine & Child Neurology, 4:119–127.

Price, L. S. (1969), The PTA and the positive approach to health. Sight Saving Review, 39(2):93–96.

Purdue Pegboard Test. Lafayette, Indiana: Lafayette Instrument Co.

Rapoport, J. L. (1978), Dextroamphetamine: cognitive and behavioral effects in normal prepubertal boys. Science, 199:560–563.

Raven, J. (1956), Colored Progressive Matrices, rev. edit. London: H. K. Lewis and Co. Ltd.

Roberts, W. L. and Banford, R. D. (1967), Evaluation of bifocal correction technique in juvenile myopia. Optometric Weekly, October 26, 1967, pp. 19–26.

Robinson, H. M. (1968), Clinical Studies in Reading. Chicago: University of Chicago Press, pp. 49–65.

Rosenbloom, A. A. (1968), Aniseikonia and achievement in reading. In: Clinical Studies in Reading III, ed. H. M. Robinson. Chicago: University of Chicago Press, pp. 109–116.

Rosner, J., Ludlam, W., and Pierce, J. (1974), Optometry and learning disabilities. Journal of the American Optometric Association, 45(5):566.

Ross, D. and Ross, S. (1976), *Hyperactivity: Research, Theory, and Action.* New York: John Wiley & Sons.

Rost, K. J. and Charles, D. C. (1967), Academic achievement of brain injured and hyperactive children in isolation. *Exceptional Children,* 34:125–126.

Roy, R. (1953), Ocular migraine and prolonged occlusion. *Optometric Weekly,* September 3, 1953; September 10, 1953; September 17, 1953.

Rubenstein, L. (1962), Continuous radio telemetry of human activity. *Nature,* 193:849–850.

Rubino, C. A. and Minden, H. A. (1973), An analysis of eye-movements in children with a reading disability. *Cortex,* 9:217–220.

Rudel, R. G. and Denckla, M. B. (1974), Relation of forward and backward digit repetition to neurological impairment in children with learning disabilities. *Neuropsychologia,* 12:109–118.

—————— (1976), Relationship of IQ and reading score to visual spatial and temporal matching tasks. *Journal of Learning Disabilities,* 9:169–178.

—————— and Broman, M. (1978), Personal communication.

—————— (1978), Rapid silent response to repeated target symbols by dyslexic and non-dyslexic children. *Brain and Language,* 6:52–62.

—————— and Hirsch, S. (1978), Word finding as a function of stimulus context: children compared with aphasic adults. *Brain and Language* (in press).

—————— and Shalten, E. (1974), The functional asymmetry of Braille letter learning in normal, sighted children. *Neurology,* 24:733–738.

—————— (1976), Paired associate learning of Morse Code and Braille letter names by dyslexic and normal children. *Cortex,* 12:61–70.

——————, Teuber, H. and Twitchell, T. (1974), Levels of impairment of sensorimotor functions in children with early brain damage. *Neuropsychologia,* 12:95–108.

Russell, E. W., Neuringer, C., and Goldstein, G. (1970), *Assessment of Brain Damage.* New York: Wiley-Interscience.

Sainsbury, P. A. (1954), A method of measuring spontaneous movements by time-sampling motion pictures. *Journal of Mental Science,* 100:742–748.

Satterfield, J. H. and Dawson, M. E. (1971), Electrodermal correlates of hyperactivity in children. *Psychophysiology,* 8:191–197.

Sattler, J. M. (1974), *Assessment of Children's Intelligence.* Philadelphia: W. B. Saunders Co.

Satz, P., Bakker, D. J., and Teunissen, J. (1975), Developmental parameters of the asymmetry: A multivariate approach. *Brain and Language,* 2:171–185.

Schain, Richard J. (1975), Minimal brain dysfunction. *Current Problems in Pediatrics,* Vol. V., No. 10. Chicago: Year Book Medical Publishers, Inc.

Schilder, P. (1950), *The Image and Appearance of the Human Body.* New York: International Universities Press.

Schulman, J. L. and Reisman, J. (1959), An objective measure of hyperactivity. *American Journal of Mental Deficiency,* 64:455–456.

Scott, T. J. (1970), The use of music to reduce hyperactivity in children. *American Journal of Orthopsychiatry,* 40(4):677–680.

Shank, K. (1964), Recognition of articulatory disorders in children. *Clinical Pediatrics*, 3:333–334.

Shankweiler, D. (1964), A study of developmental dyslexia. *Neuropsychologia*, 1:267–286.

Shearer, R. V. (1938), Eye findings in children with reading difficulties. *Journal of Pediatric Ophthalmology*, 3:10–16.

Sherman, A. (1973), Relating vision disorders to learning disability. *Journal of American Optometry Association*, 44(2):140–141.

Sherrington, C. (1951), *Man on His Nature*. Cambridge: Cambridge University Press.

Shorr, R. and Svagr, V. (1966), The relationship of perceptual and visual skills with reading accuracy and comprehension. *Journal of the American Optometric Association*, 37(7):671–677.

Sidman, M. and Kirk, B. (1974), Letter reversals in naming, writing, and matching to sample. *Child Development*, 45:616–625.

Siegel, E. (1974), *The Exceptional Child Grows Up*. New York: E. P. Dutton & Co., Inc.

Simpson, R. H. (1944), The specific meanings of certain terms indicating differing degrees of frequency. *Quarterly Journal of Speech*, 30:328–330.

Sloan, W. (1955), The Lincoln-Oseretsky motor development scale. *Genetic Psychology Monographs*, 51:183–252.

Slosson, R. L. (1963), *Slosson Intelligence Test*. East Aurora, New York: Slosson Educational Publications, Inc.

Smith, W. (1971), Clinical procedures in orthoptics, visual training, and pleoptics. *The Optical Journal and Review of Optometry*, 108(22):32–34.

Spache, G. D. (1940), The role of visual defects in spelling and reading difficulties. *American Journal of Orthopsychiatry*, 10:229–238.

Speaks, C. and Jerger, J. (1965), Method for measurement of speech identification. *Journal of Speech and Hearing Research*, 8:185–194.

Spitz, R. A. (1945), Hospitalism. *The Psychoanalytic Study of the Child*, 1:53–74. New York: International Universities Press.

——— (1946a), Anaclitic depression. *The Psychoanalytic Study of the Child*, 2:313–342. New York: International Universities Press.

——— (1946b), Hospitalism: a follow-up report. *The Psychoanalytic Study of the Child*, 2:113–117. New York: International Universities Press.

Sprague, R. L. and Toppe, L. K. (1966), Relationship between activity level and delay of reinforcement in the retarded. *Journal of Experimental Child Psychology*, 3:390–397.

Stein, N. and Mandler, J. (1974), Children's recognition of reversals of geometric figures. *Child Development*, 45:604–615.

Stone, H. S. (1959), Psychodynamics of brain-damaged children: a preliminary report. *Journal of Child Psychology and Psychiatry*, 1:203–214.

Strauss, A. A. and Kephart, N. C. (1955), *Psychopathology and Education of the Brain-Injured Child*, Vol. II. New York: Grune & Stratton.

——— and Lehtinen, L. (1947), *Psychopathology and Education of the Brain-Injured Child*, Vol. I. New York: Grune and Stratton.

Studdert-Kennedy, M. and Shankweiler, D. (1970), Hemispheric specialization for speech perception. *Journal of the Acoustics Society of America,* 48:579-594.

Swanson, W. L. (1972), Optometric vision therapy—how successful is it in the treatment of learning disorders? *Journal of Learning Disabilities,* 5(5):285-296.

Sykes, D., Douglas, V., and Morgenstern, G. (1972), The effect of methylphenidate on sustained attention in hyperactive children. *Psychopharmacologia* (Berl.), 5:262-274.

Tatara, M. (1974), Personal communication.

Taylor, E. A. and Solan, H. A. (1957), *Visual Training with the Prism Reader.* Huntington, New York: Educational Development Labs.

Taylor, S. E. (1966), *The Fundamental Reading Skill as Related to Eye Movement Photography and Visual Anomalies.* Springfield, Illinois: Charles C. Thomas.

Terman, L. M. and Merrill, M. A. (1937), *Measuring Intelligence.* Boston: Houghton Mifflin.

——————(1960), *Stanford-Binet Intelligence Scale.* Boston: Houghton Mifflin Co.

Teuber, H. L. and Weinstein, S. (1956), Ability to discover hidden figures after cerebral lesions. *AMA Archives of Neurology and Psychiatry,* 76-83.

Thomas, A., Birch, H., Chess, S., Hertig, M., and Korn, S. (1963), *Behavioral Individuality in Early Childhood.* New York: New York University Press.

Thompson, B. B. (1963), A longitudinal study of auditory discrimination. *Journal of Educational Research,* 56:376.

Touwen, B. and Prechtl, H. (1970), *The Neurological Examination of the Child with Minor Nervous Dysfunction.* Clinics in Developmental Medicine, No. 38. Philadelphia: J. B. Lippincott Co.

Towbin, A. (1971), Organic causes of minimal brain dysfunction. *Journal of the American Medical Association,* 217:1207-1214.

Turnure, J. E. (1970), Children's reaction to distractors in a learning situation. *Developmental Psychology,* 2:115-122.

——————(1971), Control of orienting behavior in children under five years of age. *Developmental Psychology,* 4:16-24.

Twitchell, T., Lecours, A., Rudel, R., and Teuber, H. (1966), Minimal cerebral dysfunction in children: motor deficits. *Transactions of the American Neurological Association,* 91:353-355.

Vernon, M. D. (1960), *Backwardness in Reading,* 2nd edit. Cambridge: Cambridge University Press.

Waldrop, M. F. and Goering, J. D. (1971), Hyperactivity and minor physical anomalies in elementary school children. *American Journal of Orthopsychiatry,* 41:602-607.

——————and Halverson, C. F. (1970), Minor physical anomalies and hyperactive behavior in young children. In: *The Exceptional Infant,* ed. J. Hellmuth, Vol. II. Seattle, Washington: Special Child Publications.

Wechsler, A. (1972), The effect of organic brain disease on recall of emotionally charged versus neutral narrative terms. *Neurology,* 23:130-135.

Wechsler, D. (1949), *Wechsler Intelligence Scale for Children.* New York: The Psychological Corp.

———— (1955), *Wechsler Adult Intelligence Scale*. New York: The Psychological Corporation.

———— (1958), *The Measurement and Appraisal of Adult Intelligence*. Baltimore: The Williams and Wilkins Co.

———— (1974), *Wechsler Intelligence Scale for Children-Revised*. New York: The Psychological Corporation.

Weinberg, J., Diller, L., Gerstmann, L., and Schulman, P. (1972), Digit span in right and left hemiplegics. *Journal of Clinical Psychology*, 28:361.

Wender, P. H. (1971), *Minimal Brain Dysfunction in Children*. New York: Wiley-Interscience.

———— and Eisenberg, L. (1974), Minimal brain dysfunction in children. In: *American Handbook of Psychiatry*, 2nd edit., ed. S. Arieti. New York: Basic Books, Inc.

Wepman, J. M. (1973), *Auditory Discrimination Test*. Palm Springs, California: Language Research Associates.

Werry, J. S. (1968), Developmental hyperactivity. *Pediatric Clinics of North America*, 15:581–599.

Wold, R. M. (1971), Vision and learning: the great puzzle. *Optometric Weekly*, October 14, 1971, pp. 33–38.

Wolfe, L. S. (1939), An experimental study of reversals in reading. *American Journal of Psychology*, 52:533–561.

Woolf, D. (1969), Dyschriescopia—syndrome of visual disability. In: *Visual and Perceptual Aspects for the Achieving and Underachieving Child*, ed. R. M. Wold. Seattle, Washington: Special Child Publications.

Wyatt, G. (1969), *Language Learning and Communication Disorders in Children*. New York: Free Press.

Yakovlev, P. and Lecours, A. (1967), The myelogenetic cycles of regional maturation of the brain. In: *Regional Development of the Brain in Early Life*, ed. A. Minkowski. Oxford and Edinburgh: Blackwell Scientific Publications.

Young, G. A. (1963), Reading, measures of intelligence and refractive errors. *American Journal of Optometry*, 40:257–264.

Zangwill, O. L. and Blakemore, C. (1972), Dyslexia: reversals of eye-movements during reading. *Neuropsychologia*, 10:371–373.

Index

443